Skills Performance Checklists

for

Clinical Nursing Skills & Techniques

Perry, Potter, Ostendorf

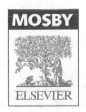

MOSBY

ELSEVIER

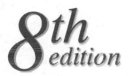

8th edition

ELSEVIER
MOSBY

3251 Riverport Lane
Maryland Heights, Missouri 63043

SKILLS PERFORMANCE CHECKLISTS FOR CLINICAL
NURSING SKILLS & TECHNIQUES   ISBN: 978-0-323-08898-5

Previous editions copyrighted 2010, 2005, 2002, 1998

Content Manager: Jean Sims Fornango
Content Coordinator: Melissa Rawe
Publishing Services Manager: Debbie Vogel and Hemamalini Rajendrababu
Senior Project Manager: Antony Prince

Printed in the United States of America

Last digit is the Print Number: 9 8 7 6 5 4 3 2 1

Contents

CHAPTER 44: DIAGNOSTIC PROCEDURES

Student _____ Date _____

Instructor _____ Date _____

PERFORMANCE CHECKLIST SKILL 2-1 **ADMITTING PATIENTS**

	S	U	NP	Comments

ROOM PREPARATION

1. Performed hand hygiene, prepared room equipment. ___ ___ ___ _____

2. Ensured equipment is in working order, assembled any special equipment in patient's room. ___ ___ ___ _____

ASSESSMENT

1. Greeted patient and family by name, introduced self and job title, explained responsibilities in patient's care. ___ ___ ___ _____

2. Identified patient using two identifiers, compared with information on patient's identification bracelet. ___ ___ ___ _____

3. Arranged for a translation service if necessary. ___ ___ ___ _____

4. Assessed patient's general appearance, noted signs or symptoms of physical distress. ___ ___ ___ _____

5. Determined patient's ability to understand and implement health information. ___ ___ ___ _____

6. Assessed patient's and family's psychological status by noting verbal and nonverbal behaviors and responses. ___ ___ ___ _____

7. Assessed vital signs and height and weight. ___ ___ ___ _____

8. Assessed for fall risk using scale with grading criteria, considered patient's risk factors. ___ ___ ___ _____

9. Had family or friends leave room unless patient wishes to have them assist with changing, provided privacy, helped patient undress, assisted patient into comfortable position. ___ ___ ___ _____

10. Obtained nursing history as soon as possible, applied standards of nursing care adopted by hospital.

    a. Assessed patient's perception of illness and health care needs. ___ ___ ___ _____

    b. Assessed patient's past medical history. ___ ___ ___ _____

    c. Assessed presenting signs and symptoms and reason for hospitalization. ___ ___ ___ _____

    d. Assessed the completed review of health status based on appropriate standards. ___ ___ ___ _____

    e. Assessed risk factors for illness. ___ ___ ___ _____

	S	U	NP	Comments

f. Assessed history of allergies.

g. Obtained detailed medication history.

h. Assessed patient's knowledge of health problems and expectations of care.

11. Conducted physical assessment of appropriate body systems.

12. Checked health care providers' orders for treatment measures to initiate immediately.

13. Oriented patient to nursing division.

   a. Introduced staff members, introduced patient appropriately.

   b. Told patient and family the name of nurse manager, explained that person's role in solving problems.

   c. Explained visiting hours and their purpose.

   d. Discussed smoking policy, identified smoking areas if available.

   e. Demonstrated use of equipment.

   f. Showed patient nurse call light, positioned it near patient, had patient demonstrate use and call for assistance if needed.

   g. Escorted patient to bathroom if appropriate.

   h. Explained hours for mealtime.

   i. Described services available.

PLANNING

1. Identified expected outcomes.

IMPLEMENTATION

1. Completed patient medication reconciliation by checking home medication list, updated medication list based on health care provider's orders for treatment.

2. Informed patient about upcoming procedures or treatments.

3. Completed learning needs assessment for patient and family.

4. Gave patient and family chance to ask questions about procedures or therapies.

5. Collected valuables patient chooses to keep at facility, completed listing sheet, had patient or family sign it, placed values in safe or sent home with family.

	S	U	NP	Comments
6. Ensured patient and family have time together alone if desired.	—	—	—	_____
7. Ensured call light is within reach and bed is in low position.	—	—	—	_____
8. Performed hand hygiene.	—	—	—	_____

EVALUATION

	S	U	NP	Comments
1. Had patient explain hospital policies, tests, and procedures.	—	—	—	_____
2. Had patient demonstrate use of call light.	—	—	—	_____
3. Monitored patient's ability to ambulate independently.	—	—	—	_____
4. Checked patient's room setup regularly.	—	—	—	_____
5. Identified unexpected outcomes.	—	—	—	_____

RECORDING AND REPORTING

	S	U	NP	Comments
1. Recorded history and assessment findings in appropriate log, began to develop nursing plan of care, conferred with patient and family as needed.	—	—	—	_____
2. Placed advanced directive in medical record if available.	—	—	—	_____
3. Notified health care provider of patient's arrival, reported unusual findings, secured admission orders if necessary.	—	—	—	_____

Student _____ Date _____

Instructor _____ Date _____

PERFORMANCE CHECKLIST SKILL 2-2   **TRANSFERRING PATIENTS**

	S	U	NP	Comments

ASSESSMENT

1. Obtained transfer order from sending health care provider. ___ ___ ___ _____

2. Assessed reason for patient's transfer in collaboration with health care provider and appropriate team members. ___ ___ ___ _____

3. Identified patient using two identifiers. ___ ___ ___ _____

4. Assessed individuals at high risk for transitional care problems. ___ ___ ___ _____

5. Explained purpose of transfer, provided time to discuss patient's and family's feelings, obtained written consent if necessary. ___ ___ ___ _____

6. Assessed patient's current physical condition, determined method for transport. ___ ___ ___ _____

7. Assessed if patient requires pain relief or other medications. ___ ___ ___ _____

8. Ensured that staff have notified patient's family of transfer as desired by patient. ___ ___ ___ _____

PLANNING

1. Identified expected outcomes. ___ ___ ___ _____

2. Arranged for patient's transport to an agency by chosen vehicle. ___ ___ ___ _____

3. Contacted new agency and arranged for bed in appropriate setting if necessary, confirmed willingness of agency to accept patient. ___ ___ ___ _____

IMPLEMENTATION

1. Ensured patient's record is complete with individualized care plan. ___ ___ ___ _____

2. Completed nursing care transfer form appropriately. ___ ___ ___ _____

3. Completed medication reconciliation appropriately, checked patient's current orders against most recent MAR and original medication list, communicated updated medication list to next provider of care. ___ ___ ___ _____

4. Had NAP gather and secure patient's personal items, checked entire room and storage areas. ___ ___ ___ _____

	S	U	NP	Comments
5. Anticipated problems patient may develop before or during transfer, performed necessary therapies.	___	___	___	_____
6. Assisted in transferring patient safely to stretcher or wheelchair.	___	___	___	_____
7. Performed and documented final assessment of patient's physical stability.	___	___	___	_____
8. Accompanied patient to transport vehicle.	___	___	___	_____
9. Called receiving agency and notified of transfer and patient's status.	___	___	___	_____

EVALUATION

	S	U	NP	Comments
1. Compared data with previous findings during final assessment.	___	___	___	_____
2. Inspected patient's alignment and positioning on wheelchair or stretcher.	___	___	___	_____
3. Ensured equipment for transfer is functioning.	___	___	___	_____
4. Confirmed patient understands transfer and procedures.	___	___	___	_____
5. Determined if receiving agency had questions about patient's care.	___	___	___	_____
6. Evaluated patient for inappropriate behaviors.	___	___	___	_____
7. Identified unexpected outcomes.	___	___	___	_____

RECORDING AND REPORTING

	S	U	NP	Comments
1. Documented pertinent information if sending patient.	___	___	___	_____
2. Documented pertinent information if receiving patient.	___	___	___	_____

Student _____ Date _____

Instructor _____ Date _____

PERFORMANCE CHECKLIST SKILL 2-3 **DISCHARGING PATIENTS**

	S	U	NP	Comments
ASSESSMENT				
1. Assessed patient's discharge needs from time of admission, used care plan to focus on ongoing assessments needed.	___	___	___	_____
2. Identified patient using two identifiers, compared with information on patient's identification bracelet.	___	___	___	_____
3. Assessed patient's and family's need for health teaching related to home therapies, home medical equipment, restrictions, and complications.	___	___	___	_____
4. Assessed for barriers to learning.	___	___	___	_____
5. Assessed for environmental factors within home that interfere with self-care.	___	___	___	_____
6. Collaborated with health care provider and interdisciplinary team in assessing need for referrals.	___	___	___	_____
7. Assessed patient's and family's perceptions of continued health care needs outside the hospital, took assessment of pertinent information.	___	___	___	_____
8. Assessed patient's acceptance of health problems and related restrictions.	___	___	___	_____
9. Consulted other health care team members about anticipated needs after discharge, made referrals in a timely manner.	___	___	___	_____
PLANNING				
1. Identified expected outcomes.	___	___	___	_____
IMPLEMENTATION				
1. Prepared before day of discharge.				
a. Suggested way to arrange home to suit patient needs.	___	___	___	_____
b. Provided patient and family with information about community health care resources.	___	___	___	_____
c. Conducted teaching lessons with patient and family as soon as possible, reviewed and gave patient discharge materials, referred patient to appropriate Internet resources.	___	___	___	_____
d. Communicated patient's and family's response to teaching and discharge plans to other team members.	___	___	___	_____

	S	U	NP	Comments

2. Performed procedures on day of discharge.

   a. Let patient and family ask questions and discuss issues, provided opportunity to demonstrate learned skills.

   b. Checked health care provider's discharge orders for prescriptions, treatment changes, or need for special equipment, arranged for delivery and setup of equipment before patient arrival.

   c. Determined whether patient or family has arranged for transportation.

   d. Provided privacy, assisted as patient dressed and packed personal belongings, checked closets and drawers, obtained copy of valuables list and had items delivered to patient.

   e. Completed medication reconciliation appropriately, checked discharge medication order against MAR and home medication list, provided patient with prescriptions or medications ordered, offered final review of information.

   f. Provided information on follow-up appointments to health care provider's office, provided phone number of unit.

   g. Contacted agency's business office to determine patient need to finalize payment arrangements.

   h. Acquired utility cart to move belongings, obtained wheelchair or stretcher for patient.

   i. Assisted patient to wheelchair or stretcher properly, escorted patient to transportation, locked wheelchair wheels, assisted patient and belongings into vehicle.

   j. Returned to divisions, notified appropriate groups of time of discharge, notified housekeeping to clean patient's room.

EVALUATION

1. Asked patient or family member to describe nature of illness, treatment, and symptoms to be reported.

2. Had patient or family members perform any treatments that will continue at home.

3. If a home care nurse, inspected home, identified obstacles, and recommended revisions.

4. Identified unexpected outcomes.

8

	S	U	NP	Comments

RECORDING AND REPORTING

1. Completed discharge summary form, provided patient with a signed copy.

2. Documented unresolved problems and description of arrangements made for resolution in appropriate log.

3. Documented patient's vitals and status of health problems at time of discharge in nurses' notes.

Student _____ Date _____

Instructor _____ Date _____

PERFORMANCE CHECKLIST SKILL 3-1 **ESTABLISHING THE NURSE–PATIENT RELATIONSHIP**

	S	U	NP	Comments
ASSESSMENT				
1. Addressed patient by name; introduced self and role; used clear, specific communication.	___	___	___	_____
2. Assessed patient's needs, coping strategies, defenses, and adaptation styles.	___	___	___	_____
3. Determined patient's need to communicate.	___	___	___	_____
4. Assessed reason patient needs health care.	___	___	___	_____
5. Assessed factors about self and patient that normally influence communication.	___	___	___	_____
6. Assessed personal barriers to communicating with patient.	___	___	___	_____
7. Assessed patient's language and ability to speak.	___	___	___	_____
8. Assessed patient's literacy level.	___	___	___	_____
9. Assessed patient's ability to hear, ensured hearing aid is functional if worn, ensured patient hears and understands words.	___	___	___	_____
10. Observed patient's pattern of communication and verbal or nonverbal behavior.	___	___	___	_____
11. Assessed resources available in selecting communication methods.	___	___	___	_____
12. Assessed patient's readiness to work toward goal attainment.	___	___	___	_____
13. Considered when patient is due to be discharged or transferred.	___	___	___	_____
PLANNING				
1. Identified expected outcomes.	___	___	___	_____
2. Planned orientation phase.	___	___	___	_____
3. Planned working phase.	___	___	___	_____
4. Planned termination phase.	___	___	___	_____
IMPLEMENTATION				
1. Established nurse-patient relationship during orientation phase.				
a. Created a climate of warmth and acceptance, was aware of nonverbal cues, provided comfort and support.	___	___	___	_____

	S	U	NP	Comments

b. Used appropriate nonverbal behaviors. _____ _____ _____ _____

c. Observed patient's nonverbal behaviors, sought clarifications if necessary. _____ _____ _____ _____

d. Explained purpose of interaction when information was being shared. _____ _____ _____ _____

e. Used active listening. _____ _____ _____ _____

f. Identified patient's expectations in seeking health care. _____ _____ _____ _____

g. Interviewed patient about health status, lifestyle, support systems, patterns of health and illness, and strengths and limitations. _____ _____ _____ _____

h. Encouraged patient to ask for clarification at any time. _____ _____ _____ _____

i. Used therapeutic communication techniques when interacting with patient. _____ _____ _____ _____

2. Set mutual goals during the working phase.

a. Used therapeutic communication skills. _____ _____ _____ _____

b. Discussed and prioritized problem areas. _____ _____ _____ _____

c. Provided information to patient, helped patient express needs and feelings. _____ _____ _____ _____

d. Used questions carefully and appropriately, asked one question at a time, used direct questions, used open-ended statements as much as possible. _____ _____ _____ _____

e. Avoided communication barriers. _____ _____ _____ _____

3. Communicated with patient during termination phase.

a. Used therapeutic communication skills to discuss discharge or termination issues, guided discussion to patient changes in thoughts and behaviors. _____ _____ _____ _____

b. Summarized with patient what was discussed during interaction. _____ _____ _____ _____

EVALUATION

1. Observed patient's verbal and nonverbal responses to communication, noted patient's willingness to share information and concerns. _____ _____ _____ _____

2. Noted your response to patient and patient's response to you, reflected on effectiveness of techniques. _____ _____ _____ _____

3. Evaluated patient's ability to work toward identifiable goals, reevaluated and identified barriers if patient goals are not met. _____ _____ _____ _____

	S	U	NP	Comments

4. Summarized and restated goals, reinforced patient strengths, outlined issues requiring work, developed an action plan.   ____ ____ ____ _____

5. Identified unexpected outcomes.   ____ ____ ____ _____

RECORDING AND REPORTING

1. Recorded pertinent communication, responses to illness or therapies, and responses that demonstrate understanding or lack thereof.   ____ ____ ____ _____

2. Reported relevant information to team members.   ____ ____ ____ _____

Student _____ Date _____

Instructor _____ Date _____

PERFORMANCE CHECKLIST SKILL 3-2 **COMMUNICATION WITH AN ANXIOUS PATIENT**

	S	U	NP	Comments
ASSESSMENT				
1. Introduced self appropriately, explained purpose of interaction.	___	___	___	_____
2. Assessed for cues indicating patient is anxious.	___	___	___	_____
3. Assessed for possible factors causing patient anxiety.	___	___	___	_____
4. Assessed factors influencing communication with patient.	___	___	___	_____
5. Discussed with family possible causes of patient's anxiety.	___	___	___	_____
PLANNING				
1. Identified expected outcomes.	___	___	___	_____
2. Prepared for communication by considering patient goals, time allocation, and resources.	___	___	___	_____
3. Recognized personal level of anxiety, tried to remain calm.	___	___	___	_____
4. Prepared quiet, calm area, allowed ample personal space.	___	___	___	_____
IMPLEMENTATION				
1. Used appropriate nonverbal behaviors and active listening skills.	___	___	___	_____
2. Used appropriate verbal techniques that are clear and concise in responses, acknowledged patient's feelings, provided direction to patient.	___	___	___	_____
3. Helped patient acquire alternative coping strategies.	___	___	___	_____
4. Provided necessary comfort measures.	___	___	___	_____
EVALUATION				
1. Observed for continuing presence of signs and behaviors reflecting anxiety.	___	___	___	_____
2. Had patient discuss ways to cope with anxiety and make decisions about own care.	___	___	___	_____
3. Evaluated patient's ability to discuss factors causing anxiety.	___	___	___	_____
4. Identified unexpected outcomes.	___	___	___	_____

	S	U	NP	Comments

RECORDING AND REPORTING

1. Recorded cause of patient's anxiety and any exhibited signs.

2. Reported methods used to relieve anxiety and patient's response.

Student _____ Date _____

Instructor _____ Date _____

PERFORMANCE CHECKLIST SKILL 3-3 **COMMUNICATING WITH THE ANGRY PATIENT**

	S	U	NP	Comments

ASSESSMENT

1. Assessed for behaviors indicating patient is angry. ___ ___ ___ _____

2. Assessed factors that influence communication, including refusal to comply, hostility, or emotional immaturity. ___ ___ ___ _____

3. Considered resources available to assist in communicating with potentially violent patient. ___ ___ ___ _____

4. Assessed for underlying medical conditions that may lead to violent behavior. ___ ___ ___ _____

PLANNING

1. Identified expected outcomes. ___ ___ ___ _____

2. Prepared for interaction with an angry patient.

   a. Paused to collect own thoughts. ___ ___ ___ _____

   b. Determined what patient is saying. ___ ___ ___ _____

   c. Attempted calm, firm, assertive approach. ___ ___ ___ _____

3. Prepared environment to de-escalate a potentially violent patient.

   a. Encouraged others to leave. ___ ___ ___ _____

   b. Maintained adequate distance. ___ ___ ___ _____

   c. Maintained open exit and did not block exit. ___ ___ ___ _____

   d. Closed door when anger began to disturb others. ___ ___ ___ _____

   e. Reduced disturbing factors in the room. ___ ___ ___ _____

   f. Took care of patient's physical and emotional needs. ___ ___ ___ _____

IMPLEMENTATION

1. Responded appropriately to a potentially violent patient.

   a. Maintained nonthreatening communication skills. ___ ___ ___ _____

   b. Used therapeutic silence, allowed patient to vent feelings. ___ ___ ___ _____

	S	U	NP	Comments

c. Answered questions as appropriate, redirected when necessary, informed patient of potential consequences, followed through with consequences. ___ ___ ___ _____

d. Set limits appropriately if patient threatens harm. ___ ___ ___ _____

e. Maintained personal space and safety if patient makes threat of violence toward others, maintained nonthreatening position. ___ ___ ___ _____

f. Explored alternatives to situation or feelings of anger if patient's anger is diffused. ___ ___ ___ _____

EVALUATION

1. Observed for continuing behaviors or verbal expressions of anger. ___ ___ ___ _____

2. Noted patient's ability to answer questions and solve problems. ___ ___ ___ _____

3. Identified unexpected outcomes. ___ ___ ___ _____

RECORDING AND REPORTING

1. Recorded cause of anger, behaviors, de-escalation techniques, and patient's response in nurses' notes. ___ ___ ___ _____

2. Reported de-escalation technique and patient's response to nurse in charge. ___ ___ ___ _____

Student _____ Date _____

Instructor _____ Date _____

PERFORMANCE CHECKLIST SKILL 3-4 **COMMUNICATING WITH A DEPRESSED PATIENT**

	S	U	NP	Comments

ASSESSMENT

1. Assessed for cues indicating patient is depressed.

2. Assessed for possible factors causing patient's depression.

3. Assessed factors influencing communication with patient.

4. Discussed possible causes of patient's depression with family members.

PLANNING

1. Identified expected outcomes.

2. Prepared for communication by considering patient goals, time allocation, and resources.

3. Maintained awareness of own nonverbal cues that affect communication with depressed patient, remained nonjudgmental.

4. Prepared environment physically.

IMPLEMENTATION

1. Introduced self, explained purpose of interaction.

2. Focused on positive aspects of patient, provided positive feedback.

3. Displayed honesty and empathy.

4. Used appropriate nonverbal behaviors and active listening skills.

5. Used appropriate verbal techniques, used observational statements to acknowledge current feelings, provided direction to patient.

6. Used open-ended questions.

7. Rewarded small decisions and independent actions, made decisions that patients are not ready to make if necessary, presented situations that require no decision making.

8. Responded to anger therapeutically, avoided becoming defensive or angry, encouraged verbal expression of anger.

9. Provided necessary comfort measures.

	S	U	NP	Comments
10. Spent time with patient who is withdrawn.	___	___	___	_____
11. Asked patient about suicidal ideation and presence of a plan.	___	___	___	_____

EVALUATION

	S	U	NP	Comments
1. Observed for continuing presence of signs or behaviors reflecting depression.	___	___	___	_____
2. Had patient discuss ways to cope with depression and make decisions about own care.	___	___	___	_____
3. Evaluated patient's ability to discuss factors causing depression.	___	___	___	_____
4. Identified unexpected outcomes.	___	___	___	_____

RECORDING AND REPORTING

	S	U	NP	Comments
1. Recorded objective and subjective behaviors in nurses' notes.	___	___	___	_____
2. Recorded and reported methods used to improve behaviors and patient's response.	___	___	___	_____

Student _____ Date _____

Instructor _____ Date _____

PERFORMANCE CHECKLIST SKILL 3-5 **COMMUNICATING WITH A COGNITIVELY IMPAIRED PATIENT**

	S	U	NP	Comments

ASSESSMENT

1. Assessed for cues indicating that a patient is cognitively impaired, assessed orientation status of the patient, performed mini-mental examination.

2. Assessed for possible factors causing cognitive impairment.

3. Assessed factors influencing communication with patient.

4. Discussed possible causes of patient's cognitive impairment with family members if necessary.

PLANNING

1. Identified expected outcomes.

2. Prepared for communication by considering type of cognitive and communication impairments, time allocation, and resources.

3. Maintained awareness of own nonverbal cues, remained nonjudgmental.

4. Prepared environment physically, reduced distractions.

IMPLEMENTATION

1. Approached patient from the front, faced patient when speaking.

2. Introduced self, explained purpose of interaction.

3. Used appropriate nonverbal behaviors and active listening skills.

4. Used clear and concise verbal techniques to respond to depressed patient, asked yes-or-no questions.

5. Asked questions one at a time, allowed time for response.

6. Repeated sentences using a steady voice, avoided being too quick to guess patient response.

7. Used assistive and augmentative devices to facilitate communication.

	S	U	NP	Comments
8. Provided assistive devices such as eyeglasses or hearing aids.	___	___	___	_____
9. Did not argue with or correct patient.	___	___	___	_____
10. Maintained meaningful interactions with patient, used creative modes of communication based on patient's comfort and ability.	___	___	___	_____

EVALUATION

	S	U	NP	Comments
1. Observed for clarity and understanding of messages sent and received.	___	___	___	_____
2. Observed verbal and nonverbal behaviors.	___	___	___	_____
3. Identified unexpected outcomes.	___	___	___	_____

RECORDING AND REPORTING

	S	U	NP	Comments
1. Recorded objective and subjective behaviors in nurses' notes.	___	___	___	_____
2. Recorded and reported methods used to communicate and patient's response.	___	___	___	_____

Student _____ Date _____

Instructor _____ Date _____

PERFORMANCE CHECKLIST PROCEDURAL GUIDELINE 4-1   **GIVING A HANDOFF REPORT**

	S	U	NP	Comments
PLANNING				
1. Gathered necessary equipment.	___	___	___	_____
PROCEDURAL STEPS				
1. Developed and organized format for delivering an appropriate description of patient's needs and problems.	___	___	___	_____
2. Gathered information from relevant documents.	___	___	___	_____
3. Prioritized information based on patient's needs and problems.	___	___	___	_____
4. Included in report:				
a. Background information	___	___	___	_____
b. Assessment data	___	___	___	_____
c. Nursing diagnoses or patient problems	___	___	___	_____
d. Interventions, outcomes, and evaluations	___	___	___	_____
e. Family information	___	___	___	_____
f. Discharge plan	___	___	___	_____
g. Current priorities	___	___	___	_____
5. Asked staff from oncoming shift if they have any questions regarding information provided.	___	___	___	_____
6. Evaluated tape for clarity, organization, rate of speaking, and volume if necessary.	___	___	___	_____

Student _____ Date _____

Instructor _____ Date _____

PERFORMANCE CHECKLIST PROCEDURAL GUIDELINE 4-2 **DOCUMENTING NURSES' PROGRESS NOTES**

	S	U	NP	Comments
PLANNING				
1. Gathered necessary equipment.	___	___	___	_____
PROCEDURAL STEPS				
1. Reviewed all necessary assessments and nursing interventions gathered or performed, evaluated patient response and status of each patient's diagnosis.	___	___	___	_____
2. Documented patient information in the proper format.	___	___	___	_____
3. Identified information to be documented after each patient contact.	___	___	___	_____
4. Documented in a timely and orderly fashion, included date and time.	___	___	___	_____
5. Documented objective data, select subjective data, nursing actions taken, patient responses, additional plans to be implemented, and to whom information was reported.	___	___	___	_____
6. Signed report appropriately, indicated level of education and school if you are a student.	___	___	___	_____
7. Reviewed previously documented entries with own entries, noted significant changes in patient's status, reported any such changes to patient's health care provider.	___	___	___	_____

Student _____ Date _____

Instructor _____ Date _____

PERFORMANCE CHECKLIST PROCEDURAL GUIDELINE 4-3 **ADVERSE EVENT/INCIDENT REPORTING**

	S	U	NP	Comments

PLANNING

1. Gathered necessary equipment.   ___ ___ ___ _____

PROCEDURAL STEPS

1. Determined what was involved in the incident and reported appropriately, notified risk management as necessary.   ___ ___ ___ _____

2. Assessed extent of injury.   ___ ___ ___ _____

3. Took steps to restore individual's safety.   ___ ___ ___ _____

4. Called health care provider immediately if patient sustained an injury.   ___ ___ ___ _____

5. Referred injured visitors or staff to emergency department.   ___ ___ ___ _____

6. Completed incident report form.

   a. Recorded objective information about the incident, included victim interpretations in quotes.   ___ ___ ___ _____

   b. Objectively described patient's condition when incident was discovered or observed.   ___ ___ ___ _____

   c. Described measures taken by caretakers at the time.   ___ ___ ___ _____

   d. Sent completed report to designated department.   ___ ___ ___ _____

7. Documented events in patient chart if necessary, entered only objective description of events and any assessments or interventions initiated.   ___ ___ ___ _____

8. Filed report properly with risk management department or designated persons.   ___ ___ ___ _____

Student _____ Date _____

Instructor _____ Date _____

PERFORMANCE CHECKLIST SKILL 5-1 **MEASURING BODY TEMPERATURE**

	S	U	NP	Comments

ASSESSMENT

1. Determined need to measure patient's body temperature.

   a. Noted patient's risks for temperature alteration. ___ ___ ___ _____

   b. Assessed for symptoms that accompany temperature alteration. ___ ___ ___ _____

   c. Assessed for factors that normally influence temperature. ___ ___ ___ _____

2. Determined appropriate measure site and device for patient. ___ ___ ___ _____

3. Determined previous baseline temperature and measurement site from patient's record. ___ ___ ___ _____

4. Assessed patient's knowledge of procedure. ___ ___ ___ _____

PLANNING

1. Identified expected outcomes. ___ ___ ___ _____

2. Explained to patient that you will measure temperature and importance of maintaining proper position. ___ ___ ___ _____

3. Verified that patient has had no food, drink, gum, or cigarettes in the past 15 minutes before measuring oral temperature. ___ ___ ___ _____

IMPLEMENTATION

1. Performed hand hygiene. ___ ___ ___ _____

2. Assisted patient to comfortable position that provides easy access to temperature site. ___ ___ ___ _____

3. Obtained temperature reading.

   a. Assessed oral temperature (electronic).

     (1) Applied clean gloves if necessary. ___ ___ ___ _____

     (2) Removed thermometer pack from charger, attached probe stem, grasped top of probe stem appropriately. ___ ___ ___ _____

     (3) Slid disposable probe cover over probe stem until cover locked in place. ___ ___ ___ _____

     (4) Asked patient to open mouth, placed thermometer probe under tongue appropriately. ___ ___ ___ _____

	S	U	NP	Comments

(5) Asked patient to hold thermometer probe with lips closed.

(6) Left thermometer in place until signal sounded and patient's temperature appeared on display, removed thermometer probe from under patient's tongue.

(7) Pushed ejection button to discard probe in the appropriate receptacle.

(8) Removed and disposed of gloves if necessary. Performed hand hygiene.

(9) Returned thermometer probe stem to storage position.

b. Assessed rectal temperature (electronic).

(1) Provided privacy, assisted patient to appropriate position, moved bed linens to expose only anal area.

(2) Perform hand hygiene. Apply clean gloves.

(3) Cleansed anal region if necessary, removed soiled gloves, reapplied clean gloves.

(4) Removed thermometer pack from charger, attached rectal probe stem to unit, grasped top of probe stem.

(5) Slid disposable probe cover over probe stem until cover locked in place.

(6) Squeezed lubricant on tissue, dipped probe cover into lubricant and covered appropriately.

(7) Exposed patient's anus with nondominant hand, asked patient to breathe and relax.

(8) Inserted thermometer appropriately into anus, did not force.

(9) Withdrew if resistance was felt.

(10) Held probe in position until signal sounded and temperature appeared on display, removed probe from anus.

(11) Discarded probe cover appropriately, wiped probe with alcohol swab.

(12) Returned thermometer stem to storage position.

	S	U	NP	Comments

(13) Wiped patient's anal area with soft tissue, discarded tissue, assisted patient to a comfortable position. ___ ___ ___ _____

(14) Removed and disposed of gloves, performed hand hygiene. ___ ___ ___ _____

c. Assessed axillary temperature (electronic).

(1) Provided privacy, assisted patient to appropriate position, moved clothing or gown away from shoulder and arm. ___ ___ ___ _____

(2) Removed thermometer pack from charger, attached oral thermometer probe stem to unit, grasped top of probe stem. ___ ___ ___ _____

(3) Slid disposable probe cover over stem until cover locked in place. ___ ___ ___ _____

(4) Raised patient's arm away from torso, inspected skin for lesions and perspiration, dried axilla if needed, inserted thermometer into center of axilla, lowered arm properly. ___ ___ ___ _____

(5) Held thermometer in place until signal sounded and temperature appeared on display, removed probe from axilla. ___ ___ ___ _____

(6) Discarded probe cover appropriately. ___ ___ ___ _____

(7) Returned thermometer stem to storage position. ___ ___ ___ _____

(8) Assisted patient to comfortable position, replaced gown. ___ ___ ___ _____

(9) Performed hand hygiene. ___ ___ ___ _____

d. Assessed tympanic membrane temperature.

(1) Assisted patient to appropriate position, obtained temperature from the appropriate ear. ___ ___ ___ _____

(2) Noted presence of earwax. ___ ___ ___ _____

(3) Removed thermometer unit from charging base. ___ ___ ___ _____

(4) Slid disposable speculum cover over lens tip until it locked in place, did not touch the lens cover. ___ ___ ___ _____

(5) Inserted speculum into ear canal, followed instructions for probe positioning. ___ ___ ___ _____

(6) Once positioned, pressed scan button, left speculum until signal sounded and patient's temperature appeared on display. ___ ___ ___ _____

	S	U	NP	Comments

(7) Removed speculum from auditory meatus, discarded speculum cover appropriately. ___ ___ ___ _____

(8) If second reading was necessary, replaced probe cover and waited 2 minutes before repeating either in same ear or in other ear, considered alternative method. ___ ___ ___ _____

(9) Returned unit to thermometer base. ___ ___ ___ _____

(10) Assisted patient to comfortable position. ___ ___ ___ _____

(11) Performed hand hygiene. ___ ___ ___ _____

e. Assessed temporal artery temperature.

(1) Ensured forehead was dry. ___ ___ ___ _____

(2) Placed sensor firmly on patient's forehead. ___ ___ ___ _____

(3) Pressed red scan button, slowly slid thermometer across forehead, kept sensor flat on skin. ___ ___ ___ _____

(4) Altered method appropriately if patient was diaphoretic. ___ ___ ___ _____

(5) Cleaned sensor with alcohol swab. ___ ___ ___ _____

4. Informed patient of temperature reading, recorded measurement. ___ ___ ___ _____

5. Returned thermometer to charger. ___ ___ ___ _____

EVALUATION

1. Established temperature as a baseline if necessary. ___ ___ ___ _____

2. Compared reading with baseline and acceptable range. ___ ___ ___ _____

3. Took temperature 30 minutes after administering antipyretics and every 4 hours until temperature stabilized. ___ ___ ___ _____

4. Identified unexpected outcomes. ___ ___ ___ _____

RECORDING AND REPORTING

1. Recorded temperature and route in appropriate record. ___ ___ ___ _____

2. Reported abnormal findings to nurse in charge or health care provider. ___ ___ ___ _____

Student _____ Date _____

Instructor _____ Date _____

PERFORMANCE CHECKLIST SKILL 5-2 **ASSESSING RADIAL PULSE**

	S	U	NP	Comments
ASSESSMENT				
1. Determined need to assess radial pulse.				
a. Assessed for any risk factors for pulse alterations.	___	___	___	_____
b. Assessed for signs of altered cardiac function.	___	___	___	_____
c. Assessed for signs of peripheral vascular disease.	___	___	___	_____
d. Assessed for factors that influence radial pulse rate and rhythm.	___	___	___	_____
2. Determined patient's previous baseline pulse rate from patient's record.	___	___	___	_____
PLANNING				
1. Identified expected outcomes.	___	___	___	_____
2. Explained to patient that you will assess HR, encouraged patient to relax, waited before assessing pulse if necessary.	___	___	___	_____
3. Collected appropriate equipment.	___	___	___	_____
IMPLEMENTATION				
1. Performed hand hygiene.	___	___	___	_____
2. Provided privacy if necessary.	___	___	___	_____
3. Assisted patient into appropriate position.	___	___	___	_____
4. Positioned patient's arms appropriately.	___	___	___	_____
5. Compressed against radius, obliterated pulse, then relaxed so pulse became palpable.	___	___	___	_____
6. Determined strength of pulse.	___	___	___	_____
7. Looked at watch to count seconds after feeling a regular pulse, counted pulse properly.	___	___	___	_____
8. Counted rate for 30 seconds if pulse was regular, and multiplied total by 2.	___	___	___	_____
9. Counted rate for 60 seconds if pulse was irregular, assessed frequency and pattern of irregularity.	___	___	___	_____
10. Compared radial pulses bilaterally when pulse was irregular.	___	___	___	_____

	S	U	NP	Comments
11. Assisted patient to comfortable position.	___	___	___	_____
12. Discussed findings with patient as needed.	___	___	___	_____
13. Performed hand hygiene.	___	___	___	_____

EVALUATION

1. Established radial pulse as baseline if necessary and within acceptable range.	___	___	___	_____
2. Compared pulse rate and character with previous baseline and acceptable range.	___	___	___	_____
3. Identified unexpected outcomes.	___	___	___	_____

RECORDING AND REPORTING

1. Recorded pulse rate and assessment site in appropriate record.	___	___	___	_____
2. Documented measurement of pulse rate after administration of specific therapies in nurses' notes.	___	___	___	_____
3. Reported abnormal findings to nurse in charge or health care provider.	___	___	___	_____

Student _____ Date _____

Instructor _____ Date _____

PERFORMANCE CHECKLIST SKILL 5-3 **ASSESSING APICAL PULSE**

	S	U	NP	Comments
ASSESSMENT				
1. Determined need to assess apical pulse.				
a. Assessed for risk factors for apical pulse alteration.	___	___	___	_____
b. Assessed for symptoms of altered cardiac function.	___	___	___	_____
c. Assessed for factors that normally influence apical pulse rate and rhythm.	___	___	___	_____
2. Determined previous baseline if available.	___	___	___	_____
3. Determined any report of latex allergy, ensured stethoscope is latex free if necessary.	___	___	___	_____
PLANNING				
1. Identified expected outcomes.	___	___	___	_____
2. Explained to patient that you will assess apical pulse rate, encouraged patient to relax, asked patient not to speak, waited if necessary.	___	___	___	_____
3. Collected appropriate supplies.	___	___	___	_____
IMPLEMENTATION				
1. Performed hand hygiene.	___	___	___	_____
2. Provided privacy if necessary.	___	___	___	_____
3. Assisted patient to appropriate position, moved bed linen and gown to expose sternum and left side of chest.	___	___	___	_____
4. Located anatomic landmarks to identify PMI.	___	___	___	_____
5. Placed diaphragm of stethoscope in palm of hand for 5 to 10 seconds.	___	___	___	_____
6. Placed diaphragm of stethoscope over PMI, auscultated for normal heart sounds.	___	___	___	_____
7. Began to count with second hand of watch when you heard heart sounds with regularity.	___	___	___	_____
8. Counted for 30 seconds if pulse was regular, multiplied total by 2.	___	___	___	_____
9. Counted for 60 seconds if pulse was irregular or patient was receiving cardiovascular medication.	___	___	___	_____
10. Note regularity of any dysrhythmia.	___	___	___	_____

	S	U	NP	Comments

11. Replaced patient's gown and linen, assisted patient to a comfortable position. ____ ____ ____ _____

12. Discussed findings with patient. ____ ____ ____ _____

13. Performed hand hygiene. ____ ____ ____ _____

14. Cleaned earpieces and diaphragm of stethoscope with alcohol swab. ____ ____ ____ _____

EVALUATION

1. Established apical rate as baseline if necessary and within acceptable range. ____ ____ ____ _____

2. Compared apical rate and character with baseline and acceptable range. ____ ____ ____ _____

3. Identified unexpected outcomes. ____ ____ ____ _____

RECORDING AND REPORTING

1. Recorded apical pulse rate and rhythm on appropriate record. ____ ____ ____ _____

2. Documented measurement of apical pulse after administration of specific therapies in nurses' notes. ____ ____ ____ _____

3. Documented location of PMI if pulse not found at fifth ICS and LMCL. ____ ____ ____ _____

4. Reported abnormal findings to nurse in charge or health care provider. ____ ____ ____ _____

Student _____ Date _____

Instructor _____ Date _____

PERFORMANCE CHECKLIST PROCEDURAL GUIDELINE 5-1 **ASSESSING APICAL–RADIAL PULSE**

	S	U	NP	Comments
PROCEDURAL STEPS				
1. Determined need to assess for pulse deficit.	___	___	___	_____
2. Performed hand hygiene.	___	___	___	_____
3. Collected appropriate supplies, provided privacy.	___	___	___	_____
4. Explained that two people will be assessing heart function at the same time.	___	___	___	_____
5. Assisted patient to appropriate position, moved bed linen and gown to expose sternum and left side of chest.	___	___	___	_____
6. Located apical and radial pulse sites.	___	___	___	_____
7. Nurse called out loud when to begin counting pulses.	___	___	___	_____
8. Completed a 60-second pulse count simultaneously with another nurse.	___	___	___	_____
9. Ascertained whether pulse deficit exists.	___	___	___	_____
10. Assessed for other signs of decreased cardiac output if a pulse deficit was noted.	___	___	___	_____
11. Discussed findings with patient.	___	___	___	_____
12. Performed hand hygiene.	___	___	___	_____
13. Recorded apical pulse, radial pulse, and pulse deficit in the nurses' notes, informed nurse in charge or health care provider if a pulse deficit exists.	___	___	___	_____

Student _____ Date _____

Instructor _____ Date _____

PERFORMANCE CHECKLIST SKILL 5-4 **ASSESSING RESPIRATIONS**

	S	U	NP	Comments
ASSESSMENT				
1. Determined need to assess patient's respirations.				
a. Assessed for risk factors of respiratory alterations.	___	___	___	_____
b. Assessed for symptoms of respiratory alterations.	___	___	___	_____
c. Assessed for factors that influence the character of respirations.	___	___	___	_____
2. Assessed pertinent laboratory values, including ABGs, pulse oximetry, and CBC.	___	___	___	_____
3. Determined previous baseline respiratory rate.	___	___	___	_____
PLANNING				
1. Identified expected outcomes.	___	___	___	_____
2. Waited before assessing respirations if necessary.	___	___	___	_____
3. Assessed respirations after pulse measurement.	___	___	___	_____
4. Ensured patient was in comfortable position.	___	___	___	_____
IMPLEMENTATION				
1. Provided privacy, performed hand hygiene.	___	___	___	_____
2. Ensured patient's chest was visible, moved linen or gown.	___	___	___	_____
3. Placed patient's arms in the appropriate position.	___	___	___	_____
4. Observed complete respiratory cycle.	___	___	___	_____
5. Counted rate properly.	___	___	___	_____
6. Counted for 30 seconds if rhythm was regular, multiplied total by 2; counted for 60 seconds if irregular (i.e., too fast or too slow).	___	___	___	_____
7. Noted depth of respirations, assessed depth after counting rate.	___	___	___	_____
8. Noted rhythm of ventilatory cycle.	___	___	___	_____
9. Replaced linen and gown.	___	___	___	_____
10. Performed hand hygiene.	___	___	___	_____
11. Discussed findings with patient if needed.	___	___	___	_____

	S	U	NP	Comments

EVALUATION

1. Established rate, rhythm, and depth as baseline if necessary.   ____   ____   ____   _____

2. Compared respirations with previous baseline.   ____   ____   ____   _____

3. Correlated respiratory rate, depth, and rhythm with data from pulse oximetry and ABG values.   ____   ____   ____   _____

4. Identified unexpected outcomes.   ____   ____   ____   _____

RECORDING AND REPORTING

1. Recorded rate in appropriate record, recorded abnormal depth and rhythm in nurses' notes.   ____   ____   ____   _____

2. Documented measurement after specific therapies in nurses' notes.   ____   ____   ____   _____

3. Recorded type and amount of oxygen therapy if necessary.   ____   ____   ____   _____

4. Reported abnormal findings to nurse in charge or health care provider.   ____   ____   ____   _____

Student _____ Date _____

Instructor _____ Date _____

PERFORMANCE CHECKLIST SKILL 5-5 **ASSESSING ARTERIAL BLOOD PRESSURE**

	S	U	NP	Comments

ASSESSMENT

1. Determined need to assess patient's blood pressure.

   a. Assessed risk factors for blood pressure alterations. ___ ___ ___ _____

   b. Assessed for symptoms of blood pressure alterations. ___ ___ ___ _____

   c. Assessed for factors that influence blood pressure. ___ ___ ___ _____

2. Determined appropriate site for blood pressure assessment. ___ ___ ___ _____

3. Determined previous baseline, determined report of latex allergy. ___ ___ ___ _____

4. Assessed patient's knowledge of procedure. ___ ___ ___ _____

PLANNING

1. Identified expected outcomes. ___ ___ ___ _____

2. Explained to patient that you will assess blood pressure, had patient rest appropriately before measuring, asked patient not to speak. ___ ___ ___ _____

3. Ensured patient has not exercised, ingested caffeine, or smoked in the last 30 minutes. ___ ___ ___ _____

4. Had patient assume appropriate position, ensured room was warm, quiet, and relaxing. ___ ___ ___ _____

5. Selected appropriate cuff size. ___ ___ ___ _____

6. Performed hand hygiene. ___ ___ ___ _____

IMPLEMENTATION

1. Assessed BP by auscultation:

   a. Positioned patient appropriately based on which extremity was to be used. ___ ___ ___ _____

   b. Exposed extremity fully. ___ ___ ___ _____

   c. Palpated artery, applied bladder of cuff properly above the artery. ___ ___ ___ _____

   d. Positioned manometer gauge vertically at eye level. ___ ___ ___ _____

   e. Measured blood pressure. ___ ___ ___ _____

	S	U	NP	Comments

(1) Two-step method:

    (a) Relocated brachial pulse, palpated artery while inflating the cuff to the appropriate pressure, slowly deflated cuff, noted where pulse reappears, deflated cuff, waited 30 seconds. ____ ____ ____ _____

    (b) Placed stethoscope ear pieces in ears, ensured sounds were clear. ____ ____ ____ _____

    (c) Relocated brachial artery, placed bell or diaphragm of stethoscope over it without touching cuff or clothing. ____ ____ ____ _____

    (d) Closed valve of pressure bulb, inflated cuff quickly to appropriate pressure. ____ ____ ____ _____

    (e) Released pressure valve slowly, allowed manometer needle to fall at appropriate rate. ____ ____ ____ _____

    (f) Noted point on manometer when you heard first clear sound. ____ ____ ____ _____

    (g) Deflated cuff gradually, noted point at which sound disappeared, listened past the last sound. ____ ____ ____ _____

(2) One-step method:

    (a) Placed stethoscope earpieces in ears, ensured sounds were clear. ____ ____ ____ _____

    (b) Relocated brachial artery, placed bell or diaphragm of stethoscope over it, did not allow bell to touch cuff or clothing. ____ ____ ____ _____

    (c) Closed valve of pressure bulb, inflated cuff quickly to appropriate pressure. ____ ____ ____ _____

    (d) Released pressure bulb slowly, allowed manometer to fall at appropriate rate, noted point on manometer when first clear sound was heard. ____ ____ ____ _____

    (e) Continued to deflate cuff, noted point at which sound disappeared, listened after last sound. ____ ____ ____ _____

  f. Took two measurements at 2 minutes apart, used second as baseline. ____ ____ ____ _____

  g. Removed cuff from patient's arm. ____ ____ ____ _____

  h. Repeated on other arm if necessary. ____ ____ ____ _____

  i. Assisted patient to a comfortable position, covered arm if necessary. ____ ____ ____ _____

	S	U	NP	Comments

j. Discussed findings with patient. ___ ___ ___ _____

k. Performed hand hygiene, cleaned stethoscope. ___ ___ ___ _____

2. Assessed systolic blood pressure by palpation.

   a. Followed steps 1a through 1d of auscultation method. ___ ___ ___ _____

   b. Located and palpated artery continuously with fingertips, inflated cuff to appropriate pressure. ___ ___ ___ _____

   c. Slowly released valve, allowed manometer to fall at appropriate rate, noted point at which pulse was palpable again. ___ ___ ___ _____

   d. Deflated cuff rapidly and completely, removed cuff from patient. ___ ___ ___ _____

   e. Assisted patient to comfortable position, covered extremity if necessary. ___ ___ ___ _____

   f. Discussed findings with patient. ___ ___ ___ _____

   g. Performed hand hygiene. ___ ___ ___ _____

EVALUATION

1. Established baseline if necessary. ___ ___ ___ _____

2. Compared reading with previous baseline and usual blood pressure for patient's age. ___ ___ ___ _____

3. Identified unexpected outcomes. ___ ___ ___ _____

RECORDING AND REPORTING

1. Recorded blood pressure and site assessed in appropriate record. ___ ___ ___ _____

2. Documented measurement after administration of specific therapies in nurses' notes. ___ ___ ___ _____

3. Recorded symptoms of blood pressure alterations in nurses' notes. ___ ___ ___ _____

4. Reported abnormal findings to nurse in charge or health care provider. ___ ___ ___ _____

Student _____ Date _____

Instructor _____ Date _____

PERFORMANCE CHECKLIST PROCEDURAL GUIDELINE 5-2 **ASSESSING BLOOD PRESSURE ELECTRONICALLY**

	S	U	NP	Comments
PROCEDURAL STEPS				
1. Determined appropriateness of using electronic blood pressure measurement.	__	__	__	_____
2. Determined best site for cuff placement.	__	__	__	_____
3. Collected appropriate equipment.	__	__	__	_____
4. Performed hand hygiene, assisted patient to comfortable position, plugged in device and placed near patient.	__	__	__	_____
5. Turned machine on.	__	__	__	_____
6. Selected appropriate cuff size and cuff.	__	__	__	_____
7. Exposed extremity.	__	__	__	_____
8. Manually squeezed all the air out, connected cuff to hose.	__	__	__	_____
9. Wrapped cuff snugly around extremity, verified that one finger fits between cuff and patient's skin, ensured artery arrow was placed correctly.	__	__	__	_____
10. Verified connector hose was not kinked.	__	__	__	_____
11. Set frequency control, pressed start.	__	__	__	_____
12. Set frequency of measurements and upper and lower alarm limits.	__	__	__	_____
13. Obtained additional readings when necessary.	__	__	__	_____
14. Removed cuff at least every 2 hours, removed and cleaned cuff after last use.	__	__	__	_____
15. Discussed findings with patient, performed hand hygiene.	__	__	__	_____
16. Compared electronic blood pressure readings with auscultatory measurements to verify accuracy.	__	__	__	_____
17. Recorded blood pressure and site assessed in appropriate record, recorded symptoms of blood pressure alterations in nurses' notes, reported abnormal findings to nurse in charge or health care provider.	__	__	__	_____

Student _____ Date _____

Instructor _____ Date _____

PERFORMANCE CHECKLIST PROCEDURAL GUIDELINE 5-3 **MEASURING OXYGEN SATURATION (PULSE OXIMETRY)**

	S	U	NP	Comments

PROCEDURAL STEPS

1. Determined need to measure patient's oxygen saturation, assessed risk factors for decreased oxygen saturation.

2. Assessed for symptoms of alterations in oxygen saturation.

3. Assessed for factors that influence measurement of SpO_2.

4. Reviewed patient's record for standard of care regarding measurement of SpO_2.

5. Determined previous baseline SpO_2 if available.

6. Determined most appropriate site for sensor probe placement by measuring capillary refill.

7. Performed hand hygiene.

8. Positioned patient comfortably, instructed patient to breathe normally.

9. Attached sensor to monitoring site, removed nail polish if necessary, instructed patient that probe will not hurt.

10. Turned oximeter on, correlated oximeter pulse rate with patient's radial pulse.

11. Left sensor in place until readout reached constant value and pulse display reached full strength, informed patient of oximeter alarm, read SpO_2 on display.

12. Determined limits for SpO_2, verified that alarms are on, assessed skin integrity under sensor probe every 2 hours, relocated if necessary.

13. Removed probe and turned oximeter off if planning to check SpO_2 intermittently, stored sensor appropriately.

14. Discussed findings with patient, performed hand hygiene.

	S	U	NP	Comments
15. Compared SpO_2 readings with baseline and acceptable SpO_2.	___	___	___	_____
16. Recorded SpO_2 in appropriate record, recorded symptoms of oxygen saturation alterations in nurses' notes, reported abnormal findings to nurse in charge or health care provider.	___	___	___	_____

Student _____ Date _____

Instructor _____ Date _____

PERFORMANCE CHECKLIST SKILL 6-1 **GENERAL SURVEY**

	S	U	NP	Comments
ASSESSMENT				
1. Noted if patient has had any acute distress, deferred general survey if necessary.	___	___	___	_____
2. Reviewed graphic sheet for previous vital signs, considered factors or conditions that may alter values.	___	___	___	_____
3. Determined patient's primary language, determined availability of interpreter if necessary, had interpreter translate verbatim.	___	___	___	_____
4. Reviewed history, confirmed primary reason patient has sought health care.	___	___	___	_____
5. Identified patient's normal height, weight, and BMI, determined amount of weight change and time period in which it occurred if necessary, assessed if patient has been dieting or exercising.	___	___	___	_____
6. Reviewed patient's past fluid I&O records.	___	___	___	_____
7. Identified patient's general perceptions about personal health.	___	___	___	_____
8. Assessed for evidence of latex allergy, asked if patient has risk factors such as food allergies.	___	___	___	_____
PLANNING				
1. Identified expected outcomes.	___	___	___	_____
2. Explained to patient that you will be doing a routine check for areas of concern, asked patient to tell you if any area hurts when touched.	___	___	___	_____
3. Performed hand hygiene, assembled necessary equipment, positioned patient appropriately.	___	___	___	_____
IMPLEMENTATION				
1. Noted patient's verbal and nonverbal behaviors, determined patient's LOC and orientation.	___	___	___	_____
2. Obtained temperature, pulse, respirations, and blood pressure if needed, informed patient of vital signs.	___	___	___	_____
3. Observed gender and race, asked age, noted patient's physical features.	___	___	___	_____

	S	U	NP	Comments
4. Rephrased or asked a similar question if necessary.	___	___	___	_____
5. Asked short questions the patient should know if responses were inappropriate.	___	___	___	_____
6. Offered simple commands if patient was unable to respond to questions of orientation.	___	___	___	_____
7. Assessed affect and mood, noted if verbal and nonverbal expressions match and were appropriate to the situation.	___	___	___	_____
8. Watched patient interact with spouse, children, or caregiver; noted any obvious physical injuries in the patient.	___	___	___	_____
9. Observed for signs of abuse.	___	___	___	_____
10. Assessed posture and position, assessed body movements.	___	___	___	_____
11. Assessed speech.	___	___	___	_____
12. Observed hygiene and grooming (i.e., hair, nails, body odor).	___	___	___	_____
13. Inspected exposed area of skin, asked if patient has noted any changes in skin.	___	___	___	_____
14. Inspected skin surfaces, compared symmetrical body parts.	___	___	___	_____
15. Inspected color of face, oral mucosa, lips, conjunctiva, sclera, palms, and nail beds.	___	___	___	_____
16. Used ungloved fingertips to palpate skin surfaces, noted texture, smoothness, and temperature.	___	___	___	_____
17. Applied gloves, inspected character of secretions, removed gloves and disposed of them.	___	___	___	_____
18. Assessed skin turgor by grasping fold of skin and releasing, noted ease and speed with which skin returned to place.	___	___	___	_____
19. Assessed condition of skin for pressure areas, applied pressure with fingertips and released over areas of redness.	___	___	___	_____
20. Used adequate lighting to inspect any lesions, used gloves if necessary, noted if patient reported tenderness, measured size of lesion with a centimeter.	___	___	___	_____

EVALUATION

1. Observed for evidence of physical and emotional distress.	___	___	___	_____
2. Compared assessment findings with previous observations.	___	___	___	_____

	S	U	NP	Comments

3. Asked patient if there was information about physical condition you have not discussed. ___ ___ ___ _____

4. Identified unexpected outcomes. ___ ___ ___ _____

RECORDING AND REPORTING

1. Recorded patient's vitals on the vital sign flow sheet. ___ ___ ___ _____

2. Recorded description of alterations in patient's general appearance. ___ ___ ___ _____

3. Described patient's behaviors using objective terms, included patient's self-reporting. ___ ___ ___ _____

4. Reported abnormalities and acute symptoms to nurse in charge or health care provider. ___ ___ ___ _____

Student _____ Date _____

Instructor _____ Date _____

PERFORMANCE CHECKLIST SKILL 6-2 **HEAD AND NECK ASSESSMENT**

	S	U	NP	Comments

ASSESSMENT

1. Assessed for history of headache, dizziness, pain, or stiffness.

2. Determined if patient has history of eye disease, diabetes mellitus, or hypertension.

3. Asked if patient has experienced blurred vision, flashing lights, halos around lights, or reduced visual field.

4. Asked if patient has experienced ear pain, itching, discharge, vertigo, tinnitus, or change in hearing.

5. Reviewed patient's occupational history.

6. Asked if patient has a history of allergies, nasal discharge, epistaxis, or postnasal drip.

7. Determined if the patient smokes or chews tobacco.

PLANNING

1. Identified expected outcomes.

2. Told patient you will be completing a routine examination of the head and neck.

IMPLEMENTATION

1. Positioned patient appropriately.

2. Inspected the head, noted position, facial features, and symmetry.

3. Assessed the eyes.

   a. Inspected position of eyes, color, condition of conjunctiva, and movement.

   b. Assessed patient's near vision and far vision.

   c. Inspected pupils for size, shape, and equality.

   d. Tested papillary reflexes properly, tested for accommodation.

4. Assessed hearing, noted patient's response to questions and presence of a hearing aid, asked patient to repeat short words if necessary.

	S	U	NP	Comments

5. Inspected nose externally, noted color of mucosa, lesions, discharge, swelling, or bleeding, consulted with health care provider if drainage was infectious. ____ ____ ____ _____

6. Inspected nares in patients with NG, NI, or nasotracheal tube, stabilized tube as needed. ____ ____ ____ _____

7. Inspected sinuses properly. ____ ____ ____ _____

8. Assessed the mouth, determined if dentures or retainers are comfortable. ____ ____ ____ _____

9. Inspected and palpated the neck, asked patient if there is history of pain or difficulty with neck movement.

   a. Inspected neck for bilateral symmetry of muscles, asked patient to flex and hyperextend neck and turn head side to side. ____ ____ ____ _____

   b. Positioned patient appropriately, inspected area where lymph nodes are distributed properly, compared both sides, noted if nodes are large, fixed, inflamed, or tender. ____ ____ ____ _____

EVALUATION

1. Compared assessment findings with previous observation. ____ ____ ____ _____

2. Asked patient to describe common symptoms of eye, ear, sinus, or mouth disease. ____ ____ ____ _____

3. Asked patient to list occupation safety precautions. ____ ____ ____ _____

4. Identified unexpected outcomes. ____ ____ ____ _____

RECORDING AND REPORTING

1. Recorded all findings, including abnormal findings, in appropriate record. ____ ____ ____ _____

2. Reported any unexpected findings to nurse in charge or health care provider. ____ ____ ____ _____

Student _____ Date _____

Instructor _____ Date _____

PERFORMANCE CHECKLIST SKILL 6-3   **THORAX AND LUNG ASSESSMENT**

	S	U	NP	Comments

ASSESSMENT

1. Assessed history of tobacco and marijuana use (i.e., type, duration, and amount in pack-years), determined length of time since smoking if patient quit.

2. Asked if patient experiences respiratory alterations.

3. Determined if patient works in environment containing pollutants, radiation, or secondhand smoke.

4. Reviewed history for risk factors and/or exposure to infectious diseases (e.g., HIV, TB).

5. Asked if patient had history of persistent cough, hemoptysis, unexplained weight loss, fatigue, night sweats, or fever.

6. Asked if patient has history of chronic hoarseness.

7. Assessed for history of allergies.

8. Reviewed family history for cancer, TB, allergies, or COPD.

PLANNING

1. Identified expected outcomes.

IMPLEMENTATION

1. Positioned patient and prepared for examination.

   a. Positioned patient appropriately.

   b. Removed gown from posterior chest, kept front of chest and legs covered, removed the gown from area being examined as you proceed.

   c. Explained all steps, encouraged patient to relax and breathe normally.

2. Inspected posterior thorax.

   a. Stood behind patient; inspected thorax for shape; noted deformities, position of spine, slope of ribs, retraction of intercostal spaces during inspiration, bulging of intercostal spaces during expiration, and symmetrical expansion.

	S	U	NP	Comments

b. Determined rate and rhythm of breathing, had patient relax. ___ ___ ___ _____

c. Palpated for lumps, masses, pulsations, unusual movement, or areas of localized tenderness; palpated suspicious mass or size, shape, and typical qualities of lesions. ___ ___ ___ _____

d. Palpated chest excursion to assess depth of patient's breathing. ___ ___ ___ _____

e. Auscultated breath sounds; had patient take slow, deep mouth breaths; listened to entire inspiration and expiration at each position; compared breath sounds over both sides; asked patient to breathe deeper if necessary. ___ ___ ___ _____

f. Had patient cough if adventitious sounds were heard, listened again to determine if sound was cleared with coughing. ___ ___ ___ _____

3. Inspected lateral thorax.

a. Instructed patient to raise arms, inspected chest wall for same characteristics as reviewed for posterior chest. ___ ___ ___ _____

b. Extended palpation and auscultation to lateral sides of chest. ___ ___ ___ _____

4. Inspected anterior thorax.

a. Inspected accessory muscles of breathing, noted effort to breathe. ___ ___ ___ _____

b. Inspected width or spread of angle made by coastal margins and tip of sternum. ___ ___ ___ _____

c. Observed patient's breathing pattern as well as symmetry and degree of chest wall and abdominal movement. ___ ___ ___ _____

d. Palpated anterior thoracic muscles and ribs for lumps, masses, tenderness, or unusual movement. ___ ___ ___ _____

e. Palpated anterior chest excursion appropriately. ___ ___ ___ _____

f. Auscultated anterior thorax properly. ___ ___ ___ _____

EVALUATION

1. Compared respiratory findings with assessment characteristics for thorax and lungs. ___ ___ ___ _____

2. Had patient identify factors leading to lung diseases. ___ ___ ___ _____

3. Identified unexpected outcomes. ___ ___ ___ _____

	S	U	NP	Comments

RECORDING AND REPORTING

1. Documented patient's respiratory rate and character in the appropriate record. ___ ___ ___ _____

2. Reported abnormalities to nurse in charge or health care provider. ___ ___ ___ _____

Student _____ Date _____

Instructor _____ Date _____

PERFORMANCE CHECKLIST SKILL 6-4 **CARDIOVASCULAR ASSESSMENT**

	S	U	NP	Comments
ASSESSMENT				
1. Assessed patient for history of smoking, alcohol intake, caffeine intake, use of "recreational" drugs, exercise habits, and dietary patterns.	___	___	___	_____
2. Determined if patient is taking medications for cardiovascular function and if patient knows their purpose, dosage, and side effects.	___	___	___	_____
3. Asked if patient has experienced the cardinal symptoms of heart disease, asked if symptoms occurred while exercising or at rest.	___	___	___	_____
4. Determined onset, factors, quality, region, severity, and radiation of any reported chest pain.	___	___	___	_____
5. Assessed family history for heart disease, diabetes, high cholesterol or lipids, hypertension, stroke, or rheumatic heart disease.	___	___	___	_____
6. Asked patient about history of preexisting heart conditions, heart surgery, or vascular disease.	___	___	___	_____
7. Determined if patient experiences leg cramps, numbness or tingling in extremities, sensation of cold hands or feet, pain in legs, or swelling or cyanosis of extremities.	___	___	___	_____
8. Asked if any leg pain or cramping was present, asked if it was relieved by walking or standing or if it occurred during sleep.	___	___	___	_____
9. Asked women if they wear tight-fitting underwear or hosiery or sit or lie in bed with legs crossed.	___	___	___	_____
PLANNING				
1. Identified expected outcomes.	___	___	___	_____
IMPLEMENTATION				
1. Assisted patient in being as relaxed and comfortable as possible.	___	___	___	_____
2. Had patient assume proper position.	___	___	___	_____
3. Explained procedure, avoided facial gestures reflecting concern.	___	___	___	_____
4. Ensured that room was quiet.	___	___	___	_____

	S	U	NP	Comments

5. Assessed the heart.

   a. Formed a mental image of the exact location of the heart. ___ ___ ___ _____

   b. Found the angle of Louis, slipped finder down each side to feel adjacent ribs. ___ ___ ___ _____

   c. Found the following anatomic landmarks:

     (1) The arotic area ___ ___ ___ _____

     (2) The pulmonic area ___ ___ ___ _____

     (3) The second pulmonic area ___ ___ ___ _____

     (4) The tricuspid area ___ ___ ___ _____

     (5) The mitral area ___ ___ ___ _____

     (6) The epigastric area ___ ___ ___ _____

   d. Stood to the patient's right, inspected and palpated the precordium, noted visible pulsations and more exaggerated lifts, palpated for pulsations at all landmarks. ___ ___ ___ _____

   e. Located PMI. ___ ___ ___ _____

   f. Turned patient onto left side if necessary. ___ ___ ___ _____

   g. Inspected epigastric area, palpated abdominal aorta, noted a localized strong beat. ___ ___ ___ _____

   h. Auscultated heart sounds properly.

     (1) Asked patient not to speak but to breathe comfortably, began with diaphragm of the stethoscope and alternated with the bell, avoided jumping from one area to another. ___ ___ ___ _____

     (2) Moved systematically around the heart sound locations in the proper order. ___ ___ ___ _____

     (3) Listened for S_2 at each site. ___ ___ ___ _____

     (4) Counted each *lub-dub* as one heartbeat, counted number of beats for 1 minute. ___ ___ ___ _____

     (5) Assessed heart rhythm by noting time between S_1 and S_2 and time between S_2 and the next S_1, listened to the full cycle at each area, noted regular intervals between each sequence. ___ ___ ___ _____

     (6) Compared apical and radial pulses when heart rate is irregular, asked a colleague for assistance if needed. ___ ___ ___ _____

	S	U	NP	Comments

i. Auscultated for extra heart sounds at each site, noted pitch, loudness, duration, timing, location on chest wall, and where heard in cardiac cycle.

   (1) Listened for low-pitched extra sounds with the bell of the stethoscope.

   (2) Positioned patient properly, asked patient to hold breath, listened for friction rubs.

j. Auscultated for heart murmurs over each auscultation site.

   (1) Noted intensity and location when you can best hear any murmur detected.

   (2) Noted pitch of the murmur.

6. Assessed neck vessels.

  a. Positioned patient appropriately.

  b. Inspected both sides of neck for obvious arterial pulsations.

  c. Palpated each carotid artery appropriately; asked patient to raise chin slightly; noted rate, rhythm, strength, and elasticity; noted if pulse changed during breathing.

  d. Auscultated for blowing sound over each carotid artery with bell of stethoscope, asked patient to hold a breath for a few heartbeats so respiratory sounds do not interfere with auscultation.

  e. Assessed JVD properly.

7. Performed peripheral vascular assessment.

  a. Inspected lower extremities for changes in color and conditions of the skin, compared skin color with patient lying and standing.

  b. Palpated edematous areas, noted mobility, consistency, and tenderness.

  c. Assessed for pitting edema properly.

  d. Checked capillary refill properly.

  e. Asked if patient experienced pain or tenderness, checked for signs on phlebitis or DVT.

  f. Palpated each peripheral artery for equality and elasticity starting at the distal end of each, noted ease with which it sprung back and strength of pulse.

  g. Palpated radial pulse properly.

	S	U	NP	Comments
h. Palpated ulnar pulse properly.	___	___	___	_____
i. Palpated brachial pulse properly.	___	___	___	_____
j. Positioned patient appropriately, palpated dorsalis pedis pulse properly.	___	___	___	_____
k. Palpated posterior tibial pulse properly.	___	___	___	_____
l. Palpated popliteal pulse properly, repositioned patient if needed.	___	___	___	_____
m. Applied gloves; positioned patient properly, palpated femoral pulse properly.	___	___	___	_____
n. Used a Doppler instrument if necessary.	___	___	___	_____
(1) Applied conducting gel to either patient's skin or transducer tip of probe, turned on Doppler.	___	___	___	_____
(2) Applied probe to skin, changed probe angle until pulsation is audible, wiped gel from patient and Doppler.	___	___	___	_____

EVALUATION

	S	U	NP	Comments
1. Compared findings with normal assessment characteristics of heart and vascular system.	___	___	___	_____
2. Asked another nurse to confirm assessment if heart sounds are not audible or pulses are not palpable.	___	___	___	_____
3. Asked patient to describe behaviors that increase risk for heart and vascular disease.	___	___	___	_____
4. Compared pulses and capillary refill bilaterally with previous assessment.	___	___	___	_____
5. Identified unexpected outcomes.	___	___	___	_____

RECORDING AND REPORTING

	S	U	NP	Comments
1. Documented quality, intensity, rate, and rhythm of heart sounds and peripheral pulses in appropriate record.	___	___	___	_____
2. Documented additional cardiac findings, JVP, and condition of extremities in appropriate record.	___	___	___	_____
3. Documented activity level and subjective data related to fatigue, shortness of breath, and chest pain.	___	___	___	_____
4. Reported any irregularities in heart function and indications of impaired arterial blood flow immediately to health care provider.	___	___	___	_____
5. Reported changes in peripheral circulation to health care provider.	___	___	___	_____

Student _____ Date _____

Instructor _____ Date _____

PERFORMANCE CHECKLIST SKILL 6-5 **ABDOMINAL ASSESSMENT**

	S	U	NP	Comments
ASSESSMENT				
1. Assessed character of any reported abdominal or lower back pain.	___	___	___	_____
2. Observed patient's movement and position.	___	___	___	_____
3. Assessed patient's normal bowel habits.	___	___	___	_____
4. Determined if patient has had abdominal surgery, trauma, or diagnostic tests of the GI tract.	___	___	___	_____
5. Assessed if patient has had recent weight changes or intolerance to diet.	___	___	___	_____
6. Assessed for indications of GI alterations.	___	___	___	_____
7. Determined if patient takes antiinflammatory medications or antibiotic.	___	___	___	_____
8. Reviewed family history of cancer, kidney disease, alcoholism, hypertension, or heart disease.	___	___	___	_____
9. Reviewed patient's history for risks of HBV exposure.	___	___	___	_____
PLANNING				
1. Identified expected outcomes.	___	___	___	_____
IMPLEMENTATION				
1. Prepared patient for abdominal assessment.				
a. Asked if patient needed to empty bladder or defecate.	___	___	___	_____
b. Kept patient's upper chest and legs draped.	___	___	___	_____
c. Ensured that room was warm.	___	___	___	_____
d. Positioned patient properly.	___	___	___	_____
e. Exposed area from just above the xiphoid process down to the symphysis pubis.	___	___	___	_____
f. Maintained conversation during assessment except during auscultation, explained steps calmly and slowly.	___	___	___	_____
g. Asked patient to point to tender areas.	___	___	___	_____
2. Performed abdominal assessment.				
a. Identified landmarks dividing abdominal region into quadrants.	___	___	___	_____

	S	U	NP	Comments

b. Inspected skin of abdomen's surface for color, scars, venous patterns, rashes, lesions, stretch marks, and artificial openings; observed lesions for characteristics described in Skill 6-1. ____ ____ ____ _____

c. Asked if patient self-administers injections if bruising was noted. ____ ____ ____ _____

d. Inspected contour, symmetry, and surface motion of the abdomen; noted masses, bulging, or distention. ____ ____ ____ _____

e. Noted if any distention was generalized, looked for flanks on each side. ____ ____ ____ _____

f. Measured size of abdominal girth if you suspected distention, used the marking pen to indicate where tape measure was applied. ____ ____ ____ _____

g. Turned off suction connected to an NG or NI tube momentarily. ____ ____ ____ _____

h. Auscultated bowel sounds appropriately, asked patient not to talk, listened at least 5 minutes before describing sounds as *absent*. ____ ____ ____ _____

i. Auscultated for vascular sounds with bell of stethoscope over the epigastric region and each quadrant. ____ ____ ____ _____

j. Positioned patient appropriately, percussed each of the four quadrants, noted areas of tympany and dullness. ____ ____ ____ _____

k. Percussed for a fluid wave properly and if necessary. ____ ____ ____ _____

l. Asked patient if abdomen feels unusually tight, determined if this was a recent development. ____ ____ ____ _____

m. Positioned patient appropriately, percussed over each CVA along scapular lines, noted if patient experienced pain. ____ ____ ____ _____

n. Lightly palpated over each quadrant, palpated painful areas last.

(1) Noted muscular resistance, distention, tenderness, and superficial masses; observed patient's face for signs of discomfort. ____ ____ ____ _____

(2) Noted if abdomen was firm or soft to touch. ____ ____ ____ _____

o. Palpated for a smooth round mass below umbilicus and above symphysis pubis, asked if patient had sensation of needing to void. ____ ____ ____ _____

	S	U	NP	Comments

p. Noted size, location, shape, consistency, tenderness, mobility, and texture of any masses palpated. ___ ___ ___ _____

q. Pressed one hand slowly into tender areas and released quickly, noted if pain was aggravated. ___ ___ ___ _____

EVALUATION

1. Compared assessment findings with previous assessment characteristics to identify changes. ___ ___ ___ _____

2. Asked patient to describe signs and symptoms of colorectal cancer. ___ ___ ___ _____

3. Identified unexpected outcomes. ___ ___ ___ _____

RECORDING AND REPORTING

1. Documented appearance of abdomen, quality of bowel sounds, presence of distention, abdominal circumference, and presence and location of tenderness in appropriate record. ___ ___ ___ _____

2. Recorded patient's ability to void and defecate, included description of output. ___ ___ ___ _____

3. Recorded content of any patient instruction. ___ ___ ___ _____

4. Reported abnormal findings to nurse in charge and health care provider. ___ ___ ___ _____

Student _____ Date _____

Instructor _____ Date _____

PERFORMANCE CHECKLIST SKILL 6-6 **GENITALIA AND RECTUM ASSESSMENT**

	S	U	NP	Comments

ASSESSMENT

1. Assessed female patient.

   a. Determined if patient has symptoms of vaginal discharge, painful or swollen perianal tissue, or genital lesions. ___ ___ ___ _____

   b. Determined if patient has symptoms or history of genitourinary problems. ___ ___ ___ _____

   c. Asked if patient has had signs of bleeding outside of normal menstruation or after menopause or has had unusual vaginal discharge. ___ ___ ___ _____

   d. Determined if patient has received HPV vaccine. ___ ___ ___ _____

   e. Determined if patient has history of HPV, first pregnancy before age 17, smoking, obesity, diet low in fruits and vegetables, or has had multiple full-term pregnancies. ___ ___ ___ _____

   f. Determined if patient is older than 63; is obese; has history of ovarian dysfunction, breast or endometrial cancer, or endometriosis; has family history of reproductive cancer; has history of infertility or nulliparity; or uses estrogen as hormone replacement therapy. ___ ___ ___ _____

   g. Determined if patient is postmenopausal, obese, or infertile; had early menarche or late menopause; has history of hypertension, diabetes, gallbladder disease, or polycystic ovary disease; has family history of endometrial, breast, or colon cancer; or has history of estrogen-related exposure. ___ ___ ___ _____

   h. Determined patient's knowledge of risk factors and signs of gynecological cancers. ___ ___ ___ _____

2. Assessed male patient.

   a. Reviewed normal elimination pattern. ___ ___ ___ _____

   b. Asked if patient has noted penile pain or swelling, genital lesions, or urethral discharge. ___ ___ ___ _____

	S	U	NP	Comments

c. Determined if patient has noted heaviness or painless enlargement or irregular lumps of testis.

d. Determined if patient reported any enlargement of inguinal area; assessed if any enlargement was intermittent, associated with straining, and painful; assessed whether coughing, lifting, or straining at stool causes pain.

e. Asked if patient has experienced weak or interrupted urine flow, difficulty with urinating, polyuria, nocturia, hematuria, or dysuria; determined if patient has continuing pain in lower back, pelvis, or upper thighs.

f. Assessed patient's knowledge of risk factors and signs of prostate and testicular cancer.

3. Assessment of all patients:

a. Determined whether patient has experienced rectal bleeding or pain, black or tarry stools, or change in bowel habits.

b. Determined whether patient has personal or family history of colorectal cancer, polyps, or chronic inflammatory bowel disease, asked if patient is over age 50.

c. Inquired about dietary habits.

d. Determined if patient is obese, physically inactive, smokes, has type 2 diabetes, or consumes alcohol.

e. Assessed medication history for use of laxatives or cathartic medications.

f. Assessed for use of codeine or iron preparations.

g. Assessed patient's knowledge of risks and signs of colorectal cancer.

PLANNING

1. Identified expected outcomes.

IMPLEMENTATION

1. Prepared patient for assessment.

a. Asked if patient needs to empty bladder or defecate.

b. Kept patient's upper chest and legs draped, kept room warm.

c. Positioned patient appropriately.

d. Applied clean gloves.

	S	U	NP	Comments

2. Performed female genitalia examination.

  a. Exposed perineal area. ___ ___ ___ _____

  b. Inspected surface characteristics of perineum; retracted labia majora; observed for inflammation, edema, lesions, or lacerations; noted if there was any discharge. ___ ___ ___ _____

3. Performed male genitalia examination.

  a. Exposed perineal area; observed genitalia for rashes, excoriations, or lesions. ___ ___ ___ _____

  b. Inspected and palpated penile surfaces. ___ ___ ___ _____

  c. Inspected and palpated testicular surfaces. ___ ___ ___ _____

  d. Palpated testes, asked if patient experiences tenderness with palpation. ___ ___ ___ _____

4. Assessed rectum.

  a. Positioned patient appropriately. ___ ___ ___ _____

  b. Viewed perianal and sacrococcygeal areas by retracting buttocks using nondominant hand. ___ ___ ___ _____

  c. Inspected anal tissue for skin characteristics, lesions, external hemorrhoids, ulcers, inflammation, rashes, and excoriation. ___ ___ ___ _____

EVALUATION

1. Compared assessment findings with previous assessment characteristics to identify change. ___ ___ ___ _____

2. Asked patient to list warning signs of appropriate cancers. ___ ___ ___ _____

3. Identified unexpected outcomes. ___ ___ ___ _____

RECORDING AND REPORTING

1. Documented results of assessment in appropriate record. ___ ___ ___ _____

2. Recorded patient's ability to void, including description of output. ___ ___ ___ _____

3. Recorded content of any patient instruction. ___ ___ ___ _____

4. Reported abnormalities to nurse in charge and health care provider. ___ ___ ___ _____

Student _____ Date _____

Instructor _____ Date _____

PERFORMANCE CHECKLIST SKILL 6-7 **MUSCULOSKELETAL AND NEUROLOGIC ASSESSMENT**

	S	U	NP	Comments

ASSESSMENT

1. Reviewed patient history for alcohol intake of more than 2 drinks per day; inadequate intake of protein, vitamin D, or calcium; thin and light body frame; family history of osteoporosis; white or Asian ancestry; sedentary lifestyle; long-term use of certain medications; certain medical conditions.

2. Determined if patient has been screened for osteoporosis.

3. Asked patient to describe history of alteration in bone, muscle, or joint function and location of alteration.

4. Assessed nature and extent of patient's musculoskeletal pain, asked if walking affects reported lower extremity pain or cramping, assessed distance walked and pain before, during, and after activity.

5. Assessed for height and weight, noted if there is a decrease in women older than 50.

6. Determined if patient uses analgesics, antipsychotics, antidepressants, nervous system stimulants, or recreational drugs.

7. Determined if patient had recent history of seizures or convulsions; clarified sequence of events; character of any symptoms; and relationship to time of day, fatigue, or stress.

8. Screened patient for headache, tremors, dizziness, vertigo, numbness or tingling, visual changes, weakness, pain, or changes in speech.

9. Discussed with spouse, family member, or friends any recent changes in behavior.

10. Assessed patient for history of change in vision, hearing, smell, taste, or touch.

11. Reviewed history for drug toxicity, serious infection, metabolic disturbances, heart failure, and severe anemia if patient displays sudden acute confusion.

12. Reviewed history for head or spinal cord injury, meningitis, congenital anomalies, neurologic disease, or psychiatric counseling.

	S	U	NP	Comments

PLANNING

1. Identified expected outcomes. ____ ____ ____ _____

IMPLEMENTATION

1. Prepared patient for assessment.

   a. Integrated musculoskeletal and neurologic assessments during other portions of assessment or care. ____ ____ ____ _____

   b. Planned time for short rest periods during assessment. ____ ____ ____ _____

2. Assessed musculoskeletal system.

   a. Observed ability to use arms for grasping objects. ____ ____ ____ _____

   b. Assessed muscle strength of upper extremities by applying gradual increase in pressure to muscle group. ____ ____ ____ _____

   c. Assessed hand grasp strength appropriately. ____ ____ ____ _____

   d. Compared strength of symmetrical muscle groups, noted weakness. ____ ____ ____ _____

   e. Measured muscle size of both muscles if muscle weakness was identified in symmetrical muscle group. ____ ____ ____ _____

   f. Observed body alignment in different positions, exposed muscles and joints. ____ ____ ____ _____

   g. Inspected gait as patient walked, had patient use assistive devices if appropriate. ____ ____ ____ _____

   h. Performed the Get Up and Go Test. ____ ____ ____ _____

   i. Stood behind patient; observed postural alignment; looked sideways at cervical, thoracic, and lumbar curves. ____ ____ ____ _____

   j. Made a general observation of extremities. ____ ____ ____ _____

   k. Palpated bones, joints, and surrounding tissue in involved areas; noted heat, tenderness, edema, or resistance to pressure. ____ ____ ____ _____

   l. Asked patient to put major joint through its full ROM, observed equality of active and passive motion in same body parts. ____ ____ ____ _____

   m. Palpated joint for swelling, stiffness, tenderness, and heat; noted any redness. ____ ____ ____ _____

   n. Assessed muscle tone in major muscle groups. ____ ____ ____ _____

	S	U	NP	Comments

3. Performed neurologic assessment.

   a. Assessed LOC and orientation. ___ ___ ___ _____

   b. Assessed CNs.

      (1) Assessed EOM for CNs III, IV, and VI. ___ ___ ___ _____

      (2) Applied light sensation with cotton ball to symmetrical areas of the face. ___ ___ ___ _____

      (3) Had patient frown, smile, puff cheeks, and raise eyebrows for CN VII, note symmetry. ___ ___ ___ _____

      (4) Had patient speak and swallow, checked midline uvula and symmetrical rise of uvula and soft palate, elicited gag reflex. ___ ___ ___ _____

   c. Assessed extremities for sensation, performed sensory test with patient's eyes closed.

      (1) Asked patient to indicate when sharp or dull sensation was felt as sharp and blunt ends of tongue blade were alternately applied to symmetrical areas. ___ ___ ___ _____

      (2) Applied light wisp of cotton in symmetrical areas. ___ ___ ___ _____

      (3) Grasped finger or toe, alternated moving up and down, asked patient to state whether digit was up or down. ___ ___ ___ _____

   d. Assessed motor and cerebellar function.

      (1) Had patient walk across the room, turn, and come back, noted use of assistive devices. ___ ___ ___ _____

      (2) Had patient stand straight first with eyes open and then closed, observed for swaying. ___ ___ ___ _____

   e. Assessed DTRs.

      (1) Determined necessity to monitor DTRs. ___ ___ ___ _____

      (2) Compared sides for each reflex tested and assigned a grade. ___ ___ ___ _____

      (3) Palpated the patellar tendon just below the patella, tapped pointed end of reflex hammer on the tendon. ___ ___ ___ _____

      (4) Stroked lateral aspect of the sole from the heel to the ball of the foot. ___ ___ ___ _____

	S	U	NP	Comments

EVALUATION

1. Compared muscle strength and ROM with previous physical assessment.

2. Compared neurologic status with previous assessment.

3. Evaluated level of patient discomfort on the appropriate pain scale.

4. Identified unexpected outcomes.

RECORDING AND REPORTING

1. Documented posture, gait, muscle strength, and ROM in appropriate record.

2. Documented LOC, orientation, papillary response, sensation, and reflex response in appropriate record.

3. Reported to nurse in charge or health care provider acute pain, sudden muscle weakness, change in LOC, or change in size or pupillary reaction.

Student _____ Date _____

Instructor _____ Date _____

PERFORMANCE CHECKLIST PROCEDURAL 6-1 **MONITORING INTAKE AND OUTPUT**

	S	U	NP	Comments

PROCEDURAL STEPS

1. Identified patients with conditions that increase fluid loss.

2. Identified patient with impaired swallowing, unconscious patients, and patients with impaired mobility.

3. Identified patients on medication that influences fluid balance.

4. Assessed signs and symptoms of dehydration and fluid overload.

5. Weighed patients daily using same scale, same time of day, and comparable clothing.

6. Monitored laboratory reports including urine specific gravity and Hct.

7. Assessed patient's and family's knowledge of purpose and process of I&O measurement.

8. Explained to patient and family the reason I&O are important.

9. Measured and recorded all intake of fluid appropriately.

10. Instructed patient and family to call you or NAP to empty contents of urinal, urine hat, or commode every time patient uses it; instructed them to monitor incontinence, vomiting, and excessive perspiration and to report it to the nurse.

11. Informed patient and family that drainage bag and tube drainage are closely monitored, measured, and recorded and who is responsible, ensured graduation container was clearly marked.

12. Applied clean gloves; measured drainage as indicated; noted color and characteristics; wore mask, eye protection, or gown if needed.

13. Removed gloves and disposed of them properly, performed hand hygiene.

14. Noted I&O balance or imbalance, reported urine output less that 30 mL/hr or significant changes in daily weight.

15. Documented on I&O form or electronic record.

Student _____ Date _____

Instructor _____ Date _____

PERFORMANCE CHECKLIST SKILL 7-1 **HAND HYGIENE**

	S	U	NP	Comments

ASSESSMENT

1. Inspected surface of hands for breaks or cuts in skin or cuticles, covered lesions with dressing before providing care, determined if lesions were too large to cover.

2. Inspected hands for visible soiling.

3. Inspected condition of nails, ensured nails were short and smooth.

PLANNING

1. Identified expected outcomes.

IMPLEMENTATION

1. Pushed wristwatch and long uniform sleeves above wrists, removed any rings.

2. Used antiseptic hand rub.

   a. Dispensed appropriate amount of product into palm of one hand.

   b. Rubbed hands together, covered all surfaces.

   c. Rubbed hands together until alcohol was dry; allowed hands to dry completely before applying gloves.

3. Used regular or antimicrobial hand soap.

   a. Stood in front of sink, kept hands and uniform away from sink surface.

   b. Turned on water; avoided splashing water against uniform.

   c. Regulated flow of water so temperature was warm.

   d. Wet hands and wrists, kept hands and forearms lower than elbows.

   e. Applied appropriate amount of antiseptic soap, rubbed hands together.

   f. Washed hands properly for at least 15 to 20 seconds.

   g. Cleaned under fingernails with nails of other hand or disposable nail cleaner.

   h. Rinsed hands and wrists, kept hands down and elbows up.

	S	U	NP	Comments
i. Dried hands and wrists thoroughly.	___	___	___	_____
j. Discarded paper towel in proper receptacle if used.	___	___	___	_____
k. Used clean, dry, paper towel to turn off hand faucet, or turned off with foot or knee pedals.	___	___	___	_____
l. Applied appropriate lotion to hands.	___	___	___	_____

EVALUATION

	S	U	NP	Comments
1. Inspected surface of hands for obvious signs of dirt and other contaminants.	___	___	___	_____
2. Identified unexpected outcomes.	___	___	___	_____

Student _____ Date _____

Instructor _____ Date _____

PERFORMANCE CHECKLIST SKILL 7-2 **CARING FOR PATIENTS UNDER ISOLATION PRECAUTIONS**

	S	U	NP	Comments

ASSESSMENT

1. Assessed patient and reviewed medical history for possible indications for isolation, reviewed precautions for appropriate isolation system.

2. Reviewed laboratory test results.

3. Considered types of care measures to be performed.

4. Reviewed nursing care plan notes or conferred with colleagues regarding patient's emotional state, determined if patient and family understood purpose of isolation procedure.

PLANNING

1. Identified expected outcomes.

IMPLEMENTATION

1. Performed hand hygiene.

2. Prepared all equipment needed in patient's room.

3. Prepared for entrance into isolation room, chose appropriate barrier protection.

   a. Applied gown and secured.

   b. Applied surgical mask or respirator around mouth and nose, had medical evaluation, and was fit-tested before using respirator.

   c. Applied goggles or eyewear if needed, used side shields if prescription glasses are worn.

   d. Applied clean gloves, brought glove cuffs over edge of gown sleeves.

4. Entered room, arranged supplies and equipment.

5. Explained purpose of isolation and precautions for patient and family to take, offered opportunity to ask questions.

6. Obtained vital signs measurements.

   a. Disinfected reusable equipment when removed from room.

	S	U	NP	Comments

b. Cleaned stethoscope thoroughly if to be reused, set aside on a clean surface. ___ ___ ___ _____

c. Used individual thermometers and blood pressure cuffs if available. ___ ___ ___ _____

7. Administered medications.

   a. Gave oral medication in wrapper or cup. ___ ___ ___ _____

   b. Disposed of wrapper or cuff in appropriate receptacle. ___ ___ ___ _____

   c. Wore gloves when administering an injection. ___ ___ ___ _____

   d. Discarded disposable syringe or needle into designated sharps container. ___ ___ ___ _____

   e. Placed reusable plastic syringe on clean towel for eventual removal and disinfection. ___ ___ ___ _____

   f. Performed hand hygiene as soon as possible if contact occurs with a contaminated article or fluid. ___ ___ ___ _____

8. Administered hygiene, encouraged patient to ask questions, provided informal teaching.

   a. Avoided allowing isolation gown to become wet. ___ ___ ___ _____

   b. Assisted patient in removing gown, discarded in impervious linen bag. ___ ___ ___ _____

   c. Removed linen from bed, avoided contact with isolation gown, placed in impervious linen bag. ___ ___ ___ _____

   d. Provided clean bed linen and towels. ___ ___ ___ _____

   e. Changed gloves, performed hand hygiene, and regloved if necessary. ___ ___ ___ _____

9. Collected specimens.

   a. Placed specimen containers on clean paper towel in patient's bathroom. ___ ___ ___ _____

   b. Followed agency procedure for collecting specimens. ___ ___ ___ _____

   c. Transferred specimen to container without soiling outside of container, placed container in labeled plastic bag, performed hand hygiene and regloved for additional procedures if necessary. ___ ___ ___ _____

   d. Checked label for accuracy, sent to laboratory, labeled with biohazard sticker. ___ ___ ___ _____

10. Disposed of linen, trash, and disposable items.

    a. Used appropriate type and number of bags. ___ ___ ___ _____

    b. Tied bags securely. ___ ___ ___ _____

	S	U	NP	Comments

11. Removed all reusable pieces of equipment, cleaned contaminated surfaces with disinfectant. ___ ___ ___ _____

12. Resupplied room as needed, had staff colleague hand new supplies to you. ___ ___ ___ _____

13. Left isolation room, removed protective barriers in the proper order.

   a. Removed gloves properly, discarded gloves in proper container. ___ ___ ___ _____

   b. Removed eyewear properly, discarded in proper container. ___ ___ ___ _____

   c. Removed gown properly, folded inside out into a bundle, discarded in laundry bag. ___ ___ ___ _____

   d. Removed mask properly, dropped into trash. ___ ___ ___ _____

   e. Performed hand hygiene. ___ ___ ___ _____

   f. Retrieved wristwatch and stethoscope, recorded vital sign values on paper. ___ ___ ___ _____

   g. Explained to patient when you plan to return, asked if patient required personal care items. ___ ___ ___ _____

   h. Disposed of contaminated supplies and equipment appropriately, performed hand hygiene. ___ ___ ___ _____

   i. Left room and provided privacy, closed door if necessary. ___ ___ ___ _____

EVALUATION

1. Asked if patient has had chance to discuss health problems, course of treatment, or other topics. ___ ___ ___ _____

2. Asked patient to describe purpose of isolation, offered chance to ask questions. ___ ___ ___ _____

3. Identified unexpected outcomes. ___ ___ ___ _____

RECORDING AND REPORTING

1. Documented procedures and patient's response to isolation, documented patient education. ___ ___ ___ _____

Student _____ Date _____

Instructor _____ Date _____

PERFORMANCE PROCEDURAL GUIDELINE 7-1 **CARING FOR PATIENTS WITH MULTIDRUG-RESISTANT ORGANISMS AND *CLOSTRIDIUM DIFFICILE***

	S	U	NP	Comments
PROCEDURAL STEPS				
1. Performed hand hygiene.	___	___	___	_____
2. Prepared all equipment needed in patient's room.	___	___	___	_____
3. Applied gown properly before entering room.	___	___	___	_____
4. Applied clean gloves.	___	___	___	_____
5. Explained purpose of contact precautions to patient and family.	___	___	___	_____
6. Provided personal care and treatments.	___	___	___	_____
7. Left room after telling patient when you will return and asking if they have questions concerning care.	___	___	___	_____
8. Removed gloves and discarded appropriately.	___	___	___	_____
9. Removed and discarded gown appropriately.	___	___	___	_____
10. Performed hand hygiene, used soap and water to clean hands if patient has *Clostridium difficile* infection.	___	___	___	_____

Student _____ Date _____

Instructor _____ Date _____

PERFORMANCE CHECKLIST SKILL 8-1 **APPLYING AND REMOVING CAP, MASK, AND PROTECTIVE EYEWEAR**

	S	U	NP	Comments
ASSESSMENT				
1. Reviewed type of sterile procedure to be performed, consulted agency's policy for use of protection.	___	___	___	_____
2. Avoided participating in procedure if you have symptoms of a respiratory infection.	___	___	___	_____
3. Assessed patient's actual or potential risk for infection when choosing barriers for surgical asepsis.	___	___	___	_____
PLANNING				
1. Identified expected outcomes.	___	___	___	_____
2. Prepared equipment, inspected packaging for integrity and exposure to sterilization.	___	___	___	_____
IMPLEMENTATION				
1. Performed hand hygiene.	___	___	___	_____
2. Applied a cap.				
a. Combed back and secured long hair.	___	___	___	_____
b. Applied cap properly, ensured all hair fit under edges of cap.	___	___	___	_____
3. Applied a mask.				
a. Ensured metal strip was along the top edge.	___	___	___	_____
b. Held mask by top strings, kept top edge above bridge of nose.	___	___	___	_____
c. Tied top strings appropriately.	___	___	___	_____
d. Tied lower ties properly with mask under chin.	___	___	___	_____
e. Pinched metal band around bridge of nose.	___	___	___	_____
4. Applied protective eyewear.				
a. Applied protective glasses, goggles, or face shield properly, checked that vision was clear.	___	___	___	_____
b. Ensured face shield fit snugly.	___	___	___	_____
5. Applied sterile gloves if needed.	___	___	___	_____

	S	U	NP	Comments

6. Removed protective barriers.

   a. Removed gloves first if worn. ___ ___ ___ _____

   b. Untied bottom strings of mask. ___ ___ ___ _____

   c. Untied top strings, removed mask while holding ties securely, discarded appropriately. ___ ___ ___ _____

   d. Removed eyewear, avoided placing hands over soiled lens. ___ ___ ___ _____

   e. Grasped outer surface of cap, lifted away from hair. ___ ___ ___ _____

   f. Discarded cap in proper receptacle, performed hand hygiene. ___ ___ ___ _____

EVALUATION

1. Assessed area of body treated for drainage, tenderness, edema, and skin changes. ___ ___ ___ _____

2. Identified unexpected outcomes. ___ ___ ___ _____

Student _____ Date _____

Instructor _____ Date _____

PERFORMANCE CHECKLIST SKILL 8-2 **PREPARING A STERILE FIELD**

	S	U	NP	Comments

ASSESSMENT

1. Verified that procedure requires surgical aseptic technique.

2. Assessed patient's comfort, oxygen requirements, and elimination needs before preparation.

3. Assessed for latex allergy.

4. Checked sterile package integrity or for sterilization indicator.

5. Anticipated number and variety of supplies needed for procedure.

PLANNING

1. Identified expected outcomes.

2. Completed all other priority tasks before procedure.

3. Asked visitors to step out, discouraged movement by assisting staff.

4. Prepared equipment at bedside.

5. Positioned patient comfortably and appropriately with assistance of NAP if necessary.

6. Explained purpose of procedure and importance of sterile technique.

IMPLEMENTATION

1. Applied PPE as needed.

2. Selected an appropriate workspace above waist level.

3. Performed hand hygiene thoroughly.

4. Prepared a sterile work surface.

   a. Using a sterile commercial kit or pack:

      (1) Placed kit or pack on workspace.

      (2) Opened outside cover, removed package and placed on surface.

      (3) Grasped outer surface or tip of outermost flap.

      (4) Opened outermost flap away from body and sterile field.

	S	U	NP	Comments

(5) Grasped outer surface of edge of first side flap.   ___ ___ ___ _____

(6) Opened side flap, allowed it to lie flat on table, kept arm away from sterile surface.   ___ ___ ___ _____

(7) Repeated for second flap.   ___ ___ ___ _____

(8) Grasped outside border of last flap, stood away from package, folded flap back, allowed it to fall on the table.   ___ ___ ___ _____

b. Opened a sterile linen-wrapped package.

(1) Placed package on workspace.   ___ ___ ___ _____

(2) Removed seal, unwrapped both layers, following same steps as with sterile kit.   ___ ___ ___ _____

(3) Used open package wrapper as sterile field.   ___ ___ ___ _____

c. Prepared a sterile drape.

(1) Placed pack containing drape on workspace and opened following same steps as with sterile kit.   ___ ___ ___ _____

(2) Applied sterile gloves.   ___ ___ ___ _____

(3) Grasped folded top edge of drape with fingertips of one hand, lifted without touching any object.   ___ ___ ___ _____

(4) Kept drape above waist and work surface and away from body as unfolded, discarded wrapper with other hand.   ___ ___ ___ _____

(5) Grasped adjacent corner of drape with other hand, held straight over work surface.   ___ ___ ___ _____

(6) Held drape, positioned bottom half over top of intended work surface.   ___ ___ ___ _____

(7) Allowed top half of drape to be placed over bottom half of work surface.   ___ ___ ___ _____

5. Added sterile items to sterile field.

a. Opened sterile item while holding outside wrapper in nondominant hand.   ___ ___ ___ _____

b. Carefully peeled wrapper over nondominant hand.   ___ ___ ___ _____

c. Placed item on field at an angle, ensured wrapper and arm are not over sterile field.   ___ ___ ___ _____

d. Disposed of outer wrapper.   ___ ___ ___ _____

	S	U	NP	Comments

6. Poured sterile solutions.

   a. Verified contents and expiration date of solution.

   b. Ensured receptacle was located near workspace edge.

   c. Removed sterile seal and cap properly.

   d. Poured needed amount of solution properly into container.

EVALUATION

1. Observed for break in sterile technique.

2. Identified unexpected outcomes.

Student _____ Date _____

Instructor _____ Date _____

PERFORMANCE CHECKLIST SKILL 8-3 **STERILE GLOVING**

	S	U	NP	Comments

ASSESSMENT

1. Considered type of procedure to be performed, consulted agency policy on use of sterile gloves. ___ ___ ___ _____

2. Considered patient's risk for infection. ___ ___ ___ _____

3. Examined glove package to determine if it was dry and intact with no water stains. ___ ___ ___ _____

4. Inspected condition of hands, determined if presence of lesions prevented participation in a procedure. ___ ___ ___ _____

5. Assessed patient for risk factors before applying latex gloves.

   a. Previous reaction to other items containing latex. ___ ___ ___ _____

   b. Personal history of asthma, contact dermatitis, eczema, urticaria, or rhinitis. ___ ___ ___ _____

   c. History of food allergies. ___ ___ ___ _____

   d. Previous history of adverse reactions during surgery or dental procedure. ___ ___ ___ _____

   e. Previous reaction to latex products. ___ ___ ___ _____

PLANNING

1. Identified expected outcomes. ___ ___ ___ _____

IMPLEMENTATION

1. Applied gloves.

   a. Performed thorough hand hygiene. ___ ___ ___ _____

   b. Removed outer glove wrapper by peeling sides apart. ___ ___ ___ _____

   c. Grasped inner package on workspace, opened package, kept gloves on inside surface of wrapper. ___ ___ ___ _____

   d. Identified right and left glove, gloved dominant hand first. ___ ___ ___ _____

   e. Grasped glove for dominant hand by touching only glove's inside surface. ___ ___ ___ _____

   f. Pulled glove over dominant hand, ensured cuff does not roll up wrist. ___ ___ ___ _____

	S	U	NP	Comments
g. Slipped fingers of gloved hand underneath second glove's cuff.	___	___	___	_____
h. Pulled second glove over nondominant hand.	___	___	___	_____
2. Disposed of gloves.				
a. Grasped outside of one cuff with other gloved hand, avoided touching wrist.	___	___	___	_____
b. Pulled glove off by turning it inside out, placed glove in gloved hand.	___	___	___	_____
c. Peeled glove off inside out and over previously removed glove, discarded both gloves in receptacle.	___	___	___	_____
d. Performed thorough hand hygiene.	___	___	___	_____

EVALUATION

	S	U	NP	Comments
1. Assessed patient for signs of infection.	___	___	___	_____
2. Evaluated patient for signs of latex allergy.	___	___	___	_____
3. Identified unexpected outcomes.	___	___	___	_____

RECORDING AND REPORTING

	S	U	NP	Comments
1. Documented specific procedure performed and patient's response and status in appropriate record.	___	___	___	_____
2. Documented any patient reaction to latex in appropriate record, noted type of response and reaction to treatment.	___	___	___	_____

Student _____ Date _____

Instructor _____ Date _____

PERFORMANCE CHECKLIST SKILL 9-1 **USING SAFE AND EFFECTIVE TRANSFER TECHNIQUES**

	S	U	NP	Comments

ASSESSMENT

1. Assessed physiologic capacity of a patient to transfer and need for special adaptive technique, including muscle strength, joint mobility and contracture formation, paralysis or paresis, and bone continuity.

2. Assessed presence of weakness, dizziness, or postural hypotension.

3. Assessed level of endurance, including level of fatigue during activity and vital signs.

4. Assessed patient's proprioceptive function.

5. Assessed patient's sensory status, including central and peripheral vision, adequacy of hearing, and presence of peripheral sensation of light.

6. Assessed patient for pain, measured level of pain, offered prescribed analgesic 30 minutes before transfer.

7. Assessed patient's cognitive status, including ability to follow verbal instructions, short-term memory, recognition of physical deficits and limitations.

8. Assessed patient's level of motivation and eagerness versus unwillingness to be mobile.

9. Assessed previous mode of transfer.

10. Determined number of people needed to assist with transfer, did not start procedure until all caregivers were available.

PLANNING

1. Identified expected outcomes.

2. Explained procedure to patient, repeated instructions simply and with continuity if necessary.

	S	U	NP	Comments

IMPLEMENTATION

1. Performed hand hygiene. _____ _____ _____ _____

2. Assisted patient to sitting position.

   a. Placed patient in supine position. _____ _____ _____ _____

   b. Faced head of bed appropriately and removed pillows. _____ _____ _____ _____

   c. Placed feet properly in a wide base of support. _____ _____ _____ _____

   d. Placed hand under shoulders, supported head and cervical vertebrae. _____ _____ _____ _____

   e. Placed other hand on bed surface. _____ _____ _____ _____

   f. Raised patient to sitting position by shifting weight. _____ _____ _____ _____

   g. Pushed against bed using arm on bed surface. _____ _____ _____ _____

3. Assisted patient to sitting position on side of bed in low position using electrical bed.

   a. Raised head of bed 30 degrees with patient in supine position. _____ _____ _____ _____

   b. Turned patient onto side facing you. _____ _____ _____ _____

   c. Stood opposite patient's hips, turned so you face the patient properly. _____ _____ _____ _____

   d. Placed feet apart in a wide base of support. _____ _____ _____ _____

   e. Placed arm under patient's shoulders, supported head and neck. _____ _____ _____ _____

   f. Placed other arm over patient's thighs. _____ _____ _____ _____

   g. Moved patient's lower legs and feet over side of bed; pivoted, allowing patient's legs to swing downward. _____ _____ _____ _____

   h. Shifted weight at the same time to rear leg and elevated patient. _____ _____ _____ _____

4. Transferred patient from bed to chair with bed in the low position.

   a. Used bariatric transfer aid with two or three caregivers if appropriate. _____ _____ _____ _____

   b. Assisted patient to sitting position, positioned chair properly, allowed patient to sit before transferring, asked if patient felt dizzy, did not leave patient unattended. _____ _____ _____ _____

   c. Applied transfer belt or used transfer board, patient's arm should be in a sling if necessary. _____ _____ _____ _____

	S	U	NP	Comments

d. Assisted patient with applying nonskid shoes, placed patient's strong leg forward. — — — _____

e. Spread your feet apart. — — — _____

f. Flexed hips and knees, aligned knees with patient's knees. — — — _____

g. Grasped transfer belt along patient's sides. — — — _____

h. Rocked patient up to standing appropriately, instructed patient to use hands to push up if applicable. — — — _____

i. Maintained stability of patient's weak leg with your knee. — — — _____

j. Pivoted on foot farther from chair. — — — _____

k. Instructed patient to use armrests to ease into chair. — — — _____

l. Flexed hips and knees while lowering patient. — — — _____

m. Assessed patient for proper alignment in sitting position, provided support for paralyzed extremities. — — — _____

n. Praised patient's progress, effort, and performance. — — — _____

5. Performed horizontal transfer from bed to stretcher using slide board or friction-reducing board.

a. Determined number of staff required to horizontally transfer patient safely. — — — _____

b. Lowered head of bed as much as patient can tolerate, ensured bed brakes are locked. — — — _____

c. Crossed patient's arms on chest. — — — _____

d. Lowered side rails, positioned nurses appropriately. — — — _____

e. Fanfolded drawsheet on both sides. — — — _____

f. Turned patient on the count of three in a smooth, continuous motion. — — — _____

g. Placed slide board under drawsheet. — — — _____

h. Gently rolled patient back onto slide board. — — — _____

i. Lined up stretcher with bed, locked brakes on stretcher. — — — _____

j. Repositioned nurses properly. — — — _____

k. Fanfolded drawsheet, two nurses pulled the drawsheet with patient under stretcher while third nurse held slide board in place. — — — _____

	S	U	NP	Comments

l. Positioned patient in center of stretcher, raised head of stretcher if not contraindicated, raised side rails, covered patient with blanket. ___ ___ ___ _____

6. Used mechanical/hydraulic lift to transfer patient from bed to chair.

   a. Brought lift to bedside or positioned ceiling lift properly. ___ ___ ___ _____

   b. Positioned chair properly. ___ ___ ___ _____

   c. Raised and flattened bed, lowered side rail. ___ ___ ___ _____

   d. Raised opposite rail if necessary. ___ ___ ___ _____

   e. Rolled patient on side away from you. ___ ___ ___ _____

   f. Placed hammock under patient to form sling, fitted edges appropriately. ___ ___ ___ _____

   g. Raised bed rail. ___ ___ ___ _____

   h. Lowered opposite side rail. ___ ___ ___ _____

   i. Rolled patient over, pulled strips through and smoothed over bed. ___ ___ ___ _____

   j. Rolled patient supine onto hammock. ___ ___ ___ _____

   k. Removed patient's glasses if appropriate. ___ ___ ___ _____

   l. Placed lift's horseshoe bar under side of bed. ___ ___ ___ _____

   m. Lowered horizontal to sling level, locked valve if required. ___ ___ ___ _____

   n. Attached hooks on strap to holes in sling. ___ ___ ___ _____

   o. Elevated head of bed. ___ ___ ___ _____

   p. Folded patient's arms over chest. ___ ___ ___ _____

   q. Pumped hydraulic handle until patient was raised off bed or turned control device to move lift. ___ ___ ___ _____

   r. Pulled lift from bed and maneuvered to chair. ___ ___ ___ _____

   s. Rolled base around chair. ___ ___ ___ _____

   t. Released check valve slowly or used control device to lower patient into chair. ___ ___ ___ _____

   u. Closed check valve or turned off control device. ___ ___ ___ _____

   v. Removed straps and mechanical/hydraulic lift. ___ ___ ___ _____

   w. Checked and corrected patient's sitting alignment. ___ ___ ___ _____

7. Performed hand hygiene. ___ ___ ___ _____

	S	U	NP	Comments

EVALUATION

1. Monitored vital signs, asked if patient felt dizzy or fatigued.

2. Noted patient's behavioral response to transfer.

3. Asked if patient experienced pain during transfer.

4. Had patient who was transferred to chair attempt to bear weight with nurse at side.

5. Identified unexpected outcomes.

RECORDING AND REPORTING

1. Documented procedure in the appropriate record.

2. Reported transfer ability and assistance need to next shift, reported progress or remission to rehabilitation staff.

Student _____ Date _____

Instructor _____ Date _____

PERFORMANCE CHECKLIST PROCEDURAL GUIDELINE 9-1 **WHEELCHAIR TRANSFER TECHNIQUES**

	S	U	NP	Comments

PROCEDURAL STEPS

1. Transferring patient from a wheelchair to bed if patient is cooperative and weight bearing:

   a. Adjusted height of bed to level of the seat of the wheelchair.

   b. Positioned and faced the wheelchair properly, locked the wheels, raised the footplates.

   c. Placed transfer belt on patient.

   d. Assisted patient to move to front of wheelchair.

   e. Positioned self properly, protected patient throughout transfer, used slide board if appropriate.

   f. Coordinated transfer with patient, had patient sit on side of mattress.

   g. Placed one arm under patient's shoulder, supported head and neck, placed other arm under patient's knees, postured self properly.

   h. Instructed patient to help lift leg when you move, raised patient as you pivoted, lowered shoulders onto bed, kept own back straight.

2. Transferred patient from a bed to wheelchair.

   a. Adjusted height of bed to the level of wheelchair seat.

   b. Positioned and faced wheelchair appropriately, locked the wheels, raised the footplates.

   c. Sat patient on side of bed.

   d. Placed transfer belt on patient.

   e. Assisted patient to move to edge of the mattress.

   f. Positioned self to guard and protect the patient.

   g. Coordinated transfer with patient.

   h. Lowered footplates after transfer, placed patient's feet on them.

	S	U	NP	Comments
i. Unlocked wheelchair.	___	___	___	_____
j. Ensured patient was positioned well back in the seat.	___	___	___	_____
3. Monitored vital signs as needed, asked if patient felt dizzy or fatigued.	___	___	___	_____
4. Noted patient's behavioral response to transfer.	___	___	___	_____

Student _____ Date _____

Instructor _____ Date _____

PERFORMANCE CHECKLIST SKILL 9-2 **MOVING AND POSITIONING PATIENTS IN BED**

	S	U	NP	Comments

ASSESSMENT

1. Assessed patient's ROM.

2. Assessed for risk factors that contribute to complications of immobility.

    a. Decreased sensation from CVA, paralysis, or neuropathy.

    b. Impaired mobility due to traction, arthritis, hip fracture, joint surgery, or other disease processes.

    c. Impaired circulation from arterial insufficiency.

    d. Age.

3. Assessed patient's LOC.

4. Assessed condition of patient's skin, especially over bony prominences.

5. Assessed patient's physical ability to help with moving and positioning.

6. Assessed for presence of tubes, incisions, and equipment.

7. Assessed motivation of patient and ability of caregivers to participate in moving and positioning.

8. Checked health care provider's orders before positioning patient.

PLANNING

1. Identified expected outcomes.

2. Raised level of bed to comfortable working height.

3. Removed all pillows and devices used in pervious position.

4. Obtained extra help as needed.

5. Explained procedure to patient.

IMPLEMENTATION

1. Performed hand hygiene.

2. Provided privacy.

	S	U	NP	Comments

3. Assisted patient in moving up in bed as necessary. ___ ___ ___ _____

4. Assisted moving up in bed using a drawsheet.

   a. Positioned patient appropriately. ___ ___ ___ _____

   b. Removed pillow from under patient. ___ ___ ___ _____

   c. Turned patient side to side to place drawsheet. ___ ___ ___ _____

   d. Returned patient to supine position. ___ ___ ___ _____

   e. Fanfolded drawsheet on both sides. ___ ___ ___ _____

   f. Positioned selves appropriately, moved patient and drawsheet into desired position on the count of three. ___ ___ ___ _____

5. Assisted moving up in bed using a friction-reducing device.

   a. Positioned patient as in steps 4a-c. ___ ___ ___ _____

   b. Placed friction-reducing device under drawsheet by having patient turn side to side. ___ ___ ___ _____

   c. Moved patient up in bed by having two nurses grasp drawsheet and one hold friction-reducing device, followed steps 4e-f to move patient. ___ ___ ___ _____

6. Positioned patient in appropriate position, protected pressure areas.

   a. Positioned patient in supported Fowler's position.

     (1) Elevated head of bed if not contraindicated. ___ ___ ___ _____

     (2) Rested head against mattress or on pillow. ___ ___ ___ _____

     (3) Used pillows to support arms if necessary. ___ ___ ___ _____

     (4) Positioned small pillow at lower back. ___ ___ ___ _____

     (5) Placed small pillow or roll under thigh. ___ ___ ___ _____

     (6) Supported calves with pillows. ___ ___ ___ _____

   b. Positioned hemiplegic patient in supported Fowler's position.

     (1) Positioned patient properly, elevated head of bed. ___ ___ ___ _____

     (2) Positioned patient in Fowler's position as straight as possible. ___ ___ ___ _____

     (3) Positioned patient's head appropriately, avoided hyperextension if patient was unable to control head movement. ___ ___ ___ _____

102

	S	U	NP	Comments

(4) Provided support for involved arm and hand appropriately.

(5) Placed a rolled blanket firmly alongside patient's legs.

(6) Supported feet in dorsiflexion with boots or splints.

c. Positioned patient in supported supine position.

(1) Placed patient supine with bed flat.

(2) Placed rolled towel under lumbar area of back.

(3) Placed pillow under upper shoulders, neck, or head.

(4) Placed rolls or sandbags parallel to lateral surface of patient's thighs.

(5) Placed patient's feet in boots or splints.

(6) Placed pillows under pronated forearms.

(7) Placed hand rolls in patient's hands.

d. Positioned hemiplegic patient in supine position.

(1) Placed head of bed flat.

(2) Placed folded towel or pillow under shoulder on affected side.

(3) Kept affected arm away from body with elbow extended and palm up, positioned affected hand in recommended position.

(4) Placed folded towel under hip of involved side.

(5) Flexed affected knee by supporting it on pillow or folded blanket.

(6) Supported feet with soft pillows at right angle to leg.

e. Positioned patient in prone position using two nurses.

(1) Rolled patient to one side while placing arm on side to be turned.

(2) Rolled patient over arm, positioned abdomen in center of bed.

(3) Turned patient's head to one side, supported with small pillow.

(4) Placed small pillow under patient's abdomen below level of diaphragm.

	S	U	NP	Comments

(5) Supported arms in flexed position level at shoulders.
    ___ ___ ___ _____

(6) Supported lower legs with pillow to elevate toes.
    ___ ___ ___ _____

f. Positioned hemiplegic patient in prone position using two nurses.

(1) Moved patient toward unaffected side.
    ___ ___ ___ _____

(2) While rolling patient onto side, placed pillow on patient's abdomen.
    ___ ___ ___ _____

(3) Rolled patient onto abdomen by positioning involved arm close to patient's body, rolled patient over arm.
    ___ ___ ___ _____

(4) Turned head toward involved side.
    ___ ___ ___ _____

(5) Positioned involved arm properly.
    ___ ___ ___ _____

(6) Flexed knees by placing pillow under legs from knees to ankles.
    ___ ___ ___ _____

(7) Kept feet at right angle to legs by using pillow.
    ___ ___ ___ _____

g. Positioned patient in 30-degree lateral position.

(1) Lowered head of bed as low as patient can tolerate.
    ___ ___ ___ _____

(2) Lowered side rail, positioned patient on side of bed opposite direction to be turned, moved upper trunk properly, then moved lower trunk properly.
    ___ ___ ___ _____

(3) Raised side rail, moved to opposite side of the bed.
    ___ ___ ___ _____

(4) Flexed patient's knee that will not be next to the mattress, placed one hand on patient's hip and one on shoulder.
    ___ ___ ___ _____

(5) Rolled patient onto side toward you.
    ___ ___ ___ _____

(6) Placed pillow under patient's head and neck.
    ___ ___ ___ _____

(7) Placed hand under patient's dependent shoulder, brought shoulder blade forward.
    ___ ___ ___ _____

(8) Positioned both arms properly, supported upper arm with pillow, supported other arm on mattress.
    ___ ___ ___ _____

(9) Placed hands under dependent hip, brought hip slightly forward.
    ___ ___ ___ _____

104

	S	U	NP	Comments

(10) Placed small tuck-back pillow behind patient's back. ___ ___   _____

(11) Placed pillow under semiflexed upper leg from groin to foot. ___ ___   _____

(12) Placed sandbags parallel to plantar surface of dependent foot, used ankle-foot orthotic on feet if available. ___ ___ ___ _____

  h. Positioned patient in Sims' position.

    (1) Lowered head of bed completely. ___ ___ ___ _____

    (2) Positioned patient appropriately. ___ ___ ___ _____

    (3) Moved to other side of bed, turned patient on side, positioned patient properly in lateral position. ___ ___ ___ _____

    (4) Placed small pillow under patient's head. ___ ___ ___ _____

    (5) Placed pillow under flexed upper arm. ___ ___ ___ _____

    (6) Placed pillow under flexed upper legs. ___ ___ ___ _____

  i. Logrolled patient with help of two nurses.

    (1) Placed small pillow between patient's knees. ___ ___ ___ _____

    (2) Crossed patient's arms to chest. ___ ___ ___ _____

    (3) Positioned two nurses on side patient was to be turned toward and one nurse where pillows were to be placed. ___ ___ ___ _____

    (4) Fanfold sheet along side of patient to be lifted. ___ ___ ___ _____

    (5) Had nurses grasp drawsheet properly; rolled patient as one unit in smooth, continuous motion on the count of three. ___ ___ ___ _____

    (6) Had nurse on opposite side place pillows along length of patient. ___ ___ ___ _____

    (7) Leaned patient as a unit back toward pillows. ___ ___ ___ _____

7. Performed hand hygiene. ___ ___ ___ _____

EVALUATION

1. Assessed patient's body alignment, position, and level of comfort. ___ ___ ___ _____

2. Measured ROM. ___ ___ ___ _____

3. Observed for areas of erythema or breakdown involving skin. ___ ___ ___ _____

4. Identified unexpected outcomes. ___ ___ ___ _____

	S	U	NP	Comments

RECORDING AND REPORTING

1. Recorded procedure and observations. ___ ___ ___ _____

2. Reported observations at change of shift, documented in nurses' notes. ___ ___ ___ _____

3. Recorded time and position change of patient throughout shift. ___ ___ ___ _____

Student _____ Date _____

Instructor _____ Date _____

PERFORMANCE CHECKLIST PROCEDURAL GUIDELINE 10-1 **PERFORMING RANGE-OF-MOTION EXERCISES**

	S	U	NP	Comments
PROCEDURAL STEPS				
1. Reviewed patient's chart for physical assessment findings, health care provider's orders, medical diagnosis, medical history, and progress.	___	___	___	_____
2. Obtained data on patient's baseline joint function.	___	___	___	_____
3. Determined patient's or caregiver's readiness to learn, explained rationales for ROM exercises, described and demonstrated exercises to be performed.	___	___	___	_____
4. Assessed patient's level of comfort, determined if patient would benefit from pain medication before beginning ROM exercises.	___	___	___	_____
5. Performed hand hygiene, wore clean gloves if wound drainage or lesions are present.	___	___	___	_____
6. Assisted patient to comfortable position.	___	___	___	_____
7. Supported joint properly when performing active-assisted or passive ROM exercises.	___	___	___	_____
8. Completed exercises in head-to-toe sequence, repeated each movement 5 times, informed patient how exercises can be incorporated into ADLs.	___	___	___	_____
9. Observed patient performing ROM activities.	___	___	___	_____
10. Measured joint motion as needed.	___	___	___	_____
11. Monitored pain throughout ROM exercise period.	___	___	___	_____

Student _____ Date _____

Instructor _____ Date _____

PERFORMANCE CHECKLIST SKILL 10-1 **PERFORMING ISOMETRIC EXERCISES**

	S	U	NP	Comments

ASSESSMENT

1. Reviewed patient's chart for contraindications to isometric exercises.

2. Assessed patient's baseline vital signs.

3. Assessed patient's baseline muscle strength.

    a. Asked patient to perform task against resistance.

    b. Assessed grasp strength, noted whether hand grasps were equal.

    c. Had patient grasp two fingers of your right hand with patient's left hand and vice versa.

    d. Observed patient's ability to do daily activities.

    e. Obtained patient's subjective statements related to muscle strength.

4. Assessed patient's nutritional status.

5. Assessed level of comfort, provided ordered analgesic before exercise if appropriate.

PLANNING

1. Identified expected outcomes.

2. Explained procedure, demonstrated exercises.

3. Assisted patient to comfortable position.

IMPLEMENTATION

1. Provided privacy.

2. Instructed patient to perform following exercises usually prescribed by a physical therapist.

    a. Quadriceps isometric exercises:

        (1) Assisted patient to appropriate position.

        (2) Instructed patient to press back of knee against mattress while trying to lift heel from bed.

        (3) Held muscles tightly contracted for 5 to 15 seconds, then relaxed completely for several seconds.

        (4) Repeated exercise.

	S	U	NP	Comments

b. Gluteal muscle isometric exercises:

   (1) Assisted patient to supine position.

   (2) Instructed patient to pinch buttocks together and hold for 5 to 15 seconds, then relax completely for several seconds.

   (3) Repeated exercise.

c. Abdominal muscle isometric exercises:

   (1) Had patient pull abdominal muscles in as tightly as possible.

   (2) Held for 5 to 15 seconds, released muscles gradually.

   (3) Repeated exercise.

d. Foot muscle isometric exercises:

   (1) Instructed patient to flex foot toward and away from knee, held muscles tightly in position for 5 to 15 seconds.

   (2) Repeated exercise.

e. Hand muscle isometric exercises:

   (1) Obtained sponge rubber ball of the appropriate size.

   (2) Had patient grip ball with entire hand 5 to 10 times.

   (3) Dig each fingertip one at a time into ball 5 to 10 times.

   (4) Gradually increased frequency of exercise until patient can grip ball and exercise once or twice a day.

f. Biceps isometric exercises:

   (1) Had patient raise arms to shoulder height and interlock fingertips of both hands.

   (2) Used arm muscles to try to pull hands apart.

   (3) Held for 5 to 15 seconds.

   (4) Relaxed muscles.

   (5) Repeated exercise.

	S	U	NP	Comments

g. Triceps muscle isometric exercises:

   (1) Arm exercises:

      (a) Had patient raise arms to shoulder height. ___ ___ ___ _____

      (b) Made fist with one hand and placed against palm of other hand. ___ ___ ___ _____

      (c) Pushed hands together as hard as possible and held for 5 to 15 seconds. ___ ___ ___ _____

      (d) Relaxed and repeated exercise. ___ ___ ___ _____

   (2) Sitting exercises:

      (a) Assisted patient to appropriate position, placed blocks under patient's hands if needed. ___ ___ ___ _____

      (b) Instructed patient to try to lift buttocks off bed by pressing down with hands. ___ ___ ___ _____

      (c) Held muscles tight for 5 to 15 seconds, then relaxed. ___ ___ ___ _____

      (d) Repeated exercise. ___ ___ ___ _____

EVALUATION

1. Observed patient's ability to perform exercises. ___ ___ ___ _____

2. Evaluated patient's level of energy, muscular strength, and comfort following exercises. ___ ___ ___ _____

3. Obtained vital signs after one or two repetitions. ___ ___ ___ _____

4. Identified unexpected outcomes. ___ ___ ___ _____

RECORDING AND REPORTING

1. Recorded all relevant information in nurses' notes. ___ ___ ___ _____

Student _____ Date _____

Instructor _____ Date _____

PERFORMANCE CHECKLIST SKILL 10-2 **CONTINUOUS PASSIVE MOTION MACHINE**

	S	U	NP	Comments
ASSESSMENT				
1. Assessed the CPM machine for electrical safety, notified electrical safety department if problem was suspected.	___	___	___	_____
2. Assessed setup of the machine before placing on bed.	___	___	___	_____
3. Assessed patient's pain before and during use.	___	___	___	_____
4. Assessed patient's baseline vital signs.	___	___	___	_____
5. Assessed patient's ability and willingness to learn about the CPM machine.	___	___	___	_____
6. Assessed the nature of the patient's condition and ROM limits prescribed.	___	___	___	_____
PLANNING				
1. Identified expected outcomes.	___	___	___	_____
2. Explained procedure, demonstrated CPM machine.	___	___	___	_____
3. Assisted patient to comfortable position.	___	___	___	_____
IMPLEMENTATION				
1. Performed hand hygiene.	___	___	___	_____
2. Identified patient using two identifiers.	___	___	___	_____
3. Provided analgesia 20 to 30 minutes before CPM machine is needed.	___	___	___	_____
4. Performed hand hygiene and applied clean gloves if necessary.	___	___	___	_____
5. Placed elastic stockings on patient if ordered.	___	___	___	_____
6. Placed CPM machine on bed.	___	___	___	_____
7. Set limits of flexion and extension as prescribed, set speed appropriately.	___	___	___	_____
8. Put machine through one full cycle.	___	___	___	_____
9. Stopped CPM machine when in extension, placed sheepskin on CPM machine.	___	___	___	_____
10. Supported patient's joints while placing extremity in CPM machine.	___	___	___	_____

	S	U	NP	Comments
11. Adjusted CPM machine to patient's extremity, lengthened and shortened appropriate sections of the frame.	___	___	___	_____
12. Centered patient's extremity on frame.	___	___	___	_____
13. Aligned patient's joint with mechanical joint of CPM.	___	___	___	_____
14. Secured patient's extremity on CPM machine with Velcro straps, applied loosely.	___	___	___	_____
15. Started machine, stopped in flexed position, checked degree of flexion.	___	___	___	_____
16. Started CPM machine, observed for two full cycles.	___	___	___	_____
17. Made sure patient was comfortable.	___	___	___	_____
18. Instructed patient to turn CPM machine off if it malfunctions or if patient experiences pain, and to notify nurse.	___	___	___	_____
19. Provided patient with on/off switch.	___	___	___	_____
20. Discarded gloves and performed hand hygiene.	___	___	___	_____

EVALUATION

	S	U	NP	Comments
1. Inspected bony prominences and areas of skin in contact with machine at least every 2 hours.	___	___	___	_____
2. Asked patient to rate pain.	___	___	___	_____
3. Checked patient's alignment and positioning at least every 2 hours.	___	___	___	_____
4. Observed patient and CPM machine with each increase in flexion and extension.	___	___	___	_____
5. Identified unexpected outcomes.	___	___	___	_____

RECORDING AND REPORTING

	S	U	NP	Comments
1. Recorded relevant information in nurses' notes.	___	___	___	_____
2. Reported resistance to ROM; increased pain; and swelling, heat, or redness in joint to nurse in charge or health care provider.	___	___	___	_____

Student _____ Date _____

Instructor _____ Date _____

PERFORMANCE CHECKLIST PROCEDURAL GUIDELINE 10-2 **APPLYING ELASTIC STOCKINGS AND SEQUENTIAL COMPRESSION DEVICE**

	S	U	NP	Comments
PROCEDURAL STEPS				
1. Assessed patient for risk factors in Virchow's triad.	___	___	___	_____
2. Observed for contraindications for use of elastic stockings or SCDs.	___	___	___	_____
3. Assessed condition of patient's skin and circulation to the legs.	___	___	___	_____
4. Obtained health care provider's orders.	___	___	___	_____
5. Performed hand hygiene.	___	___	___	_____
6. Identified patient using two identifiers.	___	___	___	_____
7. Explained procedure and reason for applying elastic stockings and SCDs.	___	___	___	_____
8. Positioned patient appropriately, elevated head of bed to comfortable position, measured patient's leg to determine stocking or SCD size.	___	___	___	_____
9. Applied small amount of powder or cornstarch to legs if patient has no sensitivity.	___	___	___	_____
10. Applied elastic stocking.				
a. Turned elastic stocking inside out, did not pull all the way through.	___	___	___	_____
b. Placed patient's toes into foot of stocking, ensured sock is smooth.	___	___	___	_____
c. Slid remaining portion of sock over patient's foot, ensured toes were covered, ensured foot fit into heel and toe positions of the sock.	___	___	___	_____
d. Slid sock over patient's calf until sock was completely extended and smooth.	___	___	___	_____
e. Instructed patient not to roll socks down.	___	___	___	_____
11. Applied SCD sleeve.				
a. Removed SCD sleeve from plastic, unfolded and flattened.	___	___	___	_____
b. Arranged SCD sleeve properly under patient's leg.	___	___	___	_____

	S	U	NP	Comments
c. Placed patient's leg on SCD sleeve, lined up ankle with ankle marking.	___	___	___	_____
d. Positioned back of knee with opening on the sleeve.	___	___	___	_____
e. Wrapped SCD sleeve securely around patient's leg, checked fit.	___	___	___	_____
12. Attached SCD sleeve connector to mechanical unit, lined up arrows on connector and mechanical unit.	___	___	___	_____
13. Turned unit on, monitored function through one full cycle of inflation and deflation.	___	___	___	_____
14. Removed elastic stockings or sleeves at least once per shift.	___	___	___	_____

Student _____ Date _____

Instructor _____ Date _____

PERFORMANCE CHECKLIST SKILL 10-3 **ASSISTING WITH AMBULATION AND USE OF CANES, CRUTCHES, AND WALKER**

	S	U	NP	Comments

ASSESSMENT

1. Reviewed patient's chart, including medical history, previous activity level, current activity order.

2. Assessed patient's physical readiness.

   a. Obtained patient's heart rate, blood pressure, and orientation.

   b. Assessed ROM, muscle strength, coordination, and presence of foot deformities.

   c. Assessed patient for any visual, perceptual, or sensory deficits.

   d. Assessed environment for threats to patient safety.

   e. Assessed patient for discomfort.

3. Determined patient's or caregiver's understanding of technique of ambulation.

4. Determined optimal time for ambulation.

5. Assessed degree of assistance patient needs.

PLANNING

1. Identified expected outcomes.

2. Prepared patient for ambulation.

   a. Explained reasons for exercise, demonstrated technique.

   b. Decided with patient how far to ambulate.

   c. Scheduled ambulation around other activities.

   d. Placed bed in low position, assisted patient to appropriate starting position.

   e. Assisted sitting patient to standing until balance was gained.

   f. Asked if patient felt dizzy or light-headed, sat patient down and rechecked blood pressure if necessary.

   g. Obtained an IV pole with wheels if necessary.

	S	U	NP	Comments

3. Determined appropriate height of ambulation device if used.

   a. Measured for crutch height in three areas with patient standing or supine, instructed patient to report tingling or numbness in upper torso, adjusted height of handgrip if necessary. ___ ___ ___ _____

   b. Positioned cane properly on stronger side of patient's body. ___ ___ ___ _____

   c. Measured for walker height properly. ___ ___ ___ _____

4. Ensured ambulation device had rubber tips. ___ ___ ___ _____

5. Ensured surface patient will walk on was clean and dry, removed obstructions from pathway. ___ ___ ___ _____

IMPLEMENTATION

1. Assisted ambulation with one nurse.

   a. Reconfirmed patient does not feel light-headed. ___ ___ ___ _____

   b. Performed hand hygiene, applied gait belt, assisted patient to standing position, observed balance. ___ ___ ___ _____

   c. Had patient take a few steps with nurse standing alongside. ___ ___ ___ _____

   d. Stood and grasped gait belt in middle of patient's back. ___ ___ ___ _____

   e. Took a few steps forward with patient, assessed for strength and balance. ___ ___ ___ _____

   f. Returned patient to bed or chair if patient became weak. ___ ___ ___ _____

   g. Eased patient onto floor by holding gait belt if patient began to fall, provided support. ___ ___ ___ _____

2. Assisted ambulation with two nurses.

   a. Followed step 1a and 1b. ___ ___ ___ _____

   b. Had a nurse stand on either side of the patient. ___ ___ ___ _____

   c. Grasped walking belt in middle of patient's back, along with other nurse. ___ ___ ___ _____

   d. Stepped forward in unison with patient. ___ ___ ___ _____

   e. Gradually increased distance walked. ___ ___ ___ _____

   f. Followed steps 1f and 1g if patient became weak or dizzy. ___ ___ ___ _____

	S	U	NP	Comments

3. Trained patient in use of assistive devices for ambulation.

   a. Chose and taught appropriate crutch gait.

     (1) Four-point gait:

	S	U	NP	Comments
(a) Began in tripod position, ensured patient's weight was on handgrips.	—	—	—	_____
(b) Moved right crutch forward.	—	—	—	_____
(c) Moved left foot forward to level of left crutch.	—	—	—	_____
(d) Moved left crutch forward.	—	—	—	_____
(e) Moved right foot forward to level of right crutch.	—	—	—	_____
(f) Repeated above sequence.	—	—	—	_____

     (2) Three-point gait:

	S	U	NP	Comments
(a) Began in tripod position.	—	—	—	_____
(b) Advanced both crutches and affected leg.	—	—	—	_____
(c) Moved stronger leg forward, stepping on foot.	—	—	—	_____
(d) Repeated sequence.	—	—	—	_____

     (3) Two-point gait:

	S	U	NP	Comments
(a) Began in tripod position.	—	—	—	_____
(b) Moved left cutch and right foot forward.	—	—	—	_____
(c) Moved right crutch and left foot forward.	—	—	—	_____
(d) Repeated sequence.	—	—	—	_____

     (4) Swing-to gait:

	S	U	NP	Comments
(a) Began in tripod position.	—	—	—	_____
(b) Moved crutches forward.	—	—	—	_____
(c) Lifted and swung legs to crutches, let crutches support body weight.	—	—	—	_____
(d) Repeated two previous steps.	—	—	—	_____

     (5) Swing-through gait:

	S	U	NP	Comments
(a) Began in tripod position.	—	—	—	_____
(b) Moved both crutches forward.	—	—	—	_____
(c) Lifted and swung legs through and beyond crutches.	—	—	—	_____

	S	U	NP	Comments

b. Assisted patient in climbing stairs with crutches.

   (1) Began in tripod position.

   (2) Transferred body weight to crutches.

   (3) Advanced strong leg to stair.

   (4) Aligned both crutches with strong leg on the stairs.

   (5) Repeated sequence until patient reaches top of stairs.

c. Assisted patient in descending stairs with crutches.

   (1) Began in tripod position.

   (2) Transferred body weight to unaffected leg, aligned with crutches.

   (3) Positioned crutches firmly on lower stairs, stepped down with affected leg, supported weight with crutches.

   (4) Brought unaffected leg to lower stair, aligned with crutches, resumed tripod position.

   (5) Repeated sequence until stairs are descended.

d. Assisting patient in ambulating with walker.

   (1) Had patient stand straight in the center of walker and grasp handgrips.

   (2) Had patient lift and move walker forward, ensured all four feet of walker are on the ground, had patient step forward with one foot and follow through with the other.

   (3) Instructed patient properly on how to advance if weakness was present.

e. Assisted patient in ambulating with cane.

   (1) Had patient place cane on side of strong leg.

   (2) Placed cane forward 15 to 25 cm (6 to 10 inches), kept weight on both legs.

   (3) Had patient stand, look straight, and move involved leg forward even with cane.

   (4) Advanced strong leg past cane.

120

	S	U	NP	Comments
(5) Moved involved leg forward even with strong leg.	——	——	——	_____
(6) Repeated these steps.	——	——	——	_____

EVALUATION

1. Obtained patient's vital signs, observed skin color, asked about patient's level of comfort and energy level.	——	——	——	_____
2. Evaluated patient's subjective statements regarding experience.	——	——	——	_____
3. Evaluated gait of patient, observed body alignment in standing position and balance.	——	——	——	_____
4. Observed patient's ability to perform self-care activities.	——	——	——	_____
5. Identified unexpected outcomes.	——	——	——	_____

RECORDING AND REPORTING

1. Recorded pertinent information in nurses' notes.	——	——	——	_____
2. Reported any injury sustained, alteration in vitals, or inability to ambulate to nurse in charge or health care provider immediately.	——	——	——	_____

Student _____ Date _____

Instructor _____ Date _____

PERFORMANCE CHECKLIST SKILL 11-1 **ASSISTING WITH CAST APPLICATION**

	S	U	NP	Comments

ASSESSMENT

1. Assessed patient's ability to cooperate and level of understanding concerning cast application process.

2. Inspected condition of skin that will be under the cast.

3. Assessed neurovascular status of area to be casted, compared with opposite extremity or surrounding tissues, paid attention to tissue distal to the cast.

4. Assessed patient's pain status on a scale of 0 to 10.

5. Determined extent to which patient will be able to use casted extremity.

PLANNING

1. Identified expected outcomes.

2. Instructed patient, parent, and other caregivers in methods they can facilitate application of cast.

IMPLEMENTATION

1. Identified patient using two identifiers.

2. Administered analgesic before cast application; if patient has a PCA, instructed patient to administer dose 2 to 5 minutes before cast application.

3. Performed hand hygiene and applied gloves, used latex-free gloves if necessary.

4. Assisted health care provider or technician in positioning patient and extremity as desired.

5. Cleansed skin to be enclosed and changed dressing, ensured skin was completely dry before application of the cast.

6. Explained that patient may experience warmth during cast application process.

7. Assisted with application of padding material around body part to be casted, applied a minimum of four layers, avoided wrinkles or unevenness.

	S	U	NP	Comments

8. Held body part(s) or assisted with preparation of cast materials.

   a. Marked end of roll properly, submerged plaster roll under water until bubbles stopped, squeezed roll, handed to person applying cast.

                   ___   ___   ___   _____

   b. Submerged cast roll in lukewarm water, squeezed roll, used a water bottle to apply water to casting material if appropriate.

                   ___   ___   ___   _____

9. Continued to hold body part(s) as cast was applied and molded, supplied additional rolls of casting tape as needed.

                   ___   ___   ___   _____

10. Compressed tape with hands when wrapping was complete.

                   ___   ___   ___   _____

11. Provided cast stabilization material as requested by health care provider.

                   ___   ___   ___   _____

12. Assisted with "finishing" cast by folding edge of stockinette over outer edge of cast, unrolled dampened plaster roll over stockinette to hold it in place, cushioned rough edges of cast with tape or moleskin.

                   ___   ___   ___   _____

13. Trimmed cast around digits if necessary.

                   ___   ___   ___   _____

14. Depending on the tissue to be casted:

   a. Elevated casted tissue properly to heart level, let cast air dry, placed ice appropriately if ordered.

                   ___   ___   ___   _____

   b. Ensured sling supported but did not encase the cast.

                   ___   ___   ___   _____

15. Removed and disposed of gloves appropriately, performed hand hygiene.

                   ___   ___   ___   _____

16. Assisted patient with transfer to wheelchair or stretcher, used additional personnel if necessary.

                   ___   ___   ___   _____

17. Repositioned patient every 2 hours, did not rest heel of cast on bed or pillow.

                   ___   ___   ___   _____

18. Informed patient to notify personnel of alteration in sensation, numbness, tingling, burning, pain on passive motion, or inability to move digits in affected extremity.

                   ___   ___   ___   _____

	S	U	NP	Comments

EVALUATION

1. Observed patient for signs of pain or anxiety.

2. Performed neurovascular assessment every 1 to 2 hours for first 24 hours, compared findings with precasting neurovascular assessment.

3. Observed for edema of tissues distal to cast.

4. Palpated temperature of tissues around casted area for signs of infection.

5. Asked patient to perform ADLs and ROM.

6. After cast dried, observed patient perform and verbalize knowledge of cast care.

7. Identified unexpected outcomes.

RECORDING AND REPORTING

1. Documented cast application, condition of skin, status of circulation, and motion of distal part.

2. Recorded instructions given to patient and family.

3. Reported abnormal or unusual findings from assessments or symptoms of compartment syndrome immediately.

4. Recorded odor and drainage from cast, reported to health care provider.

Student _____ Date _____

Instructor _____ Date _____

PERFORMANCE CHECKLIST PROCEDURAL GUIDELINE 11-1 **CARE OF PATIENT DURING CAST REMOVAL**

	S	U	NP	Comments
PROCEDURAL STEPS				
1. Assessed patient's understanding of and response to upcoming cast removal.	___	___	___	_____
2. Assisted with positioning patient.	___	___	___	_____
3. Described physical sensations to expect during cast removal.	___	___	___	_____
4. Described expected appearance of the extremity.	___	___	___	_____
5. Described and demonstrated the noise of the cast saw.	___	___	___	_____
6. Performed hand hygiene, applied PPE to self and patient.	___	___	___	_____
7. Stayed with patient, explained progress of procedure as cast and padding were removed.	___	___	___	_____
8. Inspected tissues underlying cast after removal.	___	___	___	_____
9. Applied cold-water enzyme wash if skin was intact, left for 15 to 20 minutes, used oil or soap and water to soften crusts, did not scrub.	___	___	___	_____
10. Rinsed off wash or soap, immersed tissues in basin to assist dead cell removal.	___	___	___	_____
11. Patted extremity dry, applied lotion generously to skin.	___	___	___	_____
12. Disposed of used supplies, equipment, and gloves; performed hand hygiene.	___	___	___	_____
13. Explained and provided written skin care procedures before patient discharge.	___	___	___	_____
14. Obtained health care provider order to perform active and passive ROM, clarified level of activity allowed.	___	___	___	_____
15. Instructed patient to observe for swelling and elevate extremity appropriately.	___	___	___	_____

Student _____ Date _____

Instructor _____ Date _____

PERFORMANCE CHECKLIST SKILL 11-2 **CARE OF A PATIENT IN SKIN TRACTION**

	S	U	NP	Comments
ASSESSMENT				
1. Assessed patient's knowledge of reason for traction.	___	___	___	_____
2. Assessed patient's overall health condition including degree of functional mobility, current medical conditions, and ability to perform ADLs.	___	___	___	_____
3. Assessed integrity and condition of skin before application of traction.	___	___	___	_____
4. Assessed patient's position in bed.	___	___	___	_____
5. Assessed patient's severity of pain, determined need for analgesics before application of traction.	___	___	___	_____
6. Assessed neurovascular status of extremity distal to traction.	___	___	___	_____
7. Reviewed medical record for amount of weight to be used in traction.	___	___	___	_____
PLANNING				
1. Identified expected outcomes.	___	___	___	_____
IMPLEMENTATION				
1. Identified patient using two identifiers.	___	___	___	_____
2. Prepared patient by discussing procedure.	___	___	___	_____
3. Administered analgesic or muscle relaxant in advance of traction application.	___	___	___	_____
4. Positioned patient properly in Buck's extension.	___	___	___	_____
5. Applied gloves, washed affected extremity, patted dry, did not shave extremity.	___	___	___	_____
6. Applied foam boot, moleskin, or elastic bandages to affected extremity, for Buck's extension.				
a. Wrapped leg in a soft roll prior to placing boot, ensured boot fits snugly.	___	___	___	_____
b. Seated heel properly in traction boot, did not pad heel.	___	___	___	_____
c. Did not apply traction boot over sequential pneumatic compression devices, used foot pump instead.	___	___	___	_____

	S	U	NP	Comments

7. Attached weight to boot properly at end of bed.

8. Inspected traction equipment, ensured knots were secure, ropes were in pulleys and not frayed, weights hung freely, and bed linens were not interfering, checked the four P's of traction maintenance.

9. Assessed patient's position and asked about permissible positions for patient before health care provider leaves the room.

10. Released and reapplied traction and provided skin care according to health care provider's orders. Removed traction boot every 4 to 8 hours.

11. Performed hand hygiene, returned unused materials to storage areas, performed hand hygiene.

EVALUATION

1. Observed patient's ability to perform ADLs.

2. Assessed condition of skin around traction straps or bandages frequently.

3. Observed patient for correct alignment.

4. Asked patient to rate discomfort and report muscle spasms.

5. Assessed neurovascular status at proper intervals after application of traction.

6. Observed patient's use of trapeze and ability to reposition self correctly.

7. Identified unexpected outcomes.

RECORDING AND REPORTING

1. Recorded assessment of skin underneath traction apparatus and nursing interventions to maintain skin integrity.

2. Documented neurovascular assessment on appropriate report.

3. Recorded length of time patient was in or out of specific traction.

4. Reported neurovascular deficits to health care provider immediately.

Student _____ Date _____

Instructor _____ Date _____

PERFORMANCE CHECKLIST SKILL 11-3 **CARE OF PATIENT IN SKELETAL TRACTION**

	S	U	NP	Comments
ASSESSMENT				
1. Assessed patient's knowledge of reason for traction.	___	___	___	_____
2. Inspected integrity and condition of skin over bony prominences and under devices, considered need for special bed or mattress.	___	___	___	_____
3. Assessed for proper alignment of extremity.	___	___	___	_____
4. Assessed patient's degree of mobility, ability to perform ADLs, and current medical condition.	___	___	___	_____
5. Assessed patient's level of pain, determined need for analgesics before procedure.	___	___	___	_____
6. Assessed traction setup following application.	___	___	___	_____
7. Assessed neurovascular status of extremity distal to traction, assessed patient's ability to move digits.	___	___	___	_____
8. Assessed pin sites following insertion for redness, edema, discharge, and odor.	___	___	___	_____
9. Assessed respiratory rate, depth, rhythm, and chest expansion.	___	___	___	_____
PLANNING				
1. Identified expected outcomes.	___	___	___	_____
IMPLEMENTATION				
1. Identified patient using two identifiers.	___	___	___	_____
2. Discussed procedure with patient.	___	___	___	_____
3. Initial traction setup:				
a. Applied gloves, positioned patient as ordered, supported limb, did not move distal part unnecessarily.	___	___	___	_____
b. Assisted while health care provider inserted pins, supported joints not at injury site, did not move distal portion unnecessarily.	___	___	___	_____
c. Attached weights and gently lowered until rope was taut once traction setup was applied.	___	___	___	_____

	S	U	NP	Comments

4. Inspected traction setups, ensured that knots were secure, footplate was in place, ropes and pulleys were not frayed, weights hung freely, and bedclothes were not interfering with traction apparatus.   ___ ___ ___ _____

5. Provided pin-site care according to policy or health care provider's orders.

    a. Applied gloves, removed gauze dressings from around pins, discarded appropriately.   ___ ___ ___ _____

    b. Inspected pin sites for signs of infection, removed and discarded gloves, performed hand hygiene.   ___ ___ ___ _____

    c. Prepared supplies.   ___ ___ ___ _____

    d. Applied gloves, cleansed each pin site properly, disposed of applicator, used new sterile applicator for each swipe.   ___ ___ ___ _____

    e. Repeated process for each pin site.   ___ ___ ___ _____

    f. Applied a small amount of topical antibiotic ointment to pin site using sterile applicator.   ___ ___ ___ _____

    g. Covered with appropriate gauze dressing or left site open to air.   ___ ___ ___ _____

6. Provided routine traction care.

    a. Inspected skin for signs of pressure, used pressure-relief devices as appropriate, repositioned areas under pressure if possible, did not massage if not appropriate.   ___ ___ ___ _____

7. Provided nonpharmacologic and pharmacologic pain relief as indicated.   ___ ___ ___ _____

8. Encouraged use of unaffected extremities in ADLs and active and passive exercises, encouraged use of trapeze bar for repositioning.   ___ ___ ___ _____

9. Provided fracture pan if needed.   ___ ___ ___ _____

10. Raised side rails as appropriate.   ___ ___ ___ _____

11. Returned equipment and supplies to proper storage places, performed hand hygiene.   ___ ___ ___ _____

EVALUATION

1. Inspected body part in traction for correct alignment.   ___ ___ ___ _____

2. Monitored neurovascular status and peripheral tissue perfusion regularly.   ___ ___ ___ _____

3. Evaluated presence of pain and muscle spasms.   ___ ___ ___ _____

	S	U	NP	Comments

4. Observed for signs of infection.   ___   ___   ___   _____

5. Monitored respiratory status for FES, atelectasis, and pulmonary embolism every shift.   ___   ___   ___   _____

6. Inspected skin for fracture blisters, did not rupture blister, applied hydrocolloid dressing to ruptured blister.   ___   ___   ___   _____

7. Identified unexpected outcomes.   ___   ___   ___   _____

RECORDING AND REPORTING

1. Documented all pertinent information in the appropriate record, drew diagram for chart and posted in the room if necessary.   ___   ___   ___   _____

2. Recorded site care performed and appearance of pin sites in nurses' notes.   ___   ___   ___   _____

3. Recorded specific assessments and frequency of assessments in appropriate log.   ___   ___   ___   _____

Student _____ Date _____

Instructor _____ Date _____

PERFORMANCE CHECKLIST SKILL 11-4 **CARE OF A PATIENT WITH AN IMMOBOLIZATION DEVICE**

	S	U	NP	Comments
ASSESSMENT				
1. Reviewed patient's medical history, previous and current activity level, and description of the condition requiring immobilization.	___	___	___	_____
2. Determined patient's previous experience with braces/splints/slings.	___	___	___	_____
3. Assessed patient's level of pain.	___	___	___	_____
4. Assessed patient's understanding of reason for brace/splint/sling and its care, application, and schedule of wear.	___	___	___	_____
5. Inspected areas of skin that would be in contact with support device.	___	___	___	_____
6. Referred to therapy consultation to determine type of brace to be used, desired position, and amount of activity and movement permitted.	___	___	___	_____
7. Assessed patient's additional need for an assistive device such as walker, cane, or crutches.	___	___	___	_____
PLANNING				
1. Identified expected outcomes.	___	___	___	_____
IMPLEMENTATION				
1. Identified patient using two identifiers.	___	___	___	_____
2. Explained reasons for brace/splint/sling, demonstrated how device works.	___	___	___	_____
3. Assisted patient to comfortable position appropriate to brace/splint/sling being applied.	___	___	___	_____
4. Applied gloves, prepared skin to be enclosed in brace/splint/sling with soap and water, patted dry, changed any dressings, put thin cotton shirt or gown on patient if applying a back brace, ensured there were no wrinkles to cause pressure.	___	___	___	_____
5. Inspected device for wear, damage, or rough edge.	___	___	___	_____

	S	U	NP	Comments

6. Applied brace/splint/sling as directed.

    a. Applied even tension as bandage was wrapped from distal to proximal. ___ ___ ___ _____

    b. Prevented padding from gathering or bunching. ___ ___ ___ _____

    c. Supported joints when placing a device. ___ ___ ___ _____

7. Applied sling using triangular bandage.

    a. Positioned one end of band over shoulder of unaffected arm. ___ ___ ___ _____

    b. Placed remaining bandage material against the chest, then under and over affected arm so as to cradle the arm. ___ ___ ___ _____

    c. Positioned pointed end of triangle toward the elbow. ___ ___ ___ _____

    d. Tied the two ends of the triangle at the side of the neck. ___ ___ ___ _____

    e. Folded pointed end of the sling at elbow in the front and secured with a safety pin. ___ ___ ___ _____

    f. Ensured sling supported the limb comfortably without interfering with circulation. ___ ___ ___ _____

8. Taught patient prescribed schedule of wear and activities while in brace/splint/sling. ___ ___ ___ _____

9. Reinforced instruction regarding signs of skin breakdown, pressure, or rubbing to report. ___ ___ ___ _____

10. Assisted patient in ambulating with brace/splint/sling in place. ___ ___ ___ _____

11. Had patient or caregiver apply and remove brace/splint/sling. ___ ___ ___ _____

EVALUATION

1. Inspected areas of skin underneath brace/splint/sling for signs of pressure. ___ ___ ___ _____

2. Observed patient using the brace/splint/sling. ___ ___ ___ _____

3. Asked patient to rate level of pain after application. ___ ___ ___ _____

4. Palpated temperature, pulse, and sensation of extremity distal to brace/splint/sling. ___ ___ ___ _____

5. Inspected alignment of the limb after device application. ___ ___ ___ _____

6. Identified unexpected outcomes. ___ ___ ___ _____

136

	S	U	NP	Comments

RECORDING AND REPORTING

1. Recorded pertinent specific assessments in nurses' notes. ___ ___ ___ _____

2. Documented instructions given to patient and family. ___ ___ ___ _____

3. Recorded observations regarding patient's ability to apply, ambulate with, and remove the brace/splint/sling. ___ ___ ___ _____

4. Reported immediately any injury sustained by patient while using brace/splint/sling. ___ ___ ___ _____

Student _____ Date _____

Instructor _____ Date _____

PERFORMANCE CHECKLIST PROCEDURAL GUIDELINE 12-1 **SELECTION OF PRESSURE-REDUCING SUPPORT SURFACES**

	S	U	NP	Comments
PROCEDURAL STEPS				
1. Assessed patient's risk for skin breakdown using a risk assessment tool.	___	___	___	_____
2. Assessed patient's existing pressure ulcers.	___	___	___	_____
3. Assessed patient's level of comfort using a pain scale.	___	___	___	_____
4. Determined the need for pressure-reduction surface, placed "at-risk" patient on a pressure-reduction surface.	___	___	___	_____
5. Identified patient factors when selecting appropriate surface:				
a. Assessed if patient needed pressure redistribution.	___	___	___	_____
b. Assessed if surface was needed for short- or long-term care.	___	___	___	_____
c. Assessed potential comfort level achieved by the surface.	___	___	___	_____
d. Assessed if patient, family, and caregiver were adherent to repositioning; assessed if they were aware a support surface should never replace repositioning.	___	___	___	_____
e. Assessed if support surface had potential to interfere with patient's independent functioning.	___	___	___	_____
f. Assessed patient's financial limitations.	___	___	___	_____
g. Assessed environmental limitations in the home if necessary.	___	___	___	_____
h. Assessed durability of the product.	___	___	___	_____
i. Assessed if patient needed pressure-relief surfaces in a chair/wheelchair and if caregiver had been instructed on appropriate inflation of device.	___	___	___	_____
6. Determined appropriate surface.	___	___	___	_____

	S	U	NP	Comments

7. Checked agency policy regarding implementing a support surface.

   a. Obtained a health care provider's orders. ____ ____ ____ _____

   b. Consulted with case manager or social worker to assist with patient's financial eligibility and terms and length of third-party reimbursement. ____ ____ ____ _____

   c. Consulted with agency home care or discharge planning if device was anticipated for long-term use. ____ ____ ____ _____

8. Inspected condition of the skin regularly to evaluate changes in skin and effectiveness of therapy. ____ ____ ____ _____

9. Observed existing pressure ulcers for evidence of healing. ____ ____ ____ _____

10. Observed for side effects. ____ ____ ____ _____

11. Documented assessments in patient record, documented surface selected and patient response. ____ ____ ____ _____

Student _____ Date _____

Instructor _____ Date _____

PERFORMANCE CHECKLIST SKILL 12-1 **PLACING A PATIENT ON A SUPPORTED SURFACE**

	S	U	NP	Comments
ASSESSMENT				
1. Performed hand hygiene.	___	___	___	_____
2. Determined patient's risk for pressure ulcer formation properly.	___	___	___	_____
3. Performed skin assessment, especially over dependent sites and bony prominences.	___	___	___	_____
4. Assessed patient's level of comfort.	___	___	___	_____
5. Assessed patient's understanding of purpose of support surface.	___	___	___	_____
6. Verified health care provider's orders for type of support surface.	___	___	___	_____
PLANNING				
1. Identified expected outcomes.	___	___	___	_____
2. Explained purpose of mattress and method of application to patient and caregiver.	___	___	___	_____
IMPLEMENTATION				
1. Provided privacy.	___	___	___	_____
2. Performed hand hygiene, applied clean gloves, obtained assistance as needed.	___	___	___	_____
3. Identified patient using two identifiers.	___	___	___	_____
4. Applied support surface to bed or prepared alternative bed, kept sharp objects away from air mattress.				
a. Replaced mattress:				
(1) Applied mattress to bed frame after removing hospital mattress.	___	___	___	_____
(2) Applied sheet over mattress, kept linens between surfaces to a minimum.	___	___	___	_____
b. Prepared an air mattress/overlay:				
(1) Applied deflated mattress flat over bed mattress.	___	___	___	_____
(2) Brought any plastic strips or flaps around corners of bed mattress.	___	___	___	_____

	S	U	NP	Comments

(3) Attached connector on air mattress to inflation device, inflated mattress to proper air pressure. ____ ____ ____ _____

(4) Placed sheet over air mattress, eliminated all wrinkles. ____ ____ ____ _____

(5) Checked air pumps to be sure pressure cycle alternates. ____ ____ ____ _____

(6) Assisted patient with transferring in and out of bed. ____ ____ ____ _____

  c. Used an air-surface bed.

(1) Obtained and placed linen on bed. ____ ____ ____ _____

(2) Placed switch in the "prevention" mode. ____ ____ ____ _____

5. Positioned patient comfortably as desired over support position, repositioned routinely. ____ ____ ____ _____

6. Removed gloves and performed hand hygiene. ____ ____ ____ _____

EVALUATION

1. Reassessed patient's risk for pressure ulcer formation at routine intervals. ____ ____ ____ _____

2. Inspected and compared condition of patient's skin every 8 hours to determine changes in skin integrity, pressure ulcer status, and effectiveness of support surface. ____ ____ ____ _____

3. Asked patient to rate comfort. ____ ____ ____ _____

4. Evaluated functioning of support surface periodically. ____ ____ ____ _____

5. Identified unexpected outcomes. ____ ____ ____ _____

RECORDING AND REPORTING

1. Recorded all pertinent information and patient teaching and validation of understanding in appropriate log. ____ ____ ____ _____

2. Reported evidence of pressure ulcer formation to nurse in charge or health care provider. ____ ____ ____ _____

Student _____ Date _____

Instructor _____ Date _____

PERFORMANCE CHECKLIST SKILL 12-2 **PLACING A PATIENT ON AN AIR-SUSPENSION OR AIR-FLUIDIZED BED**

	S	U	NP	Comments
ASSESSMENT				
1. Performed hand hygiene.	___	___	___	_____
2. Determined patient's risk for pressure ulcer formation, assessed for risk factors for pressure ulcers.	___	___	___	_____
3. Identified if patient would benefit from air-suspension therapy or air-fluidized therapy.	___	___	___	_____
4. Inspected condition of skin, noted appearance of existing ulcers and determined stage of ulcer.	___	___	___	_____
5. Assessed patient's comfort level.	___	___	___	_____
6. Reviewed health care provider orders.	___	___	___	_____
7. Assessed patient's level of orientation.	___	___	___	_____
8. Assessed patient's and family members' knowledge about therapy and understanding of purpose of bed.	___	___	___	_____
9. Reviewed patient's serum electrolyte levels if available.	___	___	___	_____
10. Determined if patient needed frequent weights.	___	___	___	_____
11. Assessed risk for complications from air-fluidized bed.	___	___	___	_____
PLANNING				
1. Identified expected outcomes.	___	___	___	_____
2. Reviewed instructions provided by manufacturer.	___	___	___	_____
3. Explained procedure and purpose of bed to patient and caregiver.	___	___	___	_____
4. Obtained additional personnel if needed.	___	___	___	_____
5. Premedicated approximately 30 minutes before transfer if needed.	___	___	___	_____
IMPLEMENTATION				
1. Provided privacy.	___	___	___	_____
2. Identified patient using two identifiers.	___	___	___	_____

	S	U	NP	Comments

3. Performed hand hygiene, applied clean gloves if necessary.   _____ _____ _____ _____

4. Transferred patient to bed using appropriate transfer techniques, did not attempt transfer without assistance.   _____ _____ _____ _____

5. Released Instaflate, fluidized, or turned on bed once patient had been transferred.   _____ _____ _____ _____

6. Positioned patient and performed ROM exercises as appropriate.   _____ _____ _____ _____

7. Turned on Instaflate settings to turn patient, position bedpans, or perform therapies; used foam wedges with air-fluidized bed.   _____ _____ _____ _____

8. Used bed's special features as needed.   _____ _____ _____ _____

9. Assessed effectiveness of pressure-relief mattress or seat cushion.   _____ _____ _____ _____

10. Removed gloves, performed hand hygiene.   _____ _____ _____ _____

EVALUATION

1. Inspected condition of patient's skin periodically while patient was on bed.   _____ _____ _____ _____

2. Observed existing pressure ulcers for evidence of healing.   _____ _____ _____ _____

3. Asked patient to rate level of comfort.   _____ _____ _____ _____

4. Assessed patient's level of orientation.   _____ _____ _____ _____

5. Identified unexpected outcomes.   _____ _____ _____ _____

RECORDING AND REPORTING

1. Recorded pertinent information in appropriate log, recorded patient teaching and validation of understanding in nurses' notes.   _____ _____ _____ _____

2. Reported changes in condition of skin, level of orientation, and electrolyte levels to health care provider.   _____ _____ _____ _____

Student _____ Date _____

Instructor _____ Date _____

PERFORMANCE CHECKLIST SKILL 12-3 **PLACING A PATIENT ON A BARIATRIC BED**

	S	U	NP	Comments
ASSESSMENT				
1. Performed hand hygiene.	___	___	___	_____
2. Determined patient's risk for pressure ulcer formation.	___	___	___	_____
3. Identified if patient would benefit from the bariatric bed system, assessed patient's mobility status.	___	___	___	_____
4. Assessed condition of patient's skin, obtained assistance if needed to turn patient, determined need for pressure-redistribution mattress.	___	___	___	_____
5. Assessed patient's and family members' understanding of purpose of bed.	___	___	___	_____
6. Reviewed health care provider's orders.	___	___	___	_____
7. Assessed need for patient to be weighed.	___	___	___	_____
8. Determined number of people needed to safely transfer patient from regular bed to bariatric bed.	___	___	___	_____
PLANNING				
1. Identified expected outcomes.	___	___	___	_____
2. Explained procedure and purpose of bed to patient and family.	___	___	___	_____
3. Reviewed instructions supplied.	___	___	___	_____
4. Medicated approximately 30 minutes before transfer if necessary.	___	___	___	_____
5. Obtained additional personnel needed for transfer.	___	___	___	_____
IMPLEMENTATION				
1. Provided privacy.	___	___	___	_____
2. Identified patient using two identifiers.	___	___	___	_____
3. Performed hand hygiene, applied clean gloves if necessary, used appropriate transfer techniques.	___	___	___	_____
4. Placed assistive devices, transferred safely.	___	___	___	_____
5. Covered and positioned patient, placed hand controls in reach, ensured out-of-bed alarm was on and overhead frame was attached if needed.	___	___	___	_____

	S	U	NP	Comments
6. Encouraged patient to initiate frequent position changes.	___	___	___	_____
7. Removed gloves, performed hand hygiene.	___	___	___	_____

EVALUATION

	S	U	NP	Comments
1. Inspected condition of patient's skin while patient was on bed.	___	___	___	_____
2. Asked patient to rate sense of comfort using pain scale.	___	___	___	_____
3. Evaluated patient's risk for injury.	___	___	___	_____
4. Evaluated patient's ability to move in bed.	___	___	___	_____
5. Identified unexpected outcomes.	___	___	___	_____

RECORDING AND REPORTING

	S	U	NP	Comments
1. Recorded pertinent information in the appropriate log, recorded patient teaching and validation of understanding in nurses' notes.	___	___	___	_____
2. Reported changes in condition of skin to nurse in charge or health care provider.	___	___	___	_____

Student _____   Date _____

Instructor _____   Date _____

PERFORMANCE CHECKLIST SKILL 12-4   **PLACING A PATIENT ON A ROTOKINETIC BED**

	S	U	NP	Comments
ASSESSMENT				
1. Performed hand hygiene.	___	___	___	_____
2. Determined patient's risk for pressure ulcer formation.	___	___	___	_____
3. Performed skin assessment, inspected condition of skin.	___	___	___	_____
4. Reviewed health care provider's orders.	___	___	___	_____
5. Assessed patient's level of comfort.	___	___	___	_____
6. Assessed patient's level of orientation.	___	___	___	_____
7. Performed pulmonary assessment, obtained vitals.	___	___	___	_____
8. Assessed patient's and family members' knowledge and understanding of purpose of bed.	___	___	___	_____
PLANNING				
1. Identified expected outcomes.	___	___	___	_____
2. Explained procedure and purpose of bed to patient and family.	___	___	___	_____
3. Reviewed instructions supplied by manufacturer.	___	___	___	_____
4. Premedicated approximately 30 minutes before transfer if necessary.	___	___	___	_____
5. Obtained any additional personnel needed to transfer patient.	___	___	___	_____
IMPLEMENTATION				
1. Provided privacy.	___	___	___	_____
2. Identified patient using two identifiers.	___	___	___	_____
3. Placed Rotokinetic bed in horizontal position; removed all bolsters, straps, and supports; closed posterior hatches.	___	___	___	_____
4. Unplugged electrical cord, locked latch.	___	___	___	_____
5. Performed hand hygiene, applied gloves.	___	___	___	_____
6. Maintained proper alignment of patient, transferred patient to Rotokinetic bed appropriately.	___	___	___	_____
7. Secured thoracic panels, bolsters, head and knee packs, and safety straps.	___	___	___	_____

	S	U	NP	Comments
8. Covered patient with top sheet.	___	___	___	_____
9. Plugged in bed.	___	___	___	_____
10. Had manufacturer representative set optional angle as ordered.	___	___	___	_____
11. Increased degree of rotation according to patient's tolerance.	___	___	___	_____
12. Provided space for caregivers and family to move around bed to facilitate communication.	___	___	___	_____
13. Stopped bed for assessment and procedures, manually repositioned bed if necessary.	___	___	___	_____
14. Informed patient that there would be a sensation of light-headedness or falling, reassured patient a fall would not occur.	___	___	___	_____

EVALUATION

	S	U	NP	Comments
1. Inspected condition of skin and musculoskeletal alignment as indicated by patient's condition.	___	___	___	_____
2. Inspected patient's pressure ulcers for evidence of healing.	___	___	___	_____
3. Observed alignment and ROM of all joints.	___	___	___	_____
4. Auscultated lung sounds every shift, compared with baseline.	___	___	___	_____
5. Determined patient's level of orientation at least once per shift while on bed.	___	___	___	_____
6. Asked whether patient was experiencing nausea or dizziness.	___	___	___	_____
7. Monitored blood pressure.	___	___	___	_____
8. Identified unexpected outcomes.	___	___	___	_____

RECORDING AND REPORTING

	S	U	NP	Comments
1. Recorded pertinent information in appropriate log, recorded patient teaching and validation of understanding in nurses' notes, took photograph to document skin condition and provide baseline.	___	___	___	_____
2. Recorded and reported subjective data indicating response to constant rotation and presence/absence of dizziness, nausea, or blood pressure changes.	___	___	___	_____
3. Used flow sheet to document routine assessment and care, rotated bed at appropriate time.	___	___	___	_____
4. Reported changes in condition of skin to nurse in charge or health care provider.	___	___	___	_____

Student _____ Date _____

Instructor _____ Date _____

PERFORMANCE CHECKLIST SKILL 13-1 **FALL PREVENTION IN A HEALTH CARE FACILITY**

	S	U	NP	Comments
ASSESSMENT				
1. Assessed patient's fall risks.	___	___	___	_____
2. Determined if patient had history of recent falls or other injuries in the home, assessed previous falls following SPLATT.	___	___	___	_____
3. Reviewed patient's medication history, assessed OTC medications and herbal products, assessed for polypharmacy.	___	___	___	_____
4. Assessed patient for fear of falling.	___	___	___	_____
5. Assessed risk factors in health care facility.	___	___	___	_____
6. Assessed condition of equipment.	___	___	___	_____
7. Performed TGUG test if patient is able to ambulate.	___	___	___	_____
8. Assessed patient for osteoporosis, anticoagulant therapy, history of previous fracture, and recent chest or abdominal surgery.	___	___	___	_____
9. Used a patient-centered approach, determined what patient knew about risks for falling and fall prevention.	___	___	___	_____
10. Applied color-coded wristband if patient at risk for falling.	___	___	___	_____
PLANNING				
1. Identified expected outcomes.	___	___	___	_____
IMPLEMENTATION				
1. Introduced self to patient, included name and title or role.	___	___	___	_____
2. Explained plan of care, specifically discussed the reasons patient was at risk for falling.	___	___	___	_____
3. Gathered equipment, performed hand hygiene.	___	___	___	_____
4. Provided privacy, assigned patient to bed that allowed patient exit on stronger side, positioned and draped patient as needed.	___	___	___	_____
5. Adjusted bed to low position with wheels locked, placed padded mats on the floor.	___	___	___	_____
6. Encouraged patient to wear proper footwear.	___	___	___	_____

	S	U	NP	Comments

7. Oriented patient to surroundings, call light, and bed control system:

   a. Provided patient's hearing aid and glasses. ____ ____ ____ _____

   b. Explained and demonstrated call light/ intercom system, had patient perform return demonstration. ____ ____ ____ _____

   c. Explained to patient and family when and why to use call system. ____ ____ ____ _____

   d. Consistently secured call light/bed control system to an accessible location. ____ ____ ____ _____

8. Taught use of hospital side rails:

   a. Explained to patient and family reasons for using side rails. ____ ____ ____ _____

   b. Checked agency policy regarding side rail use. ____ ____ ____ _____

9. Provided environmental interventions:

   a. Removed excess equipment, supplies, and furniture from rooms and halls. ____ ____ ____ _____

   b. Kept floors clear, coiled and secured other cords or tubing. ____ ____ ____ _____

   c. Cleaned all spills promptly, managed wet floor signs appropriately. ____ ____ ____ _____

   d. Ensured adequate glare-free lighting, used a night light. ____ ____ ____ _____

   e. Had assistive devices located on exit side of the bed. ____ ____ ____ _____

   f. Arranged necessary items within patient's reach. ____ ____ ____ _____

   g. Secured locks on beds, stretchers, and wheelchairs. ____ ____ ____ _____

10. Implemented additional interventions for high risk patients:

   a. Prioritized call light responses. ____ ____ ____ _____

   b. Monitored and assisted patient in following daily schedules. ____ ____ ____ _____

   c. Established elimination schedule, used bedside commode when appropriate. ____ ____ ____ _____

   d. Stayed with patient during toileting. ____ ____ ____ _____

   e. Placed patients in Geri chair or wheelchair with a wedge cushion. ____ ____ ____ _____

   f. Used a low bed. ____ ____ ____ _____

   g. Activated bed alarm for patient. ____ ____ ____ _____

	S	U	NP	Comments

11. Had patient wear gait belt while ambulating, walked along patient's strong side.

12. Explained to patient that hourly rounds would be conducted to reassess for fall risks, provide toileting needs, and attend to symptom management.

13. Explained to patient specific safety measures to prevent falls.

14. Consulted with therapist about possibility of gait training and muscle-strengthening exercises.

15. Discussed with health care provider and pharmacist possibility of adjusting patient's medication to reduce side effects and interactions.

16. Safe transport using a wheelchair:

   a. Positioned wheelchair on same side of bed as patient's strong side.

   b. Placed wedge cushion in chair.

   c. Locked brakes on both wheels for transfer into and out of wheelchair.

   d. Raised footplates before transfer, lowered footplates and placed feet on footplates after patient is seated.

   e. Had patient sit well back in seat.

   f. Backed wheelchair into and out of elevator or door.

EVALUATION

1. Conducted hourly rounds.

2. Observed patient's immediate environment for presence of hazards.

3. Evaluated patient's ability to use assistive device.

4. Asked patient or family member to identify safety risks.

5. Evaluated motor, sensory, and cognitive status; reviewed if any falls or injuries had occurred.

6. Identified unexpected outcomes.

	S	U	NP	Comments

RECORDING AND REPORTING

1. Recorded fall risks assessment findings and specific interventions used to prevent falls in appropriate log.   ___ ___ ___ _____

2. Reported to health care personnel specific risks to patient's safety and measures taken to minimize risks.   ___ ___ ___ _____

3. Informed primary health care provider if patient suffers fall; documented incident; included baseline assessment, injuries, tests or treatments, follow-up care, or safety precautions taken after fall.   ___ ___ ___ _____

PERFORMANCE CHECKLIST SKILL 13-2 **DESIGNING A RESTRAINT-FREE ENVIRONMENT**

	S	U	NP	Comments
ASSESSMENT				
1. Assessed patient's medical history for dementia and depression.	___	___	___	_____
2. Assessed patient's behavior, balance, gait, vision, hearing, bowel/bladder routine, level of pain, electrolyte and blood count values, and presence of orthostatic hypotension.	___	___	___	_____
3. Reviewed prescribed medications for interactions and untoward effects.	___	___	___	_____
4. Assessed patient's knowledge of condition and prescribed treatments.	___	___	___	_____
5. Assessed cognitive decline using MMSE for patients who wander or have known dementia.	___	___	___	_____
6. Assessed the degree of wandering behavior using RAWS.	___	___	___	_____
7. Asked family or friends about patient's usual communication style and cues for patients with dementia.				
PLANNING				
1. Identified expected outcomes.	___	___	___	_____
IMPLEMENTATION				
1. Oriented patient and family to surroundings, introduced staff, explained all treatments and procedures, ensured patient was able to read your name badge.	___	___	___	_____
2. Assigned same staff to care for patient as often as possible, encouraged friends and families to stay with patient.	___	___	___	_____
3. Placed patient in room that is easily accessible to caregivers.	___	___	___	_____
4. Ensured patient has sensory aid devices, ensured all devices were functioning.	___	___	___	_____
5. Provided visual and auditory stimuli meaningful to patient.	___	___	___	_____
6. Anticipated patient's basic needs as quickly as possible.	___	___	___	_____

	S	U	NP	Comments

7. Provided scheduled ambulation, chair activity, and toileting; organized treatments so patient had uninterrupted periods throughout the day. ___ ___ ___ _____

8. Positioned catheters and tubes/drains out of patient view, camouflaged IV site, covered visible catheters or feeding tubes/drains. ___ ___ ___ _____

9. Eliminated stressors that may encourage wandering. ___ ___ ___ _____

10. Used stress-reduction techniques including back rub, massage, and guided imagery. ___ ___ ___ _____

11. Used diversional activities, ensured patient had interest in the chosen activity, involved a family member in the activity if possible. ___ ___ ___ _____

12. Positioned patient on a wedge cushion, applied a wraparound belt. ___ ___ ___ _____

13. Used pressure-sensitive bed or chair pad with alarms:

    a. Explained use of device to patient and family. ___ ___ ___ _____

    b. Positioned device under patient's mid-to-low back or under buttocks. ___ ___ ___ _____

    c. Tested alarm by applying and releasing pressure. ___ ___ ___ _____

14. Used an Ambularm monitoring device:

    a. Explained use of device to patient and family. ___ ___ ___ _____

    b. Measured patient's thigh to determine appropriate size. ___ ___ ___ _____

    c. Tested battery and alarm. ___ ___ ___ _____

    d. Applied leg band just above knee, snapped battery in place. ___ ___ ___ _____

    e. Instructed patient that alarm would sound if leg was not in horizontal position. ___ ___ ___ _____

    f. Deactivated alarm to ambulate patient, unsnapped device from leg band. ___ ___ ___ _____

15. Placed patient in an enclosure bed system. ___ ___ ___ _____

16. Consulted with therapists for activities that provide stimulation and exercise. ___ ___ ___ _____

17. Minimized invasive treatments as much as possible. ___ ___ ___ _____

	S	U	NP	Comments

EVALUATION

1. Observed patient for any injuries. ___ ___ ___ _____

2. Observed patient's behavior toward staff, visitors, and other patients. ___ ___ ___ _____

3. Determined need for continuation of invasive treatments and whether less invasive treatment may be substituted. ___ ___ ___ _____

4. Identified unexpected outcomes. ___ ___ ___ _____

RECORDING AND REPORTING

1. Recorded restraint alternatives attempted, patient behaviors that related to cognitive status, and interventions in appropriate log. ___ ___ ___ _____

Student _____ Date _____

Instructor _____ Date _____

PERFORMANCE CHECKLIST SKILL 13-3 **APPLYING PHYSICAL RESTRAINTS**

	S	U	NP	Comments

ASSESSMENT

1. Assessed patient's behavior.

2. Followed agency policies regarding restraints; checked health care provider's orders for purpose, type, location, and duration of restraint; determined if signed consent was needed.

3. Reviewed manufacturer instructions for restraint application, determined most appropriate size of restraint.

4. Inspected area where restraint was to be placed; noted nearby tubing or devices; assessed condition of skin, sensation, adequacy of circulation, and ROM.

PLANNING

1. Identified expected outcomes.

IMPLEMENTATION

1. Gathered equipment, performed hand hygiene.

2. Used a calm approach, introduced self to patient using both name and title or role.

3. Identified patient using two identifiers.

4. Provided privacy, explained to patient and family purpose of restraint, ensured patient was in a correct and comfortable position.

5. Adjusted bed to proper height, lowered side rail on side of patient contact.

6. Padded skin and bony prominences that would be covered by the restraint.

7. Applied proper-size restraint:

   a. Belt restraint: Had patient sit properly, applied belt over clothes, placed restraint around waist, removed wrinkles in clothing, brought ties through slots in belt, helped patient lie down if needed.

   b. Extremity restraint: Wrapped restraint with soft part toward skin, secured with Velcro straps, ensured restraint is not too tight.

	S	U	NP	Comments

c. Mitten restraint: Placed hand in mitten, ensured straps are around wrist. ___ ___ ___ _____

   d. Elbow restraint: Inserted patient's arm so that elbow joint rested against padded area, kept joint rigid. ___ ___ ___ _____

8. Attached restraint straps to appropriate part of bedframe, ensured straps were secured. ___ ___ ___ _____

9. Secured restraints with appropriate quick-release tie, buckle, or locking device. ___ ___ ___ _____

10. Inserted two fingers under secured restraint. ___ ___ ___ _____

11. Assessed proper placement of restraint. ___ ___ ___ _____

12. Removed restraints at least every 2 hours, assessed patient each time, obtained assistance and removed restraints one at a time if necessary. ___ ___ ___ _____

13. Secured call light or intercom within reach. ___ ___ ___ _____

14. Left bed or chair with wheels locked, kept bed in lowest position. ___ ___ ___ _____

15. Performed hand hygiene. ___ ___ ___ _____

EVALUATION

1. Evaluated patient's condition for signs of injury regularly, used visual checks if needed. ___ ___ ___ _____

2. Evaluated patient for any complications of immobility. ___ ___ ___ _____

3. Observed catheters and drainage tubes routinely. ___ ___ ___ _____

4. Evaluated patient's need for restraints on an ongoing basis, obtained a health care provider's assistance if patient used restraints for violent behavior. ___ ___ ___ _____

5. Identified unexpected outcomes. ___ ___ ___ _____

RECORDING AND REPORTING

1. Recorded patient's behavior before and after restraints were applied, level of orientation, and patient's or family members' statement of understanding and consent. ___ ___ ___ _____

2. Recorded restraint alternatives tried and patient's response in nurses' notes. ___ ___ ___ _____

3. Recorded all pertinent information in the appropriate log. ___ ___ ___ _____

Student _____ Date _____

Instructor _____ Date _____

	S	U	NP	Comments

PROCEDURAL STEPS

1. Reviewed agency guidelines for rapid response to emergency, understood nursing responsibilities. ____ ____ ____ _____

2. Knew location of fire alarms, emergency equipment, MSDS forms, eyewash stations, and exit routes. ____ ____ ____ _____

3. Assessed patient's mental status and ability to ambulate, transfer, and move to anticipate evacuation procedures. ____ ____ ____ _____

4. Remained alert to situations that increase risk for fire. ____ ____ ____ _____

5. Knew which patients were on oxygen. ____ ____ ____ _____

6. Inspected equipment for current maintenance sticker, checked electrical equipment for basic safety features, knew agency policy for reporting unsafe equipment. ____ ____ ____ _____

7. Fire safety:

   a. Followed RACE acronym:

      (1) Rescued patient from immediate injury. ____ ____ ____ _____

      (2) Activated fire alarm, followed agency policy for alerting staff. ____ ____ ____ _____

      (3) Contained fire by closing doors and windows, turning off oxygen and equipment, and placing wet towels along base of doors. ____ ____ ____ _____

      (4) Evacuated patients:

         (a) Directed ambulatory patients to a safe area. ____ ____ ____ _____

         (b) Maintained respiratory status of patient on life support manually until removed from fire area. ____ ____ ____ _____

         (c) Moved bedridden patients by stretcher, bed, or wheelchair. ____ ____ ____ _____

         (d) Moved patient who cannot walk appropriately using blanket, two-person swing, or "back-strap" method. ____ ____ ____ _____

	S	U	NP	Comments

b. Extinguished fire using appropriate fire extinguisher, followed PASS acronym. ___ ___ ___ _____

8. Electrical safety:

   a. Unplugged electrical source and assessed for presence of pulse after patient received a shock, checked for presence of water on the floor. ___ ___ ___ _____

   b. Provided appropriate interventions, instituted emergency resuscitation if needed. ___ ___ ___ _____

   c. Notified emergency personnel and patient's health care provider. ___ ___ ___ _____

   d. Obtained vitals and assessed skin for signs of thermal injury if patient had pulse and remained alert. ___ ___ ___ _____

9. Chemical safety:

   a. Attended to any exposed person, treated splashes to the eyes immediately, removed contact lenses if necessary. ___ ___ ___ _____

   b. Notified persons in immediate area of spill, evacuated nonessential personnel. ___ ___ ___ _____

   c. Referred to MSDS, turned off electrical and heat sources if necessary. ___ ___ ___ _____

   d. Avoided breathing vapors, applied respirator if necessary. ___ ___ ___ _____

   e. Used appropriate PPE to clean up spill. ___ ___ ___ _____

   f. Disposed of any materials used in cleanup as hazardous waste. ___ ___ ___ _____

10. Inspected patient's room regularly for hazards. ___ ___ ___ _____

11. Followed agency policy for reporting events. ___ ___ ___ _____

Student _____ Date _____

Instructor _____ Date _____

PERFORMANCE CHECKLIST SKILL 13-4 **SEIZURE PRECAUTIONS**

	S	U	NP	Comments

ASSESSMENT

1. Assessed patient's seizure history and knowledge of precipitating factors; asked patient to describe frequency, presence and type of aura, and body parts affected; used family as a resource if needed. ___ ___ ___ _____

2. Assessed for medical and surgical conditions. ___ ___ ___ _____

3. Assessed medication history, assessed patient's adherence to drug levels if test results were available. ___ ___ ___ _____

4. Inspected patient's environment for potential safety hazards if seizure occurred; kept bed low, side rails up, and patient in side-lying position. ___ ___ ___ _____

5. Assessed patient's individual and cultural perspective about meaning of seizures and their treatment. ___ ___ ___ _____

PLANNING

1. Identified expected outcomes. ___ ___ ___ _____

IMPLEMENTATION

1. Kept bed in lowest position with side rails up, padded rails if needed, had oral suction and oxygen equipment ready for use. ___ ___ ___ _____

2. Positioned patient's room close to nurses' station or in a room with a video monitor if necessary. ___ ___ ___ _____

3. Seizure response:

   a. Positioned patient safely.

      (1) Guided patient to floor, protected head appropriately, turned patient onto side with head tilted forward, did not lift patient during seizure. ___ ___ ___ _____

      (2) Turned patient in bed on side and raised side rails. ___ ___ ___ _____

   b. Noted time seizure began, called for help, tracked duration of seizure, had health care provider notified immediately, had staff bring emergency cart, cleared surrounding area of furniture. ___ ___ ___ _____

	S	U	NP	Comments

c. Kept patient in side-lying position, supported head, and kept it flexed slightly forward.
___ ___ ___ _____

d. Provided privacy, had staff control flow of visitors.
___ ___ ___ _____

e. Did not restrain patient, held limbs loosely if necessary, loosened restrictive clothing.
___ ___ ___ _____

f. Never forced any object into patient's mouth.
___ ___ ___ _____

g. Maintained patient's airway, suctioned orally if needed, checked patient's LOC and oxygen saturation, provided oxygen if necessary.
___ ___ ___ _____

h. Observed sequence and timing of seizure activity, noted all relevant behaviors.
___ ___ ___ _____

i. Assessed vital signs and reoriented patient after patient regained consciousness, explained what happened and answered patient's questions, stayed with patient until fully awake.
___ ___ ___ _____

4. Status epilepticus:

a. Called health care provider and response team immediately.
___ ___ ___ _____

b. Inserted oral airway when jaw was relaxed.
___ ___ ___ _____

c. Accessed oxygen and suction equipment, kept airway patent.
___ ___ ___ _____

d. Prepared for IV insertion and administration of IV medications.
___ ___ ___ _____

5. Assisted patient to appropriate position with side rails up and bed in lowest position; placed call light or intercom within reach; provided quiet, nonstimulating environment; instructed patient not to get out of bed without assistance.
___ ___ ___ _____

6. Reoriented and reassured patient, explained what happened, provided time for patient to express feelings and concerns.
___ ___ ___ _____

7. Performed hand hygiene.
___ ___ ___ _____

EVALUATION

1. Checked vital signs and oxygen saturation every 15 minutes, maintained patient airway.
___ ___ ___ _____

2. Examined patient for injury, included oral cavity and extremities.
___ ___ ___ _____

3. Evaluated patient's mental status, encouraged patient to verbalize feelings.
___ ___ ___ _____

4. Identified unexpected outcomes.
___ ___ ___ _____

162

	S	U	NP	Comments

RECORDING AND REPORTING

1. Recorded observations in nurses' notes, provided detailed descriptions of type of seizure activity and sequence of events.

2. Alerted primary health care provider immediately.

Student _____   Date _____

Instructor _____   Date _____

PERFORMANCE CHECKLIST PROCEDURAL GUIDELINE 13-2 **CONDUCTING A ROOT CAUSE ANALYSIS**

	S	U	NP	Comments
PROCEDURAL STEPS				
1. Ensure that immediate needs of patient and family are met in response to a sentinel event, reported event according to agency policy.	___	___	___	_____
2. Helped to review event, identified professionals involved, ensured all professional groups were represented in analysis.	___	___	___	_____
3. Analyzed factors leading to and associated with sentinel event: what happened, why it happened, and what factors contributed to the event.	___	___	___	_____
4. Helped team decide if any element was a root cause and if action would be needed.	___	___	___	_____
5. Contributed to further analysis of HR, educational, information management, and leadership issues.	___	___	___	_____
6. Used appropriate approaches for analyzing data such as Six Sigma or Fish Diagram.	___	___	___	_____
7. Developed an action plan for risk reduction.	___	___	___	_____
8. Implemented the plan, considered if pilot testing was needed.	___	___	___	_____
9. Evaluated results.	___	___	___	_____

Student _____ Date _____

Instructor _____ Date _____

PERFORMANCE CHECKLIST SKILL 14-1 **CARE OF PATIENT AFTER BIOLOGIC EXPOSURE**

	S	U	NP	Comments
ASSESSMENT				
1. Performed hand hygiene, applied proper PPE.	___	___	___	_____
2. Conducted focused health history and physical examination, reviewed history of patient's presenting symptoms, determined whether pattern existed.	___	___	___	_____
3. Measured patient's vital signs.	___	___	___	_____
4. Reviewed results of diagnostic tests, consulted with health care provider.	___	___	___	_____
5. Assessed patient for health risks that complicated the effects of exposure to a biologic agent.	___	___	___	_____
6. Stayed calm, assessed patient's immediate psychological response after exposure.	___	___	___	_____
7. Identified all patient contacts in the waiting room.	___	___	___	_____
8. Identified resources available.	___			_____
PLANNING				
1. Identified expected outcomes.	___	___	___	_____
2. Dispensed timely and accurate information to patient and family.	___	___	___	_____
IMPLEMENTATION				
1. Performed hand hygiene.	___	___	___	_____
2. Instituted transmission-based isolation precautions, used strict isolation and appropriate precautions with smallpox.	___	___	___	_____
3. Decontaminated if indicated, had patient remove clothes and place in a biohazard bag, cut garments off instead of pulling them over the patient's head, instructed patient to shower thoroughly with soap and water.	___	___	___	_____
4. Administered appropriate antibiotics/antitoxins.	___	___	___	_____
5. Administered immunizations.	___	___	___	_____
6. Administered fluid and nutrition therapy.	___	___	___	_____
7. Administered oxygen therapy.	___	___	___	_____

	S	U	NP	Comments

8. Provided supportive care. ___ ___ ___ _____

9. Counseled patient and family on acute and potential long-term psychological effects of exposure, offered access to counselors, supported survivors of a disaster by identifying resources. ___ ___ ___ _____

EVALUATION

1. Observed for improved airway maintenance, breathing, circulation, LOC, and neurologic functioning. ___ ___ ___ _____

2. Evaluated vital signs and level of pain. ___ ___ ___ _____

3. Inspected condition of patient's skin, noted character of lesions. ___ ___ ___ _____

4. Asked patient "How do you feel right now?," checked level of orientation and ability to conduct conversation. ___ ___ ___ _____

5. Identified unexpected outcomes. ___ ___ ___ _____

RECORDING AND REPORTING

1. Reported suspected cases of biologic incident to health care provider or ED officer. ___ ___ ___ _____

2. Created checklists and utilized them in a disaster to record data regarding patient status and response to treatment. ___ ___ ___ _____

3. Reported unexpected outcome to health care provider in charge. ___ ___ ___ _____

Student _____ Date _____

Instructor _____ Date _____

PERFORMANCE CHECKLIST SKILL 14-2 **CARE OF A PATIENT AFTER CHEMICAL EXPOSURE**

	S	U	NP	Comments
ASSESSMENT				
1. Performed hand hygiene, applied proper PPE.	___	___	___	_____
2. Assessed patient's symptoms and level of pain, performed appropriate focused physical examination.	___	___	___	_____
3. Observed for presence of liquid on patient's skin or clothing and for odor.	___	___	___	_____
4. Assessed patient for preexisting medical conditions that will complicate effects of toxic exposure.	___	___	___	_____
5. Assessed patient's immediate psychological response following exposure.	___	___	___	_____
6. Identified resources available.	___	___	___	_____
PLANNING				
1. Identified expected outcomes.	___	___	___	_____
2. Explained care to patient and family, explained your role, oriented patient to location and activities, asked how patient was feeling, assured patient that a medical professional would see the patient shortly.	___	___	___	_____
IMPLEMENTATION				
1. Performed hand hygiene.	___	___	___	_____
2. If trained, applied appropriate PPE to decontaminate patient.	___	___	___	_____
3. Provided privacy.	___	___	___	_____
4. Decontaminated the patient:				
a. Acted quickly, avoided touching contaminated parts of clothing.	___	___	___	_____
b. Removed all of patient's clothing, cut garments off.	___	___	___	_____
c. Used large amounts of soap and water to wash patient thoroughly.	___	___	___	_____
d. Rinsed eyes with water if necessary, removed contacts if needed, washed eyeglasses and re-applied them.	___	___	___	_____

	S	U	NP	Comments

5. Disposed of patient's contaminated clothing in sealed biohazard bag, placed in another plastic bag and sealed.   ___ ___ ___   _____

6. Initiated treatment for chemical agent using appropriate chemical agent protocol.   ___ ___ ___   _____

7. Established airway if needed, administered oxygen therapy.   ___ ___ ___   _____

8. Controlled bleeding.   ___ ___ ___   _____

9. Administered fluid and nutritional therapy.   ___ ___ ___   _____

10. Provided supportive care.   ___ ___ ___   _____

11. Counseled patient and family on acute and potential long-term psychological effect of exposure, offered access to trained counselors.   ___ ___ ___   _____

EVALUATION

1. Observed status of airway maintenance, breathing, circulation, LOC, and neurologic functioning; assessed vital signs.   ___ ___ ___   _____

2. Asked patient to rate level of pain on scale of 0 to 10.   ___ ___ ___   _____

3. Inspected condition of skin, noted extent of blistering.   ___ ___ ___   _____

4. Evaluated patient's level of orientation, ability to problem solve, and perception of condition.   ___ ___ ___   _____

5. Identified unexpected outcomes.   ___ ___ ___   _____

RECORDING AND REPORTING

1. Reported suspected cases of a toxic chemical event to health care provider or emergency officer.   ___ ___ ___   _____

2. Recorded in nurses' notes patient's status, decontamination and treatment procedures, and response to treatment/comfort measures.   ___ ___ ___   _____

3. Reported any unexpected outcome to health care provider in charge.   ___ ___ ___   _____

Student _____ Date _____

Instructor _____ Date _____

PERFORMANCE CHECKLIST SKILL 14-3 **CARE OF A PATIENT AFTER RADIATION EXPOSURE**

	S	U	NP	Comments
ASSESSMENT				
1. Assessed patient's symptoms by performing a focused physical examination.	___	___	___	_____
2. Assessed patient for secondary traumatic wounds.	___	___	___	_____
3. Assessed patient for preexisting medical conditions that would complicate effects of radiologic exposure.	___	___	___	_____
4. Determined patient's allergies.	___	___	___	_____
5. Assessed individual psychological response to radiologic event, determined level of orientation.	___	___	___	_____
6. Identified resources available.	___	___	___	_____
PLANNING				
1. Identified expected outcomes.	___	___	___	_____
2. Explained care to patient and family, explained role, oriented to location and activities, explained what patient had experienced, asked how patient was feeling, assured patient that medical personnel would see the patient shortly.	___	___	___	_____
IMPLEMENTATION				
1. Performed hand hygiene.	___	___	___	_____
2. If trained, applied appropriate PPE to decontaminate patients.	___	___	___	_____
3. Provided privacy.	___	___	___	_____
4. Decontaminated patient:				
a. Removed patient's clothing.	___	___	___	_____
b. Washed patient's skin thoroughly with soap and water, took care not to abrade or irritate skin, did not allow radioactive material to be incorporated into wounds.	___	___	___	_____
c. Had radiation technician resurvey patient after washing, rewashed if necessary.	___	___	___	_____
d. Isolated and covered areas of skin still positive for radiation by using a plastic bag or wrap.	___	___	___	_____

	S	U	NP	Comments

5. Bagged and tagged patient's contaminated clothing for further evaluation, placed in appropriate biohazard container. ___ ___ ___ _____

6. Prepared for obtaining a CBC, urinalysis, fecal specimen, and swabs of body orifices. ___ ___ ___ _____

7. Treated symptoms according to ordinary treatment practices, provided IV fluid support, antidiarrheal therapies, antiemetic medication, and potassium iodine tablets. ___ ___ ___ _____

EVALUATION

1. Observed skin integrity, fluid balance, respiratory and GI status, LOC, and neurologic functioning, looked for improvement of other radiologic agent–specific symptoms, evaluated vital signs. ___ ___ ___ _____

2. Monitored CBC and other laboratory tests. ___ ___ ___ _____

3. Evaluated patient's LOC, orientation, and ability to relate events; asked if patient remembers what occurred; observed affect. ___ ___ ___ _____

4. Identified unexpected outcomes. ___ ___ ___ _____

RECORDING AND REPORTING

1. Recorded in nurses' notes patient's status and response to treatment/comfort measures. ___ ___ ___ _____

2. Reported presence of open wound and any suspected radioactive fragment to health care provider in charge. ___ ___ ___ _____

3. Reported any unexpected outcomes to health care provider. ___ ___ ___ _____

Student _____ Date _____

Instructor _____ Date _____

PERFORMANCE CHECKLIST SKILL 15-1   **PROVIDING PAIN RELIEF**

	S	U	NP	Comments
ASSESSMENT				
1. Assessed patient's risk for pain.	___	___	___	_____
2. Asked patient about level of pain, used terms such as *hurt* or *discomfort*.	___	___	___	_____
3. Assessed patient's response to previous pharmacologic interventions, especially ability to function.	___	___	___	_____
4. Examined site of patient's pain, inspected ROM of joints involved, percussed and auscultated to help identify abnormalities, determined cause of pain, auscultated abdomen before palpation.	___	___	___	_____
5. Assessed physical, behavioral, and emotional signs and symptoms of pain.	___	___	___	_____
6. Assessed characteristics of pain, followed agency policy regarding frequency of assessment, used PQRSTU pain assessment.	___	___	___	_____
PLANNING				
1. Identified expected outcomes.	___	___	___	_____
IMPLEMENTATION				
1. Performed hand hygiene, applied clean gloves if indicated.	___	___	___	_____
2. Identified patient using two identifiers.	___	___	___	_____
3. Prepared patient's environment.	___	___	___	_____
4. Taught patient how to use pain-rating scale.	___	___	___	_____
5. Set pain-intensity goal with patient when able.	___	___	___	_____
6. Administered pain-relieving medications per health care provider's orders.	___	___	___	_____
7. Removed or reduced painful stimuli:				
a. Assisted patient to a comfortable position.	___	___	___	_____
b. Smoothed wrinkles in bed linens.	___	___	___	_____
c. Loosened constrictive bandages or devices.	___	___	___	_____
d. Repositioned underlying tubes or equipment.	___	___	___	_____

	S	U	NP	Comments

8. Taught patient how to splint over the site of pain.

   a. Explained purpose of splinting. ___ ___ ___ _____

   b. Placed pillow or blanket over site, assisted patient to place hands firmly over area of discomfort. ___ ___ ___ _____

   c. Had patient hold area firmly while coughing, deep breathing, and turning. ___ ___ ___ _____

9. Reduced or eliminated emotional factors that increase pain experiences.

   a. Offered information that reduces anxiety. ___ ___ ___ _____

   b. Offered patient opportunity to pray. ___ ___ ___ _____

   c. Spent time to allow patient to talk about pain. ___ ___ ___ _____

10. If used, removed and disposed of gloves, performed hand hygiene. ___ ___ ___ _____

EVALUATION

1. Asked patient to describe level of relief within 1 hour of intervention. ___ ___ ___ _____

2. Compared patient's current pain with personally set pain-intensity goal. ___ ___ ___ _____

3. Compared patient's ability to function and perform ADLs before and after pain interventions. ___ ___ ___ _____

4. Observed patient's nonverbal behaviors. ___ ___ ___ _____

5. Evaluated for analgesic side effects. ___ ___ ___ _____

6. Identified unexpected outcomes. ___ ___ ___ _____

RECORDING AND REPORTING

1. Recorded and reported character of pain before intervention, therapies used, and patient response in nurses' notes. ___ ___ ___ _____

2. Recorded inadequate pain relief, reduction in patient function, adverse side effects from pain interventions, and any patient or family education. ___ ___ ___ _____

Student _____ Date _____

Instructor _____ Date _____

PERFORMANCE CHECKLIST SKILL 15-2 **PATIENT-CONTROLLED ANALGESIA**

	S	U	NP	Comments
ASSESSMENT				
1. Checked accuracy and completeness of each MAR, verified patient was not allergic to medication.	___	___	___	_____
2. Assessed patient's cognitive and physical ability to press device button.	___	___	___	_____
3. Assessed character of patient's pain, including physical, behavioral, and emotional signs.	___	___	___	_____
4. Obtained pulse oximetry or capnography reading.	___	___	___	_____
5. Assessed environment for factors that could contribute to pain.	___	___	___	_____
6. Applied clean gloves and inspected incision if patient had had surgery, palpated area for tenderness, used sterile gloves.	___	___	___	_____
7. Assessed existing IV infusion line and surrounding tissue for patency and condition of site for infiltration or inflammation.	___	___	___	_____
8. Assessed patient's knowledge and effectiveness of previous pain management strategies.	___	___	___	_____
PLANNING				
1. Identified expected outcomes.	___	___	___	_____
2. Explained purpose and demonstrated function of PCA to patient and family.	___	___	___	_____
IMPLEMENTATION				
1. Performed hand hygiene.	___	___	___	_____
2. Checked prepared analgesic, followed "six rights" for administration of medication.	___	___	___	_____
3. Identified patient using two identifiers.	___	___	___	_____
4. Compared MAR with name of medication on drug cartridge at bedside, had a second RN confirm health care provider's orders and correct setup of PCA.	___	___	___	_____
5. Explained purpose of PCA and demonstrated function of PCA to patient and family:				
a. Explained type of medication in PCA device.	___	___	___	_____

	S	U	NP	Comments

b. Explained how device works and when to use it. ____ ____ ____ _____

c. Explained lockout interval and dosage limits. ____ ____ ____ _____

d. Demonstrated how to push medication demand button on PCA device. ____ ____ ____ _____

e. Instructed patient to notify nurse for possible side effects, problems in attaining pain relief, changes in severity or location, alarms sounding, or questions. ____ ____ ____ _____

6. Checked infuser and patient-control module for accurate labeling or evidence of leaking. ____ ____ ____ _____

7. Programmed computerized PCA pump as ordered. ____ ____ ____ _____

8. Inserted drug cartridge into infusion device and primed tubing. ____ ____ ____ _____

9. Applied clean gloves, attached needleless adapter to tubing adapter of PCA module. ____ ____ ____ _____

10. Wiped injection port of main IV line with alcohol. ____ ____ ____ _____

11. Inserted needleless adapter into injection port nearest patient. ____ ____ ____ _____

12. Secured connection with tape and anchored PCA tubing, labeled tubing, and removed gloves. ____ ____ ____ _____

13. Administered loading dose of analgesia if prescribed. ____ ____ ____ _____

14. Had patient demonstrate use of PCA system if currently in pain; had patient verbally repeat instructions given earlier if not currently in pain. ____ ____ ____ _____

15. Discontinued PCA:

a. Obtained necessary information from pump for documentation. ____ ____ ____ _____

b. Applied clean gloves, turned pump off, disconnected PCA tubing but maintained IV access. ____ ____ ____ _____

c. Disposed of empty cartridge according to agency policy, removed gloves and discarded. ____ ____ ____ _____

	S	U	NP	Comments

EVALUATION

1. Established that patient is evaluating pain intensity properly.

2. Monitored patient's level of sedation, vital signs, and pulse oximetry every 1 to 2 hours for 12 hours.

3. Observed patient for adverse reactions.

4. Had patient demonstrate dose delivery.

5. Evaluated number of attempts, delivery of demand doses, and basal dose if ordered.

6. Identified unexpected outcomes.

RECORDING AND REPORTING

1. Recorded all pertinent information in appropriate log.

2. Recorded regular assessment of patient response to analgesia in appropriate logs.

PERFORMANCE CHECKLIST SKILL 15-3   **EPIDURAL ANALGESIA**

	S	U	NP	Comments
ASSESSMENT				
1. Assessed level of patient's comfort and character of patient's pain.	___	___	___	_____
2. Assessed presenting condition and appropriateness for epidural analgesia.	___	___	___	_____
3. Assessed nonverbal pain responses if necessary.	___	___	___	_____
4. Checked to see if patient recently received anticoagulants.	___	___	___	_____
5. Assessed if patient routinely takes herbal medication, documented complete list.	___	___	___	_____
6. Assessed for history of drug allergies.	___	___	___	_____
7. Assessed patient's sedation level.	___	___	___	_____
8. Assessed rate, pattern, and depth of respirations; assessed pulse oximetry; assessed blood pressure.	___	___	___	_____
9. Assessed initial motor and sensory function of lower extremities.	___	___	___	_____
10. Verified that catheter was secured to patient's skin.	___	___	___	_____
11. Assessed catheter insertion site for signs of infection, applied sterile gloves when removing occlusive dressing.	___	___	___	_____
12. Verified health care provider's order against MAR.	___	___	___	_____
13. Checked patency of IV tubing, checked infusion pump for proper calibration and operation if necessary.	___	___	___	_____
PLANNING				
1. Identified expected outcomes.	___	___	___	_____
2. Explained purpose and function of epidural analgesia and expectations of patient during procedure.	___	___	___	_____

	S	U	NP	Comments

IMPLEMENTATION

1. Prepared analgesic following "six rights" of medication administration. ___ ___ ___ _____

2. Identified patient using two identifiers. ___ ___ ___ _____

3. Attached "epidural line" label to infusion tubing, ensured there are *no Y-ports*. ___ ___ ___ _____

4. Compared MAR with medication container at bedside. ___ ___ ___ _____

5. Performed hand hygiene, applied clean gloves. ___ ___ ___ _____

6. Administered epidural analgesia:

    a. Administered dose on demand, assured patient was fully informed on method and effect of analgesia. ___ ___ ___ _____

    b. Administered continuous infusion:

        (1) Attached container of medication to pump tubing, primed tubing. ___ ___ ___ _____

        (2) Inserted tubing into infusion pump, attached distal end of tubing to catheter. ___ ___ ___ _____

        (3) Checked infusion pump for proper calibration and operation. ___ ___ ___ _____

        (4) Taped all tubing connection, gave ordered bolus or started infusion. ___ ___ ___ _____

    c. Administered bolus dose of analgesic:

        (1) Changed filter needle on prepared syringe to regular 20-gauge needleless adapter. ___ ___ ___ _____

        (2) Cleaned injection cap of epidural catheter with antiinfective swab, *not* alcohol. ___ ___ ___ _____

        (3) Dried injection cap with sterile gauze. ___ ___ ___ _____

        (4) Inserted needleless adapter of syringe into injection cap, aspirated. ___ ___ ___ _____

        (5) Injected opioid at appropriate rate. ___ ___ ___ _____

        (6) Removed syringe from injection cap. ___ ___ ___ _____

7. Explained that you would monitor patient's response to analgesia routinely, instructed patient on signs and problems to report. ___ ___ ___ _____

8. Removed and disposed of gloves, performed hand hygiene. ___ ___ ___ _____

9. Checked for presence of therapeutic anticoagulation before removal of epidural catheter, checked agency policy. ___ ___ ___ _____

	S	U	NP	Comments

EVALUATION

1. Evaluated patient's comfort level.

2. Observed sedation level; observed respiratory rate, rhythm, and pattern; observed pulse oximetry at proper times; monitored patient with risk factors.

3. Monitored blood pressure and pulse, assisted patient when changing positions to avoid postural hypotension.

4. Monitored I&O, assessed for bladder distention, observed for frequency or urgency of urination.

5. Observed for pruritus, informed patient that this is a side effect and not an allergic response.

6. Observed for nausea, vomiting, and presence of headache.

7. Evaluated catheter insertion site every 2 to 4 hours for infection, noted character of drainage.

8. Evaluated for motor weakness or numbness and tingling of lower extremities.

9. Identified unexpected outcomes.

RECORDING AND REPORTING

1. Recorded pertinent specific information in the appropriate log.

2. Obtained and recorded pump readout with appropriate frequency with continuous or demand infusion.

3. Recorded regular periodic assessments of patient's status in appropriate logs.

4. Reported any adverse reactions or complications to health care provider immediately.

Student _____ Date _____

Instructor _____ Date _____

PERFORMANCE CHECKLIST SKILL 15-4 **LOCAL ANESTHETIC INFUSION PUMP FOR ANALGESIA**

	S	U	NP	Comments
ASSESSMENT				
1. Performed hand hygiene, applied clean gloves, assessed dressing and site of catheter insertion.	___	___	___	_____
2. Assessed catheter connections, notified surgeon immediately if connections become detached.	___	___	___	_____
3. Performed a complete pain assessment.	___	___	___	_____
4. Reviewed surgeon's operative report for position of catheter.	___	___	___	_____
5. Compared label on device to MAR or health care provider.	___	___	___	_____
6. Assessed for blood backing up in tubing, stopped infusion, notified health care provider if present.	___	___	___	_____
7. Determined level of extremity activity that patient can perform.	___	___	___	_____
8. Assessed for signs of local anesthetic toxicity.	___	___	___	_____
9. Assessed patient's and caregiver's knowledge of infusion pump.	___	___	___	_____
PLANNING				
1. Identified expected outcomes.	___	___	___	_____
IMPLEMENTATION				
1. Identified patient using two identifiers.	___	___	___	_____
2. Avoided catheter dislodgement when repositioning or ambulating patient.	___	___	___	_____
3. Taught patient or caregiver how to remove catheter:				
a. Instructed patient or caregiver how to perform hand hygiene and apply clean gloves.	___	___	___	_____
b. Had patient assume a relaxed position.	___	___	___	_____
c. Removed surgical dressing.	___	___	___	_____
d. Explained to patient feeling of catheter removal.	___	___	___	_____
e. Placed gauze over site, removed catheter so as to minimize tissue trauma, notified surgeon if necessary.	___	___	___	_____
f. Observed for mark on end of catheter tip.	___	___	___	_____

	S	U	NP	Comments
g. Placed a new sterile dressing over area, applied pressure for at least 2 minutes.	___	___	___	_____
h. Placed catheter in bag using standard precautions, removed gloves, performed hand hygiene.	___	___	___	_____
4. Reminded patient or caregiver of follow-up appointment with surgeon.	___	___	___	_____

EVALUATION

1. Asked patient to rate pain intensity at rest and with activity.	___	___	___	_____
2. Observed for signs of adverse drug reactions, reported signs immediately.	___	___	___	_____
3. Observed patient's position, mobility, relaxation, participation in ADLs, and any nonverbal behaviors.	___	___	___	_____
4. Inspected condition of surgical dressing.	___	___	___	_____
5. Inspected catheter exit site during follow-up visit.	___	___	___	_____
6. Identified unexpected outcomes.	___	___	___	_____

RECORDING AND REPORTING

1. Recorded drug, concentration, date inserted, and type of demand feature in MAR.	___	___	___	_____
2. Recorded location of catheter, patient's pain rating, response to anesthetic and additional comfort measure given in nurses' notes.	___	___	___	_____
3. Recorded additional analgesics necessary to control pain.	___	___	___	_____
4. Recorded any adverse reaction to local anesthetic.	___	___	___	_____
5. Reported damp dressing/displaced catheter to surgeon.	___	___	___	_____

Student _____ Date _____

Instructor _____ Date _____

PERFORMANCE CHECKLIST SKILL 15-5 **NONPHARMACOLOGIC PAIN MANAGEMENT**

	S	U	NP	Comments
ASSESSMENT				
1. Had patient identify pain intensity using pain-rating scale.	___	___	___	_____
2. Assessed signs and symptoms of pain.	___	___	___	_____
3. Assessed characteristics of pain and possible underlying cause.	___	___	___	_____
4. Examined site of patient's pain or discomfort.	___	___	___	_____
5. Reviewed health care provider's orders for pain relief.	___	___	___	_____
6. Assessed patient's understanding of pain and willingness to receive nonpharmacologic pain-relief measures.	___	___	___	_____
7. Assessed patient's preferred activities.	___	___	___	_____
8. Assessed patient's language level, identified descriptive terms to use.	___	___	___	_____
PLANNING				
1. Identified expected outcomes.	___	___	___	_____
2. Explained purpose of technique and what was expected of patient.	___	___	___	_____
3. Planned time to perform technique when patient was able to concentrate.	___	___	___	_____
4. Administered analgesic 30 minutes before implementing a nonpharmacologic strategy.	___	___	___	_____
IMPLEMENTATION				
1. Prepared patient's environment.	___	___	___	_____
2. Massaged patient:				
a. Performed hand hygiene.	___	U	NP	_____
b. Placed patient in appropriate, comfortable position.	___	___	___	_____
c. Adjusted bed to comfortable working height, lowered side rail.	___	___	___	_____
d. Turned on music to patient's preference.	___	___	___	_____
e. Ensured patient was not allergic to lotion, warmed lotion.	___	___	___	_____
f. Chose stroke technique based on desired effect or body part.	___	___	___	_____

	S	U	NP	Comments

g. Encouraged patient to breathe deeply and relax during massage.   ___ ___ ___ _____

h. Stood behind patient, stimulated scalp and temples.   ___ ___ ___ _____

i. Used friction to rub muscles at base of head while supporting patient's head.   ___ ___ ___ _____

j. Massaged hands and arms properly with patient in supine position.   ___ ___ ___ _____

k. Massaged neck appropriately after determining patient had no neck injury that contraindicated manipulation.   ___ ___ ___ _____

l. Massaged back appropriately.   ___ ___ ___ _____

m. Massaged feet appropriately.   ___ ___ ___ _____

n. Told patient massage was ending.   ___ ___ ___ _____

o. Instructed patient to inhale deeply and exhale when procedure was complete, cautioned patient to move slowly after resting a few minutes.   ___ ___ ___ _____

p. Wiped excess lotion or oil from patient's body with bath towel.   ___ ___ ___ _____

q. Returned bed to low position, raised side rails, performed hand hygiene.   ___ ___ ___ _____

3. Performed progressive relaxation:

a. Instructed patient to take several slow, deep breaths.   ___ ___ ___ _____

b. Had patient close eyes if desired.   ___ ___ ___ _____

c. Had patient alternate tightening and relaxing of all muscle groups for 6 to 7 seconds:

(1) Instructed patient to tighten during inhalation and relax during exhalation.   ___ ___ ___ _____

(2) Asked patient to enjoy relaxed feeling and allow mind to drift, had patient breathe deeply.   ___ ___ ___ _____

d. Explained sensations patient would feel while relaxing.   ___ ___ ___ _____

e. Asked patient to continue slow, deep breaths.   ___ ___ ___ _____

f. Instructed patient to breathe deeply and move slowly after resting.   ___ ___ ___ _____

4. Instructed patient in deep breathing:

a. Instructed patient to sit comfortably.   ___ ___ ___ _____

186

	S	U	NP	Comments

b. Placed one hand on patient's chest and other on abdomen. ___ ___ ___ _____

c. Coached patient to inhale deeply through the nose allowing abdomen to rise. ___ ___ ___ _____

d. Told patient to continue to breathe and allow chest to expand when abdomen was partially expanded. ___ ___ ___ _____

e. Paused a few seconds, had patient exhale slowly through pursed lips, repeated for 4 to 6 minutes. ___ ___ ___ _____

5. Led patient through guided imagery:

   a. Directed patient through guided imagery exercise:

      (1) Instructed patient to imagine that inhaled air is a ball of healing energy. ___ ___ ___ _____

      (2) Instructed patient to imagine inhaled air travels to area of pain. ___ ___ ___ _____

   b. Directed imagery if necessary:

      (1) Asked patient to imagine a pleasant place such as beach or mountains. ___ ___ ___ _____

      (2) Directed patient to experience all sensory aspects of the restful place. ___ ___ ___ _____

      (3) Directed patient to continue slow, deep, rhythmic breathing. ___ ___ ___ _____

      (4) Directed patient to count to three, inhale, and open eyes, suggested patient initially move slowly. ___ ___ ___ _____

   c. Provided patient time to practice exercise without interruption. ___ ___ ___ _____

6. Performed distraction techniques:

   a. Directed patient's attention away from pain with distraction techniques. ___ ___ ___ _____

   b. Asked patient to close eyes or focus on a single object in the room. ___ ___ ___ _____

   c. Instructed patient to concentrate on slow, rhythmic breathing; guided breathing. ___ ___ ___ _____

   d. Continued distraction using patient's preferred technique. ___ ___ ___ _____

	S	U	NP	Comments

EVALUATION

1. Observed character of respirations, body position, facial expression, tone of voice, mood, mannerisms, or verbalization of discomfort.

2. Asked patient to rate comfort level.

3. Observed patient perform pain-control measures.

4. Identified unexpected outcomes.

RECORDING AND REPORTING

1. Recorded pertinent information in nurses' notes.

2. Reported patient's response to nonpharmacologic interventions to staff at change of shift.

3. Reported unusual responses to techniques to nurse in charge or health care provider.

Student _____ Date _____

Instructor _____ Date _____

PERFORMANCE CHECKLIST SKILL 16-1 **SUPPORTING PATIENTS AND FAMILIES IN GRIEF**

	S	U	NP	Comments
ASSESSMENT				
1. Sat near patient in a quiet, private location; established quiet presence and eye contact if appropriate.	—	—	—	_____
2. Considered individual patient while communicating.	—	—	—	_____
3. Listened carefully; observed patient responses, used open communication to develop a genuine, caring relationship.	—	—	—	_____
4. Determined meaning of loss to patient and specifics, used open-ended questions.	—	—	—	_____
5. Combined knowledge of grief theory with observation of patient behaviors, validated observations with patient.	—	—	—	_____
6. Encouraged patient to describe loss and impact on daily life.	—	—	—	_____
7. Asked patient to describe coping strategies that patient uses often.	—	—	—	_____
8. Assessed family caregiver's unique needs and resources.	—	—	—	_____
9. Assessed patient's spiritual needs and resources.	—	—	—	_____
PLANNING				
1. Identified expected outcomes.	—	—	—	_____
IMPLEMENTATION				
1. Showed empathetic understanding of patient's strengths and needs.	—	—	—	_____
2. Offered information about patient's illness, clarified misunderstandings.	—	—	—	_____
3. Encouraged patient to sustain relationships with others, included patient-identified support persons in discussions.	—	—	—	_____
4. Assisted patient in achieving short-term goals.	—	—	—	_____
5. Provided frequent opportunities for patient and family to express concerns, maintained attention.	—	—	—	_____

	S	U	NP	Comments

6. Helped patients and family identify and solve problems, encouraged use of resources. ___ ___ ___ _____

7. Instructed patient in relaxation strategies, guided imagery, meditation, hand massage, healing touch, or acupressure. ___ ___ ___ _____

8. Encouraged visits with loved ones, life review, or projects (e.g., looking at photos, journaling). ___ ___ ___ _____

9. Addressed patient's spiritual needs, made referral to spiritual care provider. ___ ___ ___ _____

EVALUATION

1. Noted patient descriptions of relationships and activities with others. ___ ___ ___ _____

2. Observed patient's behaviors during ongoing interactions. ___ ___ ___ _____

3. Elicited patient perceptions of benefit gained from coping interventions. ___ ___ ___ _____

4. Discussed progress toward performing routine activities at home. ___ ___ ___ _____

5. Identified unexpected outcomes. ___ ___ ___ _____

RECORDING AND REPORTING

1. Recorded interventions, noted patient's verbal and nonverbal responses in nurses' notes. ___ ___ ___ _____

2. Reported patient's grief reactions to interdisciplinary team, noted behaviors affecting health outcomes. ___ ___ ___ _____

PERFORMANCE CHECKLIST SKILL 16-2 **SYMPTOM MANAGEMENT AT THE END OF LIFE**

	S	U	NP	Comments
ASSESSMENT				
1. Asked patient to describe symptoms in his or her own words, used open-ended prompts.	___	___	___	_____
2. Allowed sufficient time for patient to describe symptoms, encouraged patient to say more.	___	___	___	_____
3. Assessed patient's pain severity, assessed characteristics of pain routinely and with new reports of pain.	___	___	___	_____
4. Assessed respiratory rate, breathing patterns, and lung sounds; asked patient if he or she is getting enough air, assessed for presence of airway secretions.	___	___	___	_____
5. Observed the condition of the skin.	___	___	___	_____
6. Inspected patient's oral cavity.	___	___	___	_____
7. Assessed bowel function:				
a. Determined usual bowel elimination pattern and effectiveness of bowel-management routines.	___	___	___	_____
b. Assessed for presence of fecal impaction if patient is passing liquid stool.	___	___	___	_____
c. Reviewed medication regimens known to cause constipation.	___	___	___	_____
d. Identified typical food and fluid intake over 1 week and activity levels.	___	___	___	_____
8. Assessed urinary elimination and ability to control urination, assessed for potential complications if incontinent.	___	___	___	_____
9. Assessed patient's appetite and for presence of nausea or vomiting.	___	___	___	_____
10. Assessed daily food and fluid intake in relation to patient's condition and preferences.	___	___	___	_____
11. Assessed fatigue, asked if fatigue has limited patient's ability to perform desired activities.	___	___	___	_____
12. Assessed for excessive restlessness in a patient near death:				
a. Assessed for pain, nausea, dyspnea, full bladder or bowel, poor sleep patterns, anxiety, or joint pain from immobility.	___	___	___	_____

	S	U	NP	Comments

b. Reviewed medical record for hyperglycemia, hypoglycemia, hyponatremia, or dehydration.

____ ____ ____ _____

c. Reviewed patient's medications.

____ ____ ____ _____

d. Determined if patient had unresolved emotional or spiritual issues.

____ ____ ____ _____

PLANNING
1. Identified expected outcomes.

____ ____ ____ _____

IMPLEMENTATION
1. Administered medications, initiated nonpharmacologic pain management interventions, provided education on causes of pain, explained interventions.

____ ____ ____ _____

2. Provided general comfort measures:

a. Provided bath and skin care based on patient's preferences and hygiene needs.

____ ____ ____ _____

b. Provided eye care, used artificial tears if necessary.

____ ____ ____ _____

c. Repositioned frequently, did not position on tubes or other objects.

____ ____ ____ _____

3. Provided oral hygiene after meals, at bedtime, and or more frequently in mouth-breathing or unconscious patient.

a. Used appropriate oral rinses.

____ ____ ____ _____

b. Moistened lips with nonpetroleum balm.

____ ____ ____ _____

4. Initiated a bowel-management regimen to reduce risk for constipation.

a. Increased fluid intake if medically tolerated by patient.

____ ____ ____ _____

b. Encouraged physical activity if tolerated.

____ ____ ____ _____

c. Administered daily stool softener or laxative.

____ ____ ____ _____

5. Provided low-residue diet for diarrhea, treated infections or discontinued medications.

____ ____ ____ _____

6. Addressed urinary incontinence with appropriate interventions.

____ ____ ____ _____

7. Offered patient favorite foods as desired, did not overly encourage eating.

a. Treated nausea by administering antiemetics rectally as prescribed, offered appropriate liquids and ice chips.

____ ____ ____ _____

b. Considered presence of nausea in patient receiving enteral feedings.

____ ____ ____ _____

	S	U	NP	Comments

8. Managed fatigue:

   a. Balanced activity and rest appropriately, eliminated extra steps in activities. ___ ___ ___ _____

   b. Explained care activities before performing, included patient in setting the daily schedule. ___ ___ ___ _____

   c. Assisted ambulatory patients with physical activity. ___ ___ ___ _____

9. Supported patient's ventilatory efforts.

   a. Positioned patient appropriately. ___ ___ ___ _____

   b. Positioned patient near death appropriately, suctioned only if necessary. ___ ___ ___ _____

   c. Provided ordered anticholinergic medications. ___ ___ ___ _____

   d. Stayed with patients experiencing dyspnea or air hunger, administered opioids or anxiolytics as prescribed, kept room cool with low humidity. ___ ___ ___ _____

10. Managed restlessness:

   a. Kept patient's room quiet with soft lighting and comfortable temperature, offered family opportunities to maintain close contact, encouraged music, prayer, or reading from patient's favorite book. ___ ___ ___ _____

   b. Used least-sedating pharmacologic means possible to control restlessness, consulted with interdisciplinary team, discontinued nonessential education. ___ ___ ___ _____

EVALUATION

1. Asked patient to rate pain and evaluate pain characteristics, assessed behavior in nonverbal patients. ___ ___ ___ _____

2. Asked patient to describe mouth comfort, inspected oral cavity. ___ ___ ___ _____

3. Inspected feces after patient defecated. ___ ___ ___ _____

4. Observed skin condition. ___ ___ ___ _____

5. Asked patient to rate fatigue, observed for fatigue or shortness of breath. ___ ___ ___ _____

6. Observed patient's respiratory patterns, asked patient if breathing was easy and comfortable. ___ ___ ___ _____

7. Observed patient's behavior, asked family to report on patient's behavior, noted level of restlessness. ___ ___ ___ _____

8. Identified unexpected outcomes. ___ ___ ___ _____

	S	U	NP	Comments

RECORDING AND REPORTING

1. Recorded detailed description of patient's symptoms in appropriate log. ___ ___ ___ _____

2. Recorded type of interventions used and patient's response in nurses' notes, noted successful interventions in care plan. ___ ___ ___ _____

3. Reported unexpected new symptoms or uncontrolled existing symptoms to health care provider. ___ ___ ___ _____

PERFORMANCE CHECKLIST SKILL 16-3 **CARE OF A BODY AFTER DEATH**

	S	U	NP	Comments
ASSESSMENT				
1. Asked health care provider to establish time of death, determined if autopsy had been requested, observed any special precautions required.	___	___	___	_____
2. Determined if family were present and if they had been informed of the death, identified patient's surrogate.				
3. Determined if patient's surrogate had been asked about organ and tissue donation, validated that donation request for had been signed, notified organ request team per agency policy.	___	___	___	_____
4. Gave family members and friends a private place to gather, allowed them time to ask questions or discuss grief.	___	___	___	_____
5. Asked family members if they had requests for viewing or preparation of the body, determined if they wished to be present or assist with care of the body.	___	___	___	_____
6. Contacted a support person to stay with family not assisting in preparation of the body.	___	___	___	_____
7. Consulted health care providers' orders for special care directives or specimens to be collected.	___	___	___	_____
8. Performed hand hygiene, applied PPE.	___	___	___	_____
9. Assessed the general condition of the body, noted presence of dressings, tubes, and medical equipment.	___	___	___	_____
PLANNING				
1. Identified expected outcomes.	___	___	___	_____
2. Placed body in a private room, moved roommate to another location if necessary.	___	___	___	_____
3. Directed NAP to gather needed equipment and arrange at bedside.	___	___	___	_____
IMPLEMENTATION				
1. Helped family members notify others of the death, notified mortuary, discussed plans for postmortem care.	___	___	___	_____
2. Consulted agency policy guidelines for care of the body if patient had made tissue donation.	___	___	___	_____

	S	U	NP	Comments
3. Performed hand hygiene, applied PPE.	___	___	___	_____
4. Identified patient using two identifiers, tagged body as directed.	___	___	___	_____
5. Removed indwelling devices, disconnected and capped IV lines, did not remove indwelling devices if autopsy was to be done.	___	___	___	_____
6. Placed dentures in mouth for viewing or transported dentures in a denture cup with body to mortuary, closed mouth with a rolled-up towel if appropriate.	___	___	___	_____
7. Placed pillow under head, positioned appropriately, checked agency policy regarding need to secure hands and feet.	___	___	___	_____
8. Closed eyes gently, left open if culturally appropriate.	___	___	___	_____
9. Shaved male facial hair unless prohibited by cultural practice.	___	___	___	_____
10. Washed soiled body parts, allowed family assistance if necessary.	___	___	___	_____
11. Removed soiled dressings, replaced with clean dressings, used paper tape and circular gauze.	___	___	___	_____
12. Placed absorbent pad under buttocks.	___	___	___	_____
13. Placed a clean gown on the body.	___	___	___	_____
14. Brushed and combed hair, removed hair accessories.	___	___	___	_____
15. Identified personal belongings that stay with the body and those to be given to the family.	___	___	___	_____
16. Placed clean sheet appropriately over body if family requested a viewing, removed medical equipment from room.	___	___	___	_____
17. Allowed family time alone with body, encouraged goodbyes and appropriate religious rituals.	___	___	___	_____
18. Removed linens and gown after viewing, placed body in shroud provided by agency.	___	___	___	_____
19. Placed identification label on outside of the shroud, followed policy for marking a body that poses infectious risks.	___	___	___	_____
20. Arranged prompt transportation of the body to mortuary or morgue.	___	___	___	_____

196

	S	U	NP	Comments

EVALUATION

1. Observed family members', friends', and significant others' responses to loss.

2. Noted appearance and condition of patient's skin during preparation of body.

3. Identified unexpected outcomes.

RECORDING AND REPORTING

1. Recorded time of death in appropriate log, described any resuscitative measures, noted name of professional certifying the death.

2. Recorded any special preparation of the body for autopsy or donation, noted who made the request.

3. Recorded name of mortuary and names of family consulted at time of death.

4. Recorded on appropriate log personal articles left on body, noted how belongings were handled and who received them, secured signature as required.

5. Recorded time body was transported and its destination, noted location of identification tags.

Student _____ Date _____

Instructor _____ Date _____

PERFORMANCE CHECKLIST SKILL 17-1 **BATHING A PATIENT**

	S	U	NP	Comments

ASSESSMENT

1. Assessed environment for safety.

2. Assessed patient's fall risk status if bathing out of bed or self-bath was to be performed.

3. Assessed patient's visual status, ability to sit without support, hand grasp, and ROM of extremities.

4. Assessed for presence of position of external medical equipment.

5. Assessed patient's bathing preferences.

6. Asked if patient had noticed any problems related to condition of skin and genitalia.

7. Assessed condition of patient's skin before or during bathing, noted presence of dryness or excessive moisture.

8. Identified risks for skin impairment.

9. Assessed patient's comfort using a 0–10 scale.

10. Assessed patient's knowledge of skin hygiene.

11. Reviewed orders for specific precautions concerning patient's movement or positioning.

PLANNING

1. Identified expected outcomes.

2. Gathered equipment and supplies.

3. Adjusted room temperature and ventilation.

4. Explained procedure, asked patient for suggestions on how to prepare supplies and how much of bath patient wished to complete.

5. Ensured call light was within reach of patient if you needed to leave the room.

IMPLEMENTATION

1. Provided privacy.

2. Offered patient bedpan or urinal, provided towel and moist washcloth.

3. Performed hand hygiene, applied clean gloves.

	S	U	NP	Comments

4. Placed supplies on bedside table, checked water temperature, had patient check water temperature, placed container of bath lotion in water if appropriate.

5. Raised bed to working height, lowered side rail, assisted patient to appropriate position.

6. Placed bath blanket over patient, removed top sheet while patient held blanket, placed soiled linen in laundry bag.

7. Removed patient's gown or pajamas:

   a. Unsnapped sleeves to remove gown.

   b. Began removal on unaffected side if an extremity was injured.

   c. Removed gown properly if patient had IV line and gown has no snaps.

8. Removed pillow if allowed, raised head of bed appropriately, placed towel under patient's head and over chest.

9. Washed face.

   a. Asked if patient was wearing contact lenses.

   b. Formed mitt with washcloth, immersed in water and wrung out thoroughly.

   c. Washed patient's eyes properly, used clean area of cloth for each eye, soaked crusts on eyelids before attempting removal, dried eyes.

   d. Asked if patient preferred soap on face; washed, rinsed, and dried face and neck; asked male patient if he wanted to be shaved.

   e. Provided eye care for unconscious patient.

      (1) Instilled eye drops or ointment per orders.

      (2) Kept eyelids closed in absence of blink reflex, closed eye before placing eye patch or shield, did not tape eyelid.

10. Washed upper extremities and trunk.

    a. Removed bath blanket from patient's arm closest to you, placed bath towel lengthwise under arm, bathed properly with water and soap.

	S	U	NP	Comments

b. Raised and supported arm, washed and dried axilla, applied deodorant if appropriate.

   — — — _____

c. Moved to other side of bed, repeated steps with other arm.

   — — — _____

d. Covered patient's chest with bath towel, folded bath blanket down to umbilicus, bathed chest properly, rinsed and dried well.

   — — — _____

11. Washed hands and nails.

a. Folded bath towel on bed, placed basin on towel, allowed hand to soak before cleaning nails, dried hand well, repeated on other side.

   — — — _____

12. Checked temperature of bath water, changed water if necessary.

   — — — _____

13. Washed the abdomen.

a. Placed bath towel over chest and abdomen; folded bath blanket down to just above pubic region; bathed, rinsed, and dried abdomen; paid attention to skin folds; dried well.

   — — — _____

b. Applied clean gown, dressed affected side first, waited until end of bath if appropriate.

   — — — _____

14. Washed lower extremities.

a. Covered chest and abdomen with bath blanket, exposed near leg by folding blanket toward midline, ensured other leg and perineum remain draped, placed towel under leg.

   — — — _____

b. Washed leg properly; assessed for signs of redness, swelling, or leg pain.

   — — — _____

c. Cleansed foot, made sure to bathe between toes, cleaned and filed nails, dried feet, soaked feet if appropriate.

   — — — _____

d. Raised side rail, moved to opposite side, repeated steps to wash other leg, applied lotion to both feet.

   — — — _____

e. Covered patient with bath blanket, raised side rail, changed bath water.

   — — — _____

15. Provided perineal care.

   — — — _____

16. Washed back.

a. Applied clean gloves, lowered side rail, assisted patient to proper position, placed towel along patient's side.

   — — — _____

b. Enclosed any fecal matter in toilet tissue, removed with disposable wipes.

   — — — _____

	S	U	NP	Comments

c. Kept patient draped by sliding bath blanket over shoulders and thighs during bathing; washed, rinsed, and dried back properly, paid attention to folds of buttocks and anus. ___ ___ ___ _____

d. Cleansed buttocks and anus; washed front to back; cleansed, rinsed, and dried areas thoroughly; placed clean absorbent pad under patient's buttocks if needed. ___ ___ ___ _____

17. Removed gloves, massaged back if patient desired. ___ ___ ___ _____

18. Applied body lotion and topical moisturizing agents to skin. ___ ___ ___ _____

19. Assisted patient into clean gown. Adjusted external lines as needed. ___ ___ ___ _____

20. Assisted patient in grooming, oral hygiene, shaving, hair care, and application of makeup if desired. ___ ___ ___ _____

21. Made patient's bed. ___ ___ ___ _____

22. Checked function and position of external devices. ___ ___ ___ _____

23. Removed soiled linen and placed in dirty linen bag; did not allow linen to contact uniform; cleaned and replaced equipment; replaced call light and personal possessions; placed bed in low, locked position with side rails raised appropriately; ensured patient comfort. ___ ___ ___ _____

24. Performed hand hygiene. ___ ___ ___ _____

EVALUATION

1. Observed skin, especially areas that were previously showing signs of breakdown; inspected areas normally exposed to pressure. ___ ___ ___ _____

2. Observed ROM during bathing. ___ ___ ___ _____

3. Asked patient to rate comfort. ___ ___ ___ _____

4. Asked if patient felt fatigued. ___ ___ ___ _____

5. Identified unexpected outcomes. ___ ___ ___ _____

RECORDING AND REPORTING

1. Recorded procedure, included amount of patient participation and how patient tolerated procedure in nurse's notes. ___ ___ ___ _____

2. Recorded condition of skin and significant findings in nurses' notes. ___ ___ ___ _____

3. Reported evidence of alterations in skin integrity, break in suture line, or increased wound secretions to nurse in charge or health care provider. ___ ___ ___ _____

Student _____ Date _____

Instructor _____ Date _____

	S	U	NP	Comments

PROCEDURAL STEPS

1. Assessed environment for safety.

2. Provided privacy, explained procedure and importance of preventing infection.

3. Performed hand hygiene, applied clean glove.

4. Perineal care for a female.

   a. Allowed patient to cleanse perineum on her own if able.

   b. Assisted patient in assuming proper position, noted restrictions in patient's positioning, placed waterproof pad under patient's buttocks.

   c. Draped patient with bath blanket in a diamond shape, lifted lower edge to expose perineum.

   d. Washed and dried patient's upper thighs.

   e. Washed labia majora, retracted labia from thigh with nondominant hand, used dominant hand to wash skinfolds, wiped front to back, repeated on opposite side with separate section of washcloth, rinsed and dried area thoroughly.

   f. Separated labia, washed urethral meatus and vaginal orifice front to back, used separate section of cloth for each stroke, avoided tension on indwelling catheter if present.

   g. Rinsed and dried area thoroughly, used front-to-back method.

   h. Poured warm water over perineal area and dried thoroughly if patient uses a bedpan.

   i. Folded lower corner of bath blanket down, asked patient to assume comfortable position.

5. Perineal care for a male.

   a. Allowed patient to cleanse perineum on his own if able.

	S	U	NP	Comments

b. Assisted patient to supine position, noted restrictions in mobility.

    ___   ___   ___   _____

c. Folded lower half of bath blanket up to expose upper thighs, washed and dried thighs.

    ___   ___   ___   _____

d. Covered thighs with bath towels, raised blanket to expose genitalia, raised penis, placed bath towel underneath, retracted foreskin if present, deferred procedure if patient had an erection.

    ___   ___   ___   _____

e. Washed tip of penis first, cleansed outwards, discarded washcloth, repeated until penis was clean, rinsed and dried thoroughly.

    ___   ___   ___   _____

f. Returned foreskin to natural position.

    ___   ___   ___   _____

g. Had patient abduct legs, cleansed shaft of penis and scrotum, paid attention to underlying surfaces and folds, rinsed and dried thoroughly.

    ___   ___   ___   _____

h. Folded bath blanket over patient's perineum, assisted patient to comfortable position.

    ___   ___   ___   _____

6. Observed perineal area for any irritation, redness, or drainage that persisted after hygiene.

    ___   ___   ___   _____

7. Disposed of gloves in receptacle, performed hand hygiene.

    ___   ___   ___   _____

Student _____ Date _____

Instructor _____ Date _____

PERFORMANCE CHECKLIST PROCEDURAL GUIDELINE 17-2 **USE OF DISPOSABLE BED BATH, TUB, OR SHOWER**

	S	U	NP	Comments

PROCEDURAL STEPS

1. Assessed environment for safety, provided privacy. ___ ___ ___ _____

2. Performed hand hygiene, applied clean gloves if risk of exposure to body fluids existed. ___ ___ ___ _____

3. Disposable bed bath.

   a. Positioned patient comfortably, warmed package per instructions. ___ ___ ___ _____

   b. Used single towel for each body part cleansed, followed proper order of cleansing. ___ ___ ___ _____

   c. Allowed skin to air dry, lightly covered patient if necessary. ___ ___ ___ _____

   d. Used extra cleansing pack or washcloths if there was excessive soiling. ___ ___ ___ _____

4. Tub bath or shower.

   a. Assessed patient's fall risk status, reviewed orders for precautions concerning patient's movement or positioning. ___ ___ ___ _____

   b. Scheduled use of shower or tub. ___ ___ ___ _____

   c. Checked tub or shower for cleanliness, used cleaning techniques per agency policy, placed rubber mat on tub or shower bottom, placed skid-proof bath mat or towel on floor in front of tub or shower. ___ ___ ___ _____

   d. Collected hygienic aids, toiletry items, and linens requested by patient, placed within easy reach of tub or shower. ___ ___ ___ _____

   e. Assisted patient to bathroom if necessary, had patient wear robe and skid-proof slippers. ___ ___ ___ _____

   f. Demonstrated how to use call signal, placed "occupied" sign on bathroom door. ___ ___ ___ _____

   g. Filled bathtub halfway with warm water, checked temperature, had patient test water, adjusted as necessary, explained faucet controls, *did not use bath oil*. ___ ___ ___ _____

	S	U	NP	Comments

h. Turned shower on and adjusted temperature if patient was taking a shower, used seat or tub chair if available. ___ ___ ___ _____

i. Instructed patient that he or she could stay in the tub no longer than 20 minutes. ___ ___ ___ _____

j. Checked on patient every 5 minutes. ___ ___ ___ _____

k. Returned to bathroom when patient signaled, knocked before entering. ___ ___ ___ _____

l. Drained tub for unsteady patient before patient attempted to get out, placed bath towel over patient's shoulders, assisted patient as needed, assisted with drying, had a shower chair available if possible. ___ ___ ___ _____

m. Assisted patient as needed in donning clothing. ___ ___ ___ _____

n. Assisted patient to room and comfortable position. ___ ___ ___ _____

o. Evaluated patient's tolerance and fatigue level. ___ ___ ___ _____

p. Cleaned tub or shower, removed soiled linen, placed in the dirty linen bag, discarded disposable equipment appropriately, placed "unoccupied" sign on bathroom door, returned supplies to storage. ___ ___ ___ _____

q. Performed hand hygiene. ___ ___ ___ _____

206

Student _____ Date _____

Instructor _____ Date _____

PERFORMANCE CHECKLIST SKILL 17-2 **ORAL HYGIENE**

	S	U	NP	Comments
ASSESSMENT				
1. Assessed environment for safety.	___	___	___	_____
2. Performed hand hygiene, applied clean gloves.	___	___	___	_____
3. Instructed patient not to bite down, inspected integrity of lips, teeth, buccal mucosa, gums, palate, and tongue.	___	___	___	_____
4. Identified presence of common oral problems.	___	___	___	_____
5. Removed gloves, performed hand hygiene.	___	___	___	_____
6. Reviewed medical record, assessed risk for oral hygiene problems.	___	___	___	_____
7. Determined patient's oral hygiene practices and willingness to attend to hygiene needs.	___	___	___	_____
8. Assessed patient's ability to grasp and manipulate toothbrush.	___	___	___	_____
PLANNING				
1. Identified expected outcomes.	___	___	___	_____
2. Gathered equipment and supplies.	___	___	___	_____
3. Explained procedure to patient, discussed preferences regarding use of hygiene aids.	___	___	___	_____
IMPLEMENTATION				
1. Provided privacy.	___	___	___	_____
2. Prepared and had supplies ready at bedside.	___	___	___	_____
3. Raised bed to working height, raised HOB and lowered side rail, assisted patient to appropriate position.	___	___	___	_____
4. Placed a towel over patient's chest.	___	___	___	_____
5. Performed hand hygiene, applied clean gloves.	___	___	___	_____
6. Applied toothpaste to brush, held brush over emesis basin, poured water over toothpaste.	___	___	___	_____
7. Allowed patient to assist, held brush properly, brushed teeth properly.	___	___	___	_____
8. Had patient hold brush appropriately and brush tongue, avoided initiating gag reflex.	___	___	___	_____

	S	U	NP	Comments

9. Allowed patient to rinse mouth with water and spit into basin, observed patient's brushing technique, taught importance of brushing twice a day.   ___   ___   ___   _____

10. Had patient rinse teeth with alcohol-free antiseptic mouthwash and spit in basin.   ___   ___   ___   _____

11. Assisted in wiping patient's mouth.   ___   ___   ___   _____

12. Allowed patient to floss or flossed patient properly (if not contraindicated), instructed patient on importance of flossing.   ___   ___   ___   _____

13. Allowed patient to rinse mouth with cool water and spit in basin, assisted wiping patient's mouth.   ___   ___   ___   _____

14. Assisted patient to comfortable position, removed basin and over-bed table, raised side rail and lowered bed to original position.   ___   ___   ___   _____

15. Wiped off over-bed table, discarded soiled linen, removed soiled gloves, returned equipment to proper place.   ___   ___   ___   _____

16. Performed hand hygiene.   ___   ___   ___   _____

EVALUATION

1. Asked patient if any area of oral cavity feels uncomfortable or irritated.   ___   ___   ___   _____

2. Applied clean gloves, inspected condition of oral cavity.   ___   ___   ___   _____

3. Asked patient to describe proper hygiene techniques and recommended frequency.   ___   ___   ___   _____

4. Observed patient brushing and flossing.   ___   ___   ___   _____

5. Identified unexpected outcomes.   ___   ___   ___   _____

RECORDING AND REPORTING

1. Recorded procedure and noted condition of oral cavity in nurses' notes.   ___   ___   ___   _____

2. Reported bleeding, pain, or presences of lesions to nurse in charge or health care provider.   ___   ___   ___   _____

Student _____ Date _____

Instructor _____ Date _____

PERFORMANCE CHECKLIST PROCEDURAL GUIDELINE 17-3 **CARE OF DENTURES**

	S	U	NP	Comments
PROCEDURAL STEPS				
1. Assessed environment for safety.	___	___	___	_____
2. Asked patient if dentures fit, if gum or mucous membrane tenderness or irritation occurred, asked about denture care and product preferences.	___	___	___	_____
3. Determined if patient could clean dentures independently.	___	___	___	_____
4. Filled emesis basin with tepid water or filled sink appropriately.	___	___	___	_____
5. Performed hand hygiene, applied clean gloves.	___	___	___	_____
6. Removed dentures properly if patient was unable to do so independently, placed dentures in emesis basin or sink.	___	___	___	_____
7. Applied cleaning agent to brush, brushed surfaces of dentures appropriately.	___	___	___	_____
8. Rinsed thoroughly in tepid water.	___	___	___	_____
9. Applied adhesive to undersurface if appropriate.	___	___	___	_____
10. Assisted patient with insertion of dentures if necessary, asked if dentures felt comfortable.	___	___	___	_____
11. Stored dentures properly if requested, kept denture cup in a secure place, labeled cup with patient's name.	___	___	___	_____
12. Disposed of supplies, removed and discarded gloves, performed hand hygiene.	___	___	___	_____

Student _____ Date _____

Instructor _____ Date _____

PERFORMANCE CHECKLIST SKILL 17-3   **PERFORMING MOUTH CARE FOR AN UNCONSCIOUS OR DEBILITATED PATIENT**

	S	U	NP	Comments
ASSESSMENT				
1. Assessed environment for safety.	___	___	___	_____
2. Performed hand hygiene, applied clean gloves.	___	___	___	_____
3. Tested for presence of gag reflex.	___	___	___	_____
4. Inspected condition of oral cavity.	___	___	___	_____
5. Removed gloves, performed hand hygiene.	___	___	___	_____
6. Assessed patient's risk for oral hygiene problems.	___	___	___	_____
7. Assessed patient's respirations on an ongoing basis.	___	___	___	_____
PLANNING				
1. Identified expected outcomes.	___	___	___	_____
2. Gathered equipment and supplies.	___	___	___	_____
3. Explained procedure	___	___	___	_____
IMPLEMENTATION				
1. Provided privacy.	___	___	___	_____
2. Performed hand hygiene, applied clean gloves.	___	___	___	_____
3. Placed towel on over-bed table, arranged equipment, turned on suction machine and connected tubing if necessary.	___	___	___	_____
4. Raised bed to appropriate height, lowered side rail, positioned patient appropriately.	___	___	___	_____
5. Placed towel under patient's head and basin under chin.	___	___	___	_____
6. Removed dentures or partial plates if present.	___	___	___	_____
7. Inserted oral airway if necessary, inserted when patient was relaxed if possible, did not use force.	___	___	___	_____

	S	U	NP	Comments

8. Cleaned mouth using moistened brush, applied toothpaste or used solution to loosen crusts, suctioned accumulated secretions. Moistened brush with chlorhexidine solution to rinse, brushed tongue, repeated rinsing several times. _____ _____ _____ _____

9. Used brush or sponge to apply thin layer of water-soluble moisturizer to lips. _____ _____ _____ _____

10. Informed patient that procedure was completed, returned patient to comfortable and safe position. _____ _____ _____ _____

11. Raised side rails; returned bed to locked, low position. _____ _____ _____ _____

12. Cleaned equipment and returned to proper place, placed soiled linen in proper receptacle. _____ _____ _____ _____

13. Removed and disposed gloves in proper receptacle, performed hand hygiene. _____ _____ _____ _____

EVALUATION

1. Applied clean gloves, inspected oral cavity. _____ _____ _____ _____

2. Asked debilitated patient if mouth feels clean. _____ _____ _____ _____

3. Identified unexpected outcomes. _____ _____ _____ _____

RECORDING AND REPORTING

1. Recorded procedure in appropriate log, included patient's ability to cooperate and whether suction was necessary. _____ _____ _____ _____

2. Documented and reported pertinent observations. _____ _____ _____ _____

3. Reported any unusual findings to nurse in charge or health care provider. _____ _____ _____ _____

Student _____ Date _____

Instructor _____ Date _____

PERFORMANCE CHECKLIST SKILL 17-4 **HAIR CARE—COMBING AND SHAVING**

	S	U	NP	Comments
ASSESSMENT				
1. Assessed environment for safety.	—	—	—	_____
2. Inspected condition of hair and scalp, inspected for presence of infestation, applied clean gloves if necessary.	—	—	—	_____
3. Assessed patient's hair-care and shaving product preferences.	—	—	—	_____
4. Assessed if patient had bleeding tendency before shaving, reviewed history, medications, and laboratory values.	—	—	—	_____
5. Assessed patient's ability to manipulate razor.	—	—	—	_____
PLANNING				
1. Identified expected outcomes.	—	—	—	_____
2. Gathered equipment and supplies.	—	—	—	_____
3. Explained procedure.	—	—	—	_____
4. Asked patient to explain steps that he or she uses to comb/shave during procedure, asked patient to indicate if uncomfortable.	—	—	—	_____
5. Positioned patient properly.	—	—	—	_____
IMPLEMENTATION				
1. Combed and brushed hair.				
a. Provided privacy.	—		—	_____
b. Arranged supplies at bedside table, adjusted lighting.	—	—	—	_____
c. Performed hand hygiene and applied clean gloves if necessary.	—	—	—	_____
d. Separated hair into four sections.	—	—	—	_____
e. Moistened hair with water, conditioner, or detangler before combing.	—	—	—	_____
f. Brushed or combed hair from scalp to ends.	—		—	_____
g. Moved fingers through hair to loosen larger tangles.	—	—	—	_____
h. Combed hair appropriately, shaped and styled hair.	—	—	—	_____

	S	U	NP	Comments

2. Shaved patient with a disposable razor.

  a. Applied clean gloves.

  b. Placed bath towel over patient's chest and shoulders.

  c. Ran warm water in washbasin, checked temperature.

  d. Placed washcloth in basin, wrung thoroughly, applied cloth over patient's face for several seconds.

  e. Applied shaving cream to patient's face; smoothed evenly over sides of face, chin, and under nose.

  f. Held razor properly in dominant hand, shaved patient properly, checked if patient felt comfortable.

  g. Dipped razor blade in water as shaving cream accumulated.

  h. Rinsed face with warm, moist washcloth after all facial hair was shaved.

  i. Dried face thoroughly, applied aftershave lotion if desired.

  j. Assisted patient to comfortable position.

  k. Returned equipment to proper place, discarded soiled linen appropriately, performed hand hygiene.

3. Shaving with electric razor.

  a. Applied clean gloves if necessary.

  b. Placed bath towel over patient's chest and shoulders.

  c. Applied skin conditioner or preshave preparation.

  d. Turned razor on, shaved patient appropriately.

  e. Applied aftershave lotion as desired after completing shave.

  f. Performed steps 2j and 2k for disposable razor.

4. Performed mustache and beard care.

  a. Placed bath towel over patient's chest and shoulders.

214

	S	U	NP	Comments

b. Gently combed mustache and beard. ___ ___ ___ _____

c. Allowed patient to use mirror and direct trimming. ___ ___ ___ _____

EVALUATION

1. Asked patient how hair and scalp felt. ___ ___ ___ _____

2. Inspected condition of shaved areas and skin underneath beard or mustache. ___ ___ ___ _____

3. Asked patient if face felt clean and comfortable. ___ ___ ___ _____

4. Asked if patient was satisfied with degree of participation. ___ ___ ___ _____

5. Identified unexpected outcomes. ___ ___ ___ _____

RECORDING AND REPORTING

1. Recorded procedure in the appropriate log, indicated if there was no area for shaving, noted how patient tolerated procedure and any complications. ___ ___ ___ _____

Student _____ Date _____

Instructor _____ Date _____

PERFORMANCE CHECKLIST PROCEDURAL GUIDELINE 17-4 **HAIR CARE—SHAMPOOING**

	S	U	NP	Comments

PROCEDURAL STEP

1. Assessed environment for safety.

2. Explained procedure, provided privacy.

3. Determined that there were no contraindications to procedure before washing patient's hair.

4. Performed hand hygiene, applied clean gloves.

5. Inspected hair and scalp before shampooing, determined if special treatments were necessary, wore gown if necessary.

6. Shampooed bed-bound patient with shampoo board.

   a. Placed waterproof pad under patient's shoulders, neck, and head; positioned patient properly; placed shampoo board under patient's head and washbasin under end of spout; ensured spout extends beyond edge of mattress.

   b. Placed towel under patient's neck and bath towel over patient's shoulders.

   c. Brushed and combed patient's hair.

   d. Obtained pitcher with warm water.

   e. Asked patient to hold towel or washcloth over eyes.

   f. Poured water over hair until completely wet, applied hydrogen peroxide to dissolve any blood clots, rinsed hair with saline, applied small amount of shampoo.

   g. Worked up lather with both hands, started at hairline and worked toward neck, lifted head slightly to wash back of head, shampooed sides of head, massaged scalp by applying pressure with fingertips.

   h. Rinsed hair with water, ensured water drained into basin, repeated rinsing until free of soap.

   i. Applied conditioner or crème rinse if requested, rinsed hair thoroughly.

	S	U	NP	Comments

j. Wrapped patient's head in bath towel, dried patient's face with cloth, dried off any moisture along neck or shoulders. ___ ___ ___ _____

k. Dried patient's hair and scalp, used second towel if necessary. ___ ___ ___ _____

l. Combed hair to remove tangles, dried hair with a dryer if desired. ___ ___ ___ _____

m. Applied oil preparation or conditioner to hair if desired. ___ ___ ___ _____

n. Handled patient with coarse, curly hair properly. ___ ___ ___ _____

o. Assisted patient to comfortable position, completed styling of hair. ___ ___ ___ _____

p. Disposed and stored supplies, removed gloves and performed hand hygiene. ___ ___ ___ _____

7. Shampooed using a disposable shampoo cap product.

a. Positioned patient properly. ___ ___ ___ _____

b. Combed hair to remove tangles or debris. ___ ___ ___ _____

c. Opened package, applied cap, secured all hair beneath cap. ___ ___ ___ _____

d. Massaged head through cap, checked fitting of cap. ___ ___ ___ _____

e. Massaged according to directions on package, added time to massage as necessary. ___ ___ ___ _____

f. Discarded cap in trash. ___ ___ ___ _____

g. Towel dried hair if desired. ___ ___ ___ _____

h. Brushed or combed patient's hair. ___ ___ ___ _____

i. Performed hand hygiene. ___ ___ ___ _____

Student _____ Date _____

Instructor _____ Date _____

PERFORMANCE CHECKLIST SKILL 17-5 **PERFORMING NAIL AND FOOT CARE**

	S	U	NP	Comments
ASSESSMENT				
1. Assessed environment for safety.	___	___	___	_____
2. Inspected all surfaces of fingers, toes, feet, and nails; paid attention to areas of dryness, inflammation, or cracking; inspected socks for stains.	___	___	___	_____
3. Observed patient's walking gait if appropriate.	___	___	___	_____
4. Asked if patient had history of leg pain upon walking that is relieved by rest.	___	___	___	_____
5. Asked patients about use of nail polish and polish remover.	___	___	___	_____
6. Assessed type of footwear patient wears.	___	___	___	_____
7. Identified patient's risk for foot or nail problems.	___	___	___	_____
8. Assessed types of home remedies patient uses for existing foot problems.	___	___	___	_____
9. Assessed patient's ability to care for nails or feet.	___	___	___	_____
10. Assessed patient's knowledge of proper foot and nail care practices.	___	___	___	_____
PLANNING				
1. Identified expected outcomes.	___	___	___	_____
2. Gathered equipment and supplies.	___	___	___	_____
3. Explained procedure to patient.	___	___	___	_____
4. Obtained health care provider's orders for cutting nails, obtained order for podiatry consult if needed.	___	___	___	_____
IMPLEMENTATION				
1. Performed hand hygiene, applied gloves, arranged equipment on over-bed table.	___	___	___	_____
2. Provided privacy.	___	___	___	_____
3. Assisted patient to appropriate position, placed bath mat on floor under patient's feet or placed waterproof pad on mattress as appropriate.	___	___	___	_____
4. Filled washbasin with warm water, tested temperature, placed basin on floor or on pad, had patient immerse feet.	___	___	___	_____

	S	U	NP	Comments

5. Adjusted over-bed table to low position, placed over patient's lap.

6. Filled emesis basin with warm water, placed basin on towel on over-bed table, tested water temperature.

7. Instructed patient to place fingers in basin, placed arms in comfortable position.

8. Allowed patient's feet and nails to soak for 10 minutes unless contraindicated.

9. Cleaned under fingernails with plastic applicator stick while fingers are immersed.

10. Cleaned around cuticles with a soft brush.

11. Removed emesis basin, dried fingers thoroughly.

12. Trimmed nails properly, filed sharp corners off nails.

13. Moved over-bed table away from patient, scrubbed callused areas of feet with washcloth.

14. Cleaned between toes, used washcloth.

15. Dried feet, trimmed nails following Step 12.

16. Applied lotion to feet and hands, assisted patient to comfortable position in bed.

17. Cleaned clippers with soap and water, cleaned appropriately if soiled with blood or fluids, returned equipment to proper place, disposed of equipment and soiled linen properly, removed gloves, performed hand hygiene.

EVALUATION

1. Inspected nails, areas between fingers and toes, and skin surfaces.

2. Asked patient to explain or demonstrate nail care.

3. Observed patient's walk after foot and nail care.

4. Identified unexpected outcomes.

RECORDING AND REPORTING

1. Recorded procedure and observations in medical record.

2. Reported any breaks in skin or ulcerations to nurse in charge or health care provider.

Student _____ Date _____

Instructor _____ Date _____

PERFORMANCE CHECKLIST PROCEDURAL GUIDELINE 17-5 **MAKING AN UNOCCUPIED BED**

	S	U	NP	Comments
PROCEDURAL STEPS				
1. Performed hand hygiene, applied gloves if necessary.	___	___	___	_____
2. Assessed environment for safety, checked position of chair for transfer, provided privacy.	___	___	___	_____
3. Assessed activity orders or restrictions in planning, assisted patient to bedside chair or recliner.	___	___	___	_____
4. Lowered side rails, raised bed to working position.	___	___	___	_____
5. Removed soiled linen, held away from uniform, placed in dirty laundry bag, avoided shaking or fanning linen.	___	___	___	_____
6. Repositioned mattress, wiped off moisture using washcloth moistened in antiseptic, dried thoroughly.	___	___	___	_____
7. Applied all bottom linen on one side of bed before moving to opposite side.				
a. Ensured fitted sheet was smoothed over mattress and edges, fitted corners on one end and then the other.	___	___	___	_____
b. Fitted flat sheet properly under mattress.	___	___	___	_____
8. Applied drawsheet if necessary, smoothed drawsheet over mattress, kept palms down.	___	___	___	_____
9. Moved to opposite side of bed, spread bottom sheet over edge of mattress from head to foot.				
a. Ensured fitted sheet was placed smoothly over mattress.	___	___	___	_____
b. Mitered top corners of bottom flat sheet, tucked remaining edge under mattress tightly.	___	___	___	_____
10. Smoothed the folded drawsheet over bottom sheet, tucked under mattress properly.	___	___	___	_____
11. Applied waterproof pad over bottom sheet or drawsheet if necessary.	___	___	___	_____

	S	U	NP	Comments

12. Placed top sheet over bed properly, opened sheet out, ensured top edges of sheet and mattress were even.

13. Tucked in remaining portion of sheet under foot of mattress, placed blanket over bed properly.

14. Made cuff properly.

15. Stood on one side at foot of bed; lifted mattress corner slightly; tucked top sheet, blanket, and spread under mattress; ensured toe plates were not pulled out.

16. Made modified mitered corner with top sheet, blanket, and spread; did not tuck tip of triangle.

17. Spread sheet, blanket, and spread out evenly from other side of bed, made cuff, made modified corner at foot of bed or left bed open.

18. Applied clean pillowcase.

19. Placed call light within patient's reach, returned bed to lowest position, assisted patient to bed.

20. Placed linen bag in appropriate receptacle, removed and disposed of gloves.

21. Arranged and organized patient's room, performed hand hygiene.

Student _____ Date _____

Instructor _____ Date _____

PERFORMANCE CHECKLIST PROCEDURAL GUIDELINE 17-6 **MAKING AN OCCUPIED BED**

	S	U	NP	Comments

PROCEDURAL STEPS

1. Assessed environment for safety, ensured equipment was working properly; put bed in low, locked position; provided privacy. ___ ___ ___ _____

2. Determined if patient had been incontinent or if excess drainage was on linen. ___ ___ ___ _____

3. Assessed restrictions in mobility/positioning, explained procedure to patient, noted patient would be asked to turn over layers of linen. ___ ___ ___ _____

4. Performed hand hygiene, applied clean gloves if necessary. ___ ___ ___ _____

5. Assembled all equipment on bedside table. ___ ___ ___ _____

6. Raised bed to working height, lowered HOB as tolerated, kept patient comfortable, removed call light, lowered side rail. ___ ___ ___ _____

7. Loosened top linen at foot of bed. ___ ___ ___ _____

8. Removed bedspread and blanket separately, placed in linen bag if soiled or folded into square and placed over chair if to be reused. ___ ___ ___ _____

9. Covered patient with bath blanket, placed over top sheet, had patient hold bath blanket, removed bath sheet, discarded in dirty linen bag. ___ ___ ___ _____

10. Assisted patient to appropriate position, adjusted pillow under patient's head. ___ ___ ___ _____

11. Assessed to ensure there was no tension on any external medical devices. ___ ___ ___ _____

12. Stood on one side of bed; loosened bottom linens; fanfolded or rolled bottom sheet, drawsheet, and cloth pads toward and under patient; tucked edges alongside patient's body. ___ ___ ___ _____

13. Cleaned, disinfected, and dried mattress surface if needed. ___ ___ ___ _____

14. Applied clean linens properly to exposed half of bed. ___ ___ ___ _____

15. Fit fitted and bottom sheets to bed properly. ___ ___ ___ _____

	S	U	NP	Comments

16. Mitered top corner of sheet at HOB if necessary, tucked sheets under properly.
    ____   ____   ____   _____

17. Mitered corner properly if necessary.
    ____   ____   ____   _____

18. Tucked lower edge of sheet, held sheet in place with other hand, tucked in properly.
    ____   ____   ____   _____

19. Tucked remaining portion of sheet under mattress, kept linen smooth.
    ____   ____   ____   _____

20. Placed over drawsheet along middle of bed, tucked remainder under patient's body, kept linen flat, placed waterproof pad under drawsheet if necessary.
    ____   ____   ____   _____

21. Raised side rail, asked patient to turn toward you, assisted as needed, told patient that he or she would be rolling over layers of linen, ensured patient kept body in correct alignment.
    ____   ____   ____   _____

22. Moved to opposite side of bed, lowered side rail, assisted patient in positioning on other side over folds of linen.
    ____   ____   ____   _____

23. Loosened edges of soiled linen, removed soiled linen by folding into bundle.
    ____   ____   ____   _____

24. Held linen away from body, placed soiled linen in laundry bag.
    ____   ____   ____   _____

25. Cleaned, disinfected, and dried other half of mattress.
    ____   ____   ____   _____

26. Pulled linen, mattress pad, and drawsheet over edge of bed, pulled up bottom sheet appropriately.
    ____   ____   ____   _____

27. Grasped remaining edge of bottom sheet, leaned back and pulled while tucking excess linen under mattress properly.
    ____   ____   ____   _____

28. Ensured sheets and pad were smooth and wrinkle-free.
    ____   ____   ____   _____

29. Assisted patient in rolling back to appropriate position.
    ____   ____   ____   _____

30. Placed top sheet over patient properly, opened sheet out over patient, ensured top edges of sheet and mattress were even.
    ____   ____   ____   _____

31. Placed bed blanket over patient, ensured top edge was placed appropriately.
    ____   ____   ____   _____

32. Spread sheet and blanket out evenly from other side of bed.
    ____   ____   ____   _____

33. Had patient hold onto sheet and blanket while you removed bath blanket.
    ____   ____   ____   _____

	S	U	NP	Comments
34. Made cuff properly.	___	___	___	_____
35. Made horizontal toe pleat appropriately.	___	___	___	_____
36. Tucked in remaining portion under mattress, tucked top sheet and blanket together, ensured toe pleats were not pulled out.	___	___	___	_____
37. Made modified mitered corner with top sheet and blanket, did not tuck tip of triangle.	___	___	___	_____
38. Repeated steps 36 and 37 from other side of bed.	___	___	___	_____
39. Applied clean pillowcase.	___	___	___	_____
40. Placed call light within patient's reach; returned bed to low, locked position.	___	___	___	_____
41. Placed linen in appropriate receptacle, removed and disposed of gloves.	___	___	___	_____
42. Arranged and organized patient's room, performed hand hygiene.	___	___	___	_____

Student _____ Date _____

Instructor _____ Date _____

PERFORMANCE CHECKLIST SKILL 18-1 **RISK ASSESSMENT, SKIN ASSESSMENT, AND PREVENTION STRATEGIES**

	S	U	NP	Comments
ASSESSMENT				
1. Identified patient characteristics that might be risk factors for pressure ulcer formation.	___	___	___	_____
2. Selected risk assessment tool, performed risk assessment when patient entered health care setting, repeated on a regular basis or with significant change in patient's condition.	___	___	___	_____
3. Obtained risk score, evaluated meaning based on patient's unique characteristics.	___	___	___	_____
4. Assessed condition of patient's skin over regions of pressure.	___	___	___	_____
5. Assessed patient for additional areas of potential pressure injury.	___	___	___	_____
6. Observed patient for preferred positions when in bed or chair.	___	___	___	_____
7. Observed ability of patient to initiate and assist with position changes.	___	___	___	_____
8. Assessed patient's and caregiver's understanding of risks for development of pressure ulcers.	___	___	___	_____
PLANNING				
1. Identified expected outcomes.	___	___	___	_____
2. Explained procedure(s) and purpose to patient and caregiver.	___	___	___	_____
IMPLEMENTATION				
1. Implemented prevention guidelines adapted from WOCN Society's *Guideline for Prevention and Management of Pressure Ulcers.*	___	___	___	_____
2. Provided privacy, performed hand hygiene.	___	___	___	_____
3. Applied clean gloves if necessary.	___	___	___	_____
4. Inspected skin at least once a day.				
a. Observed patient's skin, paying particular attention to bony prominences, gently pressed any reddened area to check for blanching, rechecked in 1 hour any area that does not blanch.	___	___	___	_____
b. Looked for color changes that differ from the patient's normal skin color in patient with darkly pigmented skin.	___	___	___	_____

	S	U	NP	Comments

5. Checked all treatment and assistive devices for potential pressure points, removed gloves. ___ ___ ___ _____

6. Reviewed patient's pressure ulcer score. ___ ___ ___ _____

7. Considered appropriate intervention if patient's immobility, inactivity, or poor sensory perception was a risk factor. ___ ___ ___ _____

8. Considered appropriate intervention if friction and shear were identified as risk factors. ___ ___ ___ _____

9. Considered appropriate intervention if patient received a low score on a moisture subscale. ___ ___ ___ _____

10. Educated patient and family caregiver regarding pressure ulcer risk and prevention. ___ ___ ___ _____

11. Removed gloves, discarded appropriately, performed hand hygiene. ___ ___ ___ _____

EVALUATION

1. Observed patient's skin for areas at risk for tissue damage, noted change in color, appearance, or texture. ___ ___ ___ _____

2. Observed tolerance of patient for position change. ___ ___ ___ _____

3. Compared subsequent risk assessment scores and skin assessments. ___ ___ ___ _____

4. Identified unexpected outcomes. ___ ___ ___ _____

RECORDING AND REPORTING

1. Recorded skin changes, risk score, and skin assessment; described pertinent information and patient's response to interventions in appropriate log. ___ ___ ___ _____

2. Reported need for additional consultations to health care provider. ___ ___ ___ _____

Student _____ Date _____

Instructor _____ Date _____

PERFORMANCE CHECKLIST SKILL 18-2 **TREATMENT OF PRESSURE ULCERS**

	S	U	NP	Comments
ASSESSMENT				
1. Assessed patient's level of comfort and need for pain medication.				
2. Determined if patient had allergies to topical agents.				
3. Reviewed the order for topical agent(s) or dressings.				
4. Provided privacy, performed hand hygiene, applied clean gloves.				
5. Positioned patient to allow dressing removal, positioned plastic bag for dressing removal.				
6. Removed wound dressing; assessed patient's wounds using wound parameters; location, stage, size, presence of undermining, presence of sinus tracts, presence of tunnels, condition of wound bed, volume of exudate, condition of periwound skin, and wound edges.				
7. Removed gloves, discarded appropriately, performed hand hygiene.				
8. Assessed for factors affecting wound healing (i.e., poor perfusion, immunosuppression, preexisting infection)				
9. Assessed patient's nutritional status.				
10. Assessed patient's and caregiver's understanding of prevention, treatment, and factors contributing to recurrence of pressure ulcers.				
PLANNING				
1. Identified expected outcomes.				
2. Explained procedure to patient and caregiver, individualized teaching.				
3. Prepared all necessary equipment and supplies.				
IMPLEMENTATION				
1. Identified patient using two identifiers.				
2. Assembled supplies at bedside, provided privacy.				

	S	U	NP	Comments

3. Performed hand hygiene, applied gloves, opened sterile packages and topical containers, kept dressings sterile, wore PPE if necessary.

4. Removed bed linens, arranged patient's gown to expose ulcer and surrounding skin only.

5. Removed dressing, assessed condition of wound and quality of drainage, removed and discarded gloves.

6. Performed hand hygiene, changed gloves.

7. Cleansed wound thoroughly with saline or prescribed agent from least contaminated to most contaminated area.

8. Applied topical agents if prescribed:

   a. Applied enzymes:

      (1) Applied small amount of enzyme debridement ointment directly to necrotic areas, *did not apply enzyme to surrounding skin.*

      (2) Placed moist gauze directly over ulcer, taped in place, followed manufacturer's recommendation for type of dressing material.

   b. Applied antimicrobials.

9. Applied prescribed wound dressing:

   a. Applied hydrogel:

      (1) Covered surface of ulcer with hydrogel or cut a sheet to fit wound base.

      (2) Applied secondary dressing such as dry gauze, taped in place.

      (3) Packed impregnated gauze loosely into wound if used, covered with secondary gauze dressing and tape.

   b. Applied calcium alginate:

      (1) Packed wound with alginate properly.

      (2) Applied secondary dressing over alginate, taped in place.

   c. Applied transparent film dressing, hydrocolloid, and foam dressings

10. Repositioned patient comfortably off pressure ulcer.

11. Removed gloves, disposed of soiled supplies, performed hand hygiene.

	S	U	NP	Comments

EVALUATION

1. Observed skin surrounding ulcer for inflammation, edema, and tenderness.

2. Inspected dressings and exposed ulcers; observed for drainage, foul odor, and tissue necrosis; monitored patient for signs of infection.

3. Compared subsequent ulcer measurements.

4. Identified unexpected outcomes.

RECORDING AND REPORTING

1. Recorded all pertinent information in the appropriate log.

2. Reported any deterioration in ulcer appearance to nurse in charge or health care provider.

Student _____ Date _____

Instructor _____ Date _____

PERFORMANCE CHECKLIST PROCEDURAL GUIDELINE 19-1 **EYE CARE FOR COMATOSE PATIENTS**

	S	U	NP	Comments
PROCEDURAL STEPS				
1. Performed hand hygiene.	___	___	___	_____
2. Observed patient's eyes for drainage, irritation, redness, and lesions; applied clean gloves if drainage is present.	___	___	___	_____
3. Explained each step of the procedure continually.	___	___	___	_____
4. Assessed for blink reflex.	___	___	___	_____
5. Performed papillary examination.	___	___	___	_____
6. Observed patient's eye movements, noted symmetry of eye movement.	___	___	___	_____
7. Explained procedure to patient and family members.	___	___	___	_____
8. Positioned patient properly.	___	___	___	_____
9. Used clean washcloth or cotton balls moistened with water or saline, wiped each eye properly, used separate cotton ball or corner of washcloth for each eye.	___	___	___	_____
10. Used eyedropper to instill prescribed lubricant, wiped away any excess lubricant.	___	___	___	_____
11. Closed patient's eyes and applied patches or a moisture chamber if blink reflex is absent, secured patch without taping eyes.	___	___	___	_____
12. Disposed of excess material, removed gloves, performed hand hygiene.	___	___	___	_____
13. Removed eye patches every 4 hours; observed condition of patient's eyes for drainage, irritation, redness, and lesions.	___	___	___	_____
14. Notified health care provider if signs of irritation or infection were present.	___	___	___	_____

Student _____   Date _____

Instructor _____   Date _____

PERFORMANCE CHECKLIST PROCEDURAL GUIDELINE 19-2   **TAKING CARE OF CONTACT LENSES**

	S	U	NP	Comments
PROCEDURAL GUIDELINE				
1. Observed patient's eye, asked patient if contact lens were in place.	___	___	___	_____
2. Determined if patient was able to manipulate and hold contact lens and if glasses were available, determined patient's usual contact lens routine.	___	___	___	_____
3. Assessed patient for any unusual visual signs or symptoms.	___	___	___	_____
4. Reviewed types of medication prescribed for patient, especially medications that decrease blink reflexes or lubrication of corneas.	___	___	___	_____
5. Explained procedure to patient.	___	___	___	_____
6. Performed hand hygiene.	___	___	___	_____
7. Verified expiration dates of all solutions, assembled equipment at bedside.	___	___	___	_____
8. Ensured fingernails were short and smooth.	___	___	___	_____
9. Positioned patient appropriately.	___	___	___	_____
10. Identified patient using two identifiers.	___	___	___	_____
11. Applied clean gloves, placed towel just below patient's face.	___	___	___	_____
12. Removed lenses:				
a. Removed soft lenses, completed for each eye.				
(1) Shined a penlight sideways onto eye to locate lens if necessary.	___	___	___	_____
(2) Added 2 to 3 drops of sterile saline to patient's eye.	___	___	___	_____
(3) Asked patient to look straight ahead, retracted lower eyelid to expose lower edge of lens.	___	___	___	_____
(4) Used pad of index finger to slide lens down off cornea.	___	___	___	_____

	S	U	NP	Comments

(5) Pulled upper eyelid down with thumb of other hand, compressed lens slightly between thumb and index finger. ___ ___ ___ _____

(6) Pinched lens and lifted out without allowing edges to stick together, placed lens in storage case. ___ ___ ___ _____

b. Removed hard lenses, completed for each eye.

(1) Inspected eye to ensure lens was positioned directly over cornea, shined penlight sideways to locate lens if necessary. ___ ___ ___ _____

(2) Placed index finder on outer corner of patient's eye, drew skin back toward ear. ___ ___ ___ _____

(3) Asked patient to blink, did not release pressure until blink was completed. ___ ___ ___ _____

(4) Retracted eyelid beyond edge of lens if necessary, pressed lower eyelid against lens to dislodge. ___ ___ ___ _____

(5) Allowed both eyelids to close slightly, grasped lens as it rose, cupped lens in hand. ___ ___ ___ _____

(6) Inspected lens to ensure it was intact, placed lens in storage container. ___ ___ ___ _____

c. Inspected eye after lens removal for redness, pain, swelling, discharge, or tearing. ___ ___ ___ _____

13. Cleaned and disinfected contact lenses:

a. Applied 1 or 2 drops of cleaning solution to lens in palm of hand. ___ ___ ___ _____

b. Held lens over emesis basin, rinsed using recommended solution. ___ ___ ___ _____

c. Placed lens in proper storage compartment, placed lenses inside up. ___ ___ ___ _____

d. Filled with disinfectant or storage solution. ___ ___ ___ _____

e. Secured cover(s) over storage case, labeled case properly. ___ ___ ___ _____

	S	U	NP	Comments

14. Inserted lens:

   a. Inserted soft lens, repeated for each eye:

      (1) Removed lens from storage case, rinsed with recommended solution, inspected for foreign materials, tears, and other damage.

      (2) Held lens on tip of index finger concave side up.

      (3) Inspected lens properly to ensure lens is not inverted.

      (4) Retracted upper lid properly, pulled lower lid down properly.

      (5) Instructed patient to look straight, placed lens on cornea, released lids slowly.

   b. Inserted rigid lens, repeated for each eye:

      (1) Removed lens from storage case properly.

      (2) Held lens on tip of index finger with concave side up.

      (3) Inspected lens to ensure it was moist, clean, clear, and free of cracks.

      (4) Wet lens surfaces using solution.

      (5) Pulled lower lid down properly.

      (6) Instructed patient to look straight, placed lens on cornea, released lids slowly.

   c. Asked patient to close eyes and avoid blinking.

15. Inspected eye to ensure lens is on cornea.

16. Asked patient to cover other eye with hand and report if vision was clear and lens was comfortable.

17. Repeated procedure to insert lens in other eye.

18. Discarded solution from case, rinsed case with sterile solution, sterilized or replaced case, allowed case to air dry, disposed of towel, removed gloves, performed hand hygiene.

19. Asked patient if lens felt comfortable.

20. Observed for unexpected outcomes.

Student _____ Date _____

Instructor _____ Date _____

	S	U	NP	Comments

PROCEDURAL STEPS

1. Performed hand hygiene.

2. Asked patient or inspected eyes to determine which eye was artificial.

3. Assessed patient's frequency and method of cleaning and length of time since last cleaning.

4. Assessed patient's ability to remove, clean, and reinsert prosthesis.

5. Assessed eyelids and socket for inflammation, tenderness, swelling, drainage, or odor before and after removal; paid attention to implant peg; assessed patient's pain.

6. Discussed procedure with patient.

7. Assembled supplies at bedside, placed one towel over work area.

8. Removed prosthesis:

   a. Positioned patient properly, provided privacy.

   b. Performed hand hygiene, applied clean gloves.

   c. Placed towel just below patient's face.

   d. Retracted lower eyelid against lower orbital ridge.

   e. Exerted slight pressure below eyelid, slid out prosthesis.

   f. Noted presence and orientation or colored dot.

   g. Placed prosthesis in palm of hand.

   h. Cleaned prosthesis appropriately, did not use alcohol.

   i. Inspected prosthesis for rough edges or surfaces, set aside on towel.

9. Stored in sterile saline in a labeled case if necessary.

	S	U	NP	Comments

10. Cleaned eyelid margins and socket:

    a. Washed and rinsed eyelid margins with mild soap and water, wiped from inner to outer canthus. ___ ___ ___ _____

    b. Retracted patient's upper and lower eyelid margins properly. ___ ___ ___ _____

    c. Irrigated socket with sterile saline solution, noted presence of discharge or odor. ___ ___ ___ _____

    d. Removed excess moisture with gauze, wiped from inner to outer canthus. ___ ___ ___ _____

11. Inserted prosthesis:

    a. Moistened prosthesis in water or sterile saline. ___ ___ ___ _____

    b. Retracted patient's upper eyelid. ___ ___ ___ _____

    c. Held prosthesis so dot was oriented properly. ___ ___ ___ _____

    d. Slid prosthesis up under upper eyelid, pushed lower lid down to allow prosthesis to slip in place. ___ ___ ___ _____

    e. Asked patient if prosthesis fit comfortably and without pain. ___ ___ ___ _____

12. Inspected eyelids and socket for signs of infection; excessive tearing or discharge, itching, or lashes turned toward prosthesis. ___ ___ ___ _____

13. Observed patient removing, cleaning, and reinserting prosthesis. ___ ___ ___ _____

14. Taught patient and family how to inspect socket for redness, drainage, or excessive dryness. ___ ___ ___ _____

15. Taught patient and family how to inspect artificial eye for damage, alerted patient to report any odor noted to health care provider. ___ ___ ___ _____

Student _____ Date _____

Instructor _____ Date _____

PERFORMANCE CHECKLIST SKILL 19-1 **EYE IRRIGATION**

	S	U	NP	Comments

ASSESSMENT

1. Reviewed medication order, including solution and affected eye(s).

2. Obtained history about injury to assess reason for irrigation.

3. Determined patient's ability to open affected eye.

4. Performed a complete eye examination if time allowed.

5. Assessed eye for redness, excessive tearing, discharge, and swelling; asked patient about symptoms of itching, burning, pain, blurred vision, or photophobia.

6. Asked patient to rate level of pain.

7. Assessed patient's ability to cooperate.

PLANNING

1. Identified expected outcomes.

2. Discussed procedure with patient.

3. Checked accuracy and completeness of MAR with written orders.

4. Assembled supplies at bedside.

5. Assisted patient to appropriate position.

IMPLEMENTATION

1. Identified patient using two identifiers.

2. Performed hand hygiene, applied clean gloves.

3. Removed any contact lens if possible, removed gloves, reapplied new gloves.

4. Explained to patient that eye could be closed and no object would touch it.

5. Placed towel or waterproof pad under patient's face and emesis basin below patient's cheek on side of affected eye.

6. Cleaned visible secretions and foreign material from eyelid margins and lashes, using moistened gauze; wiped from inner to outer canthus.

	S	U	NP	Comments

7. Explained next steps to patient, encouraged relaxation:

   a. Retracted upper and lower eyelids to expose conjunctival sacs.   ____ ____ ____ _____

   b. Held lids open properly, did not apply pressure over eye.   ____ ____ ____ _____

8. Held irrigating syringe, dropper, or IV tubing in appropriate position.   ____ ____ ____ _____

9. Asked patient to look toward brow, irrigated with steady stream toward conjunctival sac, moved from inner to outer canthus.   ____ ____ ____ _____

10. Reinforced importance of procedure, encouraged patient appropriately.   ____ ____ ____ _____

11. Allowed patient to blink periodically.   ____ ____ ____ _____

12. Continued irrigation until secretions were clear.   ____ ____ ____ _____

13. Blotted excess moisture from eyelids and face with gauze or towel.   ____ ____ ____ _____

14. Disposed of soiled supplies, removed gloves, performed hand hygiene.   ____ ____ ____ _____

EVALUATION

1. Observed for verbal and nonverbal signs of anxiety during irrigation.   ____ ____ ____ _____

2. Assessed patient's comfort level after irrigation.   ____ ____ ____ _____

3. Inspected eye for movement and PERRLA.   ____ ____ ____ _____

4. Asked patient about improved visual acuity.   ____ ____ ____ _____

5. Identified unexpected outcomes.   ____ ____ ____ _____

RECORDING AND REPORTING

1. Recorded condition of eye and patient's report of pain and symptoms, recorded amount and type of irrigation on MAR.   ____ ____ ____ _____

2. Reported continuing symptoms of pain or blurred vision.   ____ ____ ____ _____

Student _____ Date _____

Instructor _____ Date _____

PERFORMANCE CHECKLIST SKILL 19-2 **EAR IRRIGATION**

	S	U	NP	Comments

ASSESSMENT

1. Reviewed medication order including solution and affected ear.

2. Reviewed medical record for history of ruptured tympanic membrane, placement of myringotomy tubes, or surgery of the auditory canal.

3. Inspected pinna and external auditory meatus for redness, swelling, drainage, abrasions, and presence of cerumen or foreign objects; attempted to remove objects by first straightening the ear canal.

4. Used otoscope to inspect deeper portions of auditory canal and tympanic membrane.

5. Asked if patient was experiencing discomfort, noted patient's ability to hear clearly.

6. Reviewed patient's knowledge of purpose for irrigation and normal care of ear.

PLANNING

1. Identified expected outcomes.

2. Checked accuracy and completeness of each MAR.

3. Identified patient using two identifiers.

4. Instilled softener into ear for 2 to 3 days before irrigation if patient had impacted cerumen.

5. Explained procedure, warned that irrigation may cause sensation of dizziness, ear fullness, and warmth.

IMPLEMENTATION

1. Identified patient using two identifiers.

2. Performed hand hygiene, arranged supplies at bedside.

3. Provided privacy.

4. Assisted patient to appropriate position, placed towel under patient's head and shoulder, had patient hold emesis basin under ear if able.

	S	U	NP	Comments

5. Poured irrigating solution into basin, checked temperature properly. ___ ___ ___ _____

6. Applied gloves, cleaned auricle and outer ear canal with gauze or cotton ball, did not force drainage or cerumen into ear canal. ___ ___ ___ _____

7. Filled irrigating syringe with solution. ___ ___ ___ _____

8. Pulled pinna back appropriately based on patient's age, placed tip of device just inside external meatus, left space around irrigating tip and canal. ___ ___ ___ _____

9. Instilled solution properly, allowed fluid to drain out into basin during instillation, continued until canal was cleaned or solution was used. ___ ___ ___ _____

10. Maintained flow of irrigation in steady stream until pieces of cerumen flowed from canal. ___ ___ ___ _____

11. Asked if patient was experiencing pain, nausea, or vertigo. ___ ___ ___ _____

12. Drained excessive fluid from ear by having patient tilt head. ___ ___ ___ _____

13. Dried outer ear canal gently with cotton ball, left in place for 5 to 10 minutes. ___ ___ ___ _____

14. Assisted patient to a sitting position. ___ ___ ___ _____

15. Removed gloves, disposed of supplies, performed hand hygiene. ___ ___ ___ _____

EVALUATION

1. Asked patient if discomfort was noted during instillation. ___ ___ ___ _____

2. Asked patient about sensations of light-headedness or dizziness. ___ ___ ___ _____

3. Reinspected condition of meatus and canal. ___ ___ ___ _____

4. Measured patient's hearing acuity. ___ ___ ___ _____

5. Asked patient to describe purpose of irrigation and proper techniques for ear care. ___ ___ ___ _____

6. Identified unexpected outcomes. ___ ___ ___ _____

	S	U	NP	Comments

RECORDING AND REPORTING

1. Recorded procedure, amount of solution instilled, time of administration, and irrigated ear in appropriate log. ⎯ ⎯ ⎯ ⎯⎯⎯⎯⎯⎯

2. Recorded appearance of external ear and patient's hearing acuity in nurses' notes. ⎯ ⎯ ⎯ ⎯⎯⎯⎯⎯⎯

3. Reported adverse effects/patient response/ withheld drugs to nurse in charge or health care provider. ⎯ ⎯ ⎯ ⎯⎯⎯⎯⎯⎯

Student _____ Date _____

Instructor _____ Date _____

PERFORMANCE CHECKLIST SKILL 19-3 **CARE OF HEARING AIDS**

	S	U	NP	Comments
ASSESSMENT				
1. Determined whether patient could hear clearly with hearing aid.	___	___	___	_____
2. Asked if patient was able to manipulate and hold hearing aid, observed patient insert aid independently.	___	___	___	_____
3. Assessed if hearing aid was working by removing from ear, turning volume up, and observing for squealing tone.	___	___	___	_____
4. Determined patient's usual hearing aid care practices.	___	___	___	_____
5. Assessed patient for unusual physical or auditory signs/symptoms.	___	___	___	_____
6. Inspected earmold for cracked or rough edges.	___	___	___	_____
7. Inspected for accumulation of cerumen around aid and plugging of opening in aid.	___	___	___	_____
8. Assessed patient's knowledge of and routines for cleansing and caring for hearing aid.	___	___	___	_____
PLANNING				
1. Identified expected outcomes.	___	___	___	_____
2. Discussed procedure with patient, explained all steps before removing aid.	___	___	___	_____
3. Assembled supplies at bedside, placed towel over work area.	___	___	___	_____
4. Had patient assume appropriate position.	___	___	___	_____
IMPLEMENTATION				
1. Removed and cleaned hearing aid, performed steps for both ears if necessary.				
a. Performed hand hygiene, applied clean gloves if drainage was present.	___	___	___	_____
b. Turned hearing aid off, grasped aid securely, removed device following natural ear contour.	___	___	___	_____

	S	U	NP	Comments

c. Held aid over towel, wiped exterior with tissue to remove cerumen.

d. Inspected all openings in aid for cerumen, removed cerumen with wax loop or device supplied with aid.

e. Inspected earmold for rough edges or frays in cords.

f. Opened battery door, placed hearing aid in labeled case, allowed it to air dry.

g. Assessed ear for redness, tenderness, discharge, or odor.

h. Placed towel beneath patient's ear(s); washed canal(s) with washcloth, soap, and water; rinsed and dried.

i. Disposed of towels, removed gloves, performed hand hygiene.

j. Placed in storage container with desiccant material if stored, labeled case appropriately, indicated in records where aid was stored.

2. Inserted hearing aid, performed steps for both ears if necessary:

a. Performed hand hygiene, applied gloves if patient had ear drainage.

b. Removed hearing aid from storage case, checked battery, ensured volume was off.

c. Identified hearing aid as right or left.

d. Allowed patient to insert aid when possible, or held hearing aid properly with canal at the bottom, inserted following natural contours to guide into place.

e. Anchored any separate pieces.

f. Adjusted or had patient adjust volume to comfortable level.

g. Closed and stored case, performed hand hygiene.

EVALUATION

1. Asked patient to rate comfort after removal or insertion.

2. Observed patient during normal conversation and in response to environmental sounds.

	S	U	NP	Comments

3. Observed patient removing, cleaning, and reinserting aid.   ___ ___ ___ _____

4. Identified unexpected outcomes.   ___ ___ ___ _____

RECORDING AND REPORTING

1. Recorded removal of aid, storage location, and patient's preferred communication techniques, ensured information was in patient's record.   ___ ___ ___ _____

2. Reported any signs of infection, injury, or sudden decrease in hearing.   ___ ___ ___ _____

Student _____ Date _____

Instructor _____ Date _____

PERFORMANCE CHECKLIST SKILL 21-1 **ADMINISTERING ORAL MEDICATIONS**

	S	U	NP	Comments
ASSESSMENT				
1. Checked accuracy and completeness of MAR, clarified incomplete or unclear orders.	___	___	___	_____
2. Reviewed pertinent information related to medication.	___	___	___	_____
3. Assessed for any contraindications to receiving oral medication, notified health care provider if contraindications were present.	___	___	___	_____
4. Assessed risk for aspiration, protected patient by assessing swallowing ability.	___	___	___	_____
5. Assessed patient's medical history, history of allergies, medication history, and diet history; listed drug allergies on MAR and medical record.	___	___	___	_____
6. Gathered and reviewed physical assessment findings and laboratory data that influence drug administration.	___	___	___	_____
7. Assessed patient's knowledge regarding health and medication use.	___	___	___	_____
8. Assessed patient's preference for fluids, determined if medication could be given with these fluids, maintained fluid restrictions.	___	___	___	_____
PLANNING				
1. Identified expected outcomes.	___	___	___	_____
2. Explained procedure to patient, explained specifically if patient wanted to self-administer.	___	___	___	_____
IMPLEMENTATION				
1. Prepared medications:				
a. Performed hand hygiene.	___	___	___	_____
b. Planned medication administration to avoid interruptions.	___	___	___	_____
c. Arranged medication tray and cups in preparation area or on cart outside of room.	___	___	___	_____
d. Accessed automated dispensing system or unlocked medicine drawer or cart.	___	___	___	_____

	S	U	NP	Comments

e. Prepared medication for *one patient at a time*, followed the six rights of medication administration, kept all pages of MARs for one patient together.   _____ _____ _____ _____

f. Selected correct drug, compared name of medication on label with MAR, exited ADS after removing drug(s).   _____ _____ _____ _____

g. Checked or calculated drug dose as necessary, double-checked calculation, checked expiration date on all medications, returned outdated medication to pharmacy.   _____ _____ _____ _____

h. Checked record for medication count and compared current count with supply available if preparing a controlled substance.   _____ _____ _____ _____

i. Prepared solid forms of oral medications:

  (1) Placed unit-dose medication directly into cup without removing wrapper.   _____ _____ _____ _____

  (2) "Popped" medications through foil or paper backing into a medication cup when using a blister pack.   _____ _____ _____ _____

  (3) Had pharmacy split dosage if necessary or split properly if tablets were pre-scored.   _____ _____ _____ _____

  (4) Placed all medication in one cup, placed medication requiring preadministration assessments in separate cups.   _____ _____ _____ _____

  (5) Crushed medications separately if patient has difficulty swallowing, used pill-crushing device properly, mixed medication with soft food.   _____ _____ _____ _____

j. Prepared liquids:

  (1) Mixed by shaking before administration unless drug is in unit-dose container, placed cap of multidose bottle upside down on work surface.   _____ _____ _____ _____

  (2) Held bottle with label against palm of hand while pouring.   _____ _____ _____ _____

  (3) Placed medication cap at eye level, filled to desired level on the scale, ensured scale was even with fluid level at surface or base of meniscus.   _____ _____ _____ _____

  (4) Wiped lip of bottle with paper towel and recapped.   _____ _____ _____ _____

	S	U	NP	Comments

(5) Prepared medication in oral syringe if appropriate.

(6) Administered liquid medication packaged in single-dose cup directly from the cup.

k. Compared MAR with labels on prepared drugs before going into patient's room.

l. Returned stock containers or unused medication to shelf or drawer, labeled cups and poured medications before leaving preparation area, did not leave drugs unattended.

2. Administered medications:

a. Took medication to patient at correct time, applied the six rights of medication administration.

b. Identified patient using two identifiers.

c. Compared MAR with medication labels at bedside.

d. Performed necessary preadministration assessment, asked patient if he or she has any allergies.

e. Discussed purpose of each medication, action, and possible side effects; allowed patient to ask any questions.

f. Assisted patient to appropriate position.

g. Allowed patient to hold cup or tablets if desired, offered preferred liquid.

h. Removed tablets or strips from packet just before use, did not push tablet through foil, placed medication on top of patient's tongue, cautioned against chewing medication.

i. Had patient place sublingually administered medication under tongue and allowed it to dissolve completely.

j. Had patient place buccal-administered medication against mucous membranes of the cheek and gums until medication dissolved.

k. Mixed powdered medication with liquids at bedside, gave mixture to patient to drink.

l. Gave each crushed medication separately with a teaspoon of food.

	S	U	NP	Comments
m. Cautioned patient against chewing or swallowing lozenges.	___	___	___	_____
n. Gave effervescent powders and tablets immediately after dissolving.	___	___	___	_____
o. Placed medication cup to patient's lips if unable to hold cup, introduced each drug to mouth, did not rush or force medication.	___	___	___	_____
p. Stayed until patient completely took all medication by the prescribed route, asked patient to open mouth if necessary.	___	___	___	_____
q. Offered patient a nonfat snack if necessary and if not contraindicated.	___	___	___	_____
r. Assisted patient in returning to comfortable position.	___	___	___	_____
s. Disposed of soiled supplies, performed hand hygiene.	___	___	___	_____

EVALUATION

	S	U	NP	Comments
1. Returned within appropriate time, evaluated patient's response to medications.	___	___	___	_____
2. Asked patient or caregiver to identify drug and explain purpose, action, schedule, and side effects.	___	___	___	_____
3. Identified unexpected outcomes.	___	___	___	_____

RECORDING AND REPORTING

	S	U	NP	Comments
1. Recorded pertinent information on MAR, included initials or signature, recorded patient teaching and validation of understanding in nurses' notes.	___	___	___	_____
2. Recorded reason for withholding doses in nurses' notes if necessary.	___	___	___	_____
3. Reported adverse effects/patient response/withheld drugs to nurse in charge or health care provider.	___	___	___	_____

PERFORMANCE CHECKLIST SKILL 21-2 **ADMINSTERING MEDICATIONS THROUGH AN ENTERAL FEEDING TUBE**

	S	U	NP	Comments

ASSESSMENT

1. Checked accuracy and completeness of each MAR against medication order, clarified incomplete or unclear orders with health care provider.

2. Reviewed pertinent information related to medication.

3. Assessed for contraindications to receiving medications enterally.

4. Assessed patient's medical history, history of allergies, medication history, and diet history; withheld medication and informed health care provider if contraindicated.

5. Reviewed postoperative orders for type of enteral tube care if necessary.

6. Gathered and reviewed physical assessment data and laboratory data that may influence drug administration.

7. Assessed for potential drug-food interactions.

8. Checked with pharmacy for availability of liquid preparation.

9. Verified placement of feeding tube before administration.

PLANNING

1. Identified expected outcomes.

2. Explained procedure to patient.

IMPLEMENTATION

1. Determined if medication interacts with enteral feeding, held feeding for 30 minutes before administration if necessary.

2. Performed hand hygiene, prepared medications for instillation, checked label against MAR twice, filled graduated container with water, used sterile water if necessary.

   a. Crushed tablets into a fine powder, dissolved each tablet in separate cup.

	S	U	NP	Comments

b. Ensured contents of capsule could be expressed from covering, opened capsule and emptied contents into water, dissolved gel caps. ___ ___ ___ _____

3. Took medication to patient at correct time, applied the six rights of medication administration. ___ ___ ___ _____

4. Identified patient using two identifiers. ___ ___ ___ _____

5. Compared MAR with medication labels at patient's bedside, asked patient if he or she has allergies. ___ ___ ___ _____

6. Discussed purpose of each medication, action, and possible adverse effects, allowed patient to ask any questions. ___ ___ ___ _____

7. Positioned patient appropriately. ___ ___ ___ _____

8. Adjusted infusion pump to hold the tube feeding if continuous enteric tube feeding is infusing. ___ ___ ___ _____

9. Applied clean gloves, checked placement of feeding tube. ___ ___ ___ _____

10. Check for GRV, returned aspirated contents to stomach if appropriate, held medication and contacted health care provider when GVR was excessive. ___ ___ ___ _____

11. Irrigated tubing:

a. Pinched enteral tube and removed syringe, drew water into syringe, reinserted tip of syringe into tube, released clamp, flushed tubing, clamped tube again, removed syringe. ___ ___ ___ _____

b. Attached tip of syringe to port on stopcock if present, turned "off" setting of stopcock away from patient and toward infusion tubing, flushed tube and set stopcock "off," removed syringe. ___ ___ ___ _____

12. Removed bulb or plunger of syringe and reinserted syringe into tip of feeding tube. ___ ___ ___ _____

13. Administered first dose by pouring into syringe, allowed to flow by gravity.

a. Flushed with water if giving only one dose. ___ ___ ___ _____

b. Gave each medication separately, flushed with water between each dose. ___ ___ ___ _____

c. Followed last dose with appropriate amount of water. ___ ___ ___ _____

256

	S	U	NP	Comments

14. Clamped proximal end of feeding tube if feeding was not being administered, capped end of tube.

15. Followed steps 1 to 12 if tube feeding was administered by an infusion pump, held feeding if medications were not compatible with feeding solution.

16. Assisted patient to comfortable position, kept head of bed elevated.

17. Disposed of soiled supplies, rinsed graduated container and syringe, removed and disposed of gloves, performed hand hygiene.

EVALUATION

1. Returned within 30 minutes to evaluate patient's response to medications.

2. Identified unexpected outcomes.

RECORDING AND REPORTING

1. Recorded all pertinent information in the appropriate logs, included initials or signature, recorded patient teaching and validation of understanding in nurses' notes.

2. Recorded total amount of water used on proper I&O form.

3. Reported adverse effects/patient response/withheld drugs to nurse in charge or health care provider.

Student _____ Date _____

Instructor _____ Date _____

PERFORMANCE CHECKLIST SKILL 21-3 **APPLYING TOPICAL MEDICATIONS TO THE SKIN**

	S	U	NP	Comments
ASSESSMENT				
1. Checked accuracy and completeness of MAR with medication order, clarified incomplete or unclear orders with health care provider before administration.	___	___	___	_____
2. Reviewed pertinent information related to medication.	___	___	___	_____
3. Assessed condition of skin or membrane where medication was to be applied; applied clean gloves if necessary; washed, rinsed, and dried site; ensured to remove previously applied medication, debris, or fluids; assessed for symptoms of skin irritation.	___	___	___	_____
4. Assessed patient's medical history, history of allergies, and medication history; asked if patient has had reaction to cream or lotion.	___	___	___	_____
5. Determined amount of topical agent required, assessed skin site, reviewed health care provider's order, read application directions carefully.	___	___	___	_____
6. Assessed patient's knowledge of action and purpose of medication and willingness to adhere to drug regimen.	___	___	___	_____
7. Determined if patient or caregiver was physically able to apply medication.	___	___	___	_____
PLANNING				
1. Identified expected outcomes.	___	___	___	_____
IMPLEMENTATION				
1. Prepared medications for application, checked label against MAR twice, checked expiration date.	___	___	___	_____
2. Took medication to patient at correct time, applied the six rights of medication administration.	___	___	___	_____
3. Performed hand hygiene, assisted patient to comfortable position.	___	___	___	_____
4. Identified patient using two identifiers.	___	___	___	_____

	S	U	NP	Comments

5. Compared MAR with medication labels at patient's bedside, asked patient if he or she had allergies. ___ ___ ___ _____

6. Discussed the purpose of each medication, action, and possible adverse effects; allowed patient to ask any questions. ___ ___ ___ _____

7. If skin was broken, applied sterile gloves. ___ ___ ___ _____

8. Applied topical creams, ointments, and oil-based lotion:

   a. Exposed affected area, kept unaffected areas covered. ___ ___ ___ _____

   b. Washed, rinsed, and dried affected area before applying medication. ___ ___ ___ _____

   c. Applied topical agent to dry and flaking skin if necessary. ___ ___ ___ _____

   d. Removed gloves, performed hand hygiene, applied new gloves. ___ ___ ___ _____

   e. Placed required amount of medication in hand, softened medication. ___ ___ ___ _____

   f. Told patient initial application of agent may feel cold, spread properly over skin surface, applied to appropriate thickness. ___ ___ ___ _____

   g. Explained to patient that skin may feel greasy after application. ___ ___ ___ _____

9. Applied antianginal ointment:

   a. Removed previous dose paper, folded used paper, and disposed in biohazard container, wiped off residual medication with tissue. ___ ___ ___ _____

   b. Wrote date, time, and nurse's initials on new application paper. ___ ___ ___ _____

   c. Applied desired number of inches of ointment to paper-measuring guide. ___ ___ ___ _____

   d. Selected application site, did not apply to hairy surfaces or over scar tissue. ___ ___ ___ _____

   e. Ensured application sites were rotated. ___ ___ ___ _____

   f. Applied ointment to skin surface by placing wrapper directly on skin, did not rub ointment into skin. ___ ___ ___ _____

   g. Secured ointment and paper with tape or dressing, used plastic wrap if necessary. ___ ___ ___ _____

	S	U	NP	Comments

10. Applied transdermal patches:

   a. Removed old patch if necessary, cleansed area, checked between skin folds for patch.

   b. Disposed of old patch in biohazard trash bag.

   c. Dated and initialed outer side of new patch, noted time of administration.

   d. Chose appropriate new site, did not apply to irritated or oily skin.

   e. Removed the patch from covering, held patch without touching adhesive edges.

   f. Applied patch, ensured edges stick well, applied overlay if provided.

   g. Did not apply patch to previously used sites for at least a week.

   h. Instructed patient not to cut patches.

   i. Instructed patient to always remove old patch before applying new one.

11. Administered aerosol sprays:

   a. Shook container vigorously, read label for recommended spray distance.

   b. Asked patient to turn face away from spray.

   c. Sprayed medication evenly over affected site.

12. Applied suspension-based lotion:

   a. Shook container vigorously.

   b. Applied lotion to gauze dressing, applied to skin properly.

   c. Explained to patient that area would feel cool and dry.

13. Applied a powder:

   a. Ensured skin was thoroughly dry, dried between skin folds.

   b. Asked patient to turn face away from powder.

   c. Dusted skin site with fine, thin layer of powder.

	S	U	NP	Comments

14. Assisted patient to comfortable position, reapplied gown, covered with bed linen as desired.   ____ ____ ____ _____

15. Disposed of soiled supplies properly, removed and disposed of gloves, performed hand hygiene.   ____ ____ ____ _____

EVALUATION

1. Asked patient or caregiver to name medication, action, purpose, dose, schedule, and side effects.   ____ ____ ____ _____

2. Had patient keep a diary of doses taken.   ____ ____ ____ _____

3. Observed patient or caregiver applying topical medication.   ____ ____ ____ _____

4. Inspected condition of skin between applications.   ____ ____ ____ _____

5. Identified unexpected outcomes.   ____ ____ ____ _____

RECORDING AND REPORTING

1. Recorded pertinent information in the appropriate record, recorded reasons for withholding doses if necessary.   ____ ____ ____ _____

2. Described condition of skin before each application in nurse's notes.   ____ ____ ____ _____

3. Reported adverse effects/patient response/withheld drugs to nurse in charge or health care provider.   ____ ____ ____ _____

Student _____ Date _____

Instructor _____ Date _____

PERFORMANCE CHECKLIST SKILL 21-4 **INSTILLING EYE AND EAR MEDICATIONS**

	S	U	NP	Comments

ASSESSMENT

1. Checked accuracy and completeness of MAR with medication order, clarified incomplete or unclear orders with health care provider.

2. Reviewed pertinent information related to medication.

3. Assessed condition of external eye or ear structures.

4. Determined whether patient had any symptoms of eye or ear discomfort or visual or hearing impairment.

5. Assessed patient's medical history, history of allergies, and medication history.

6. Assessed patient's LOC and ability to follow directions.

7. Assessed patient's knowledge regarding drug therapy and desire to self-administer medication.

8. Assessed patient's ability to manipulate and hold dropper or disk.

PLANNING

1. Identified expected outcomes.

2. Explained procedure to patient.

IMPLEMENTATION

1. Prepared medications for instillation, checked label of medication against MAR twice, checked expiration date on container.

2. Took medication(s) to patient at correct time, applied the six rights of medication administration.

3. Performed hand hygiene, arranged supplies at bedside.

4. Identified patient using two identifiers.

5. Compared MAR with medication labels at bedside, asked patient if he or she had allergies.

	S	U	NP	Comments

6. Discussed purpose of each medication, action, and possible adverse side effects; allowed patient to ask any questions; told patients receiving eyedrops that vision would be blurred and light sensitivity may occur.   ___ ___ ___ _____

7. Instilled eye medications:

   a. Applied clean gloves, asked patient to assume appropriate position.   ___ ___ ___ _____

   b. Washed away drainage or crusting along margins, soaked dried crusts, wiped clean from inner to outer canthus, removed gloves, performed hand hygiene.   ___ ___ ___ _____

   c. Explained there may be burning sensation from the drops.   ___ ___ ___ _____

   d. Instilled eye drops:

      (1) Applied clean gloves, held cotton ball or tissue below lower eyelid.   ___ ___ ___ _____

      (2) Pressed downward against bony orbit, did not press directly against patient's eyeball.   ___ ___ ___ _____

      (3) Asked patient to look at ceiling, held eyedropper appropriately above conjunctival sac.   ___ ___ ___ _____

      (4) Dropped prescribed number of drops into conjunctival sac.   ___ ___ ___ _____

      (5) Repeated procedure if patient blinked or closed eyes during administration.   ___ ___ ___ _____

      (6) Applied gentle pressure with tissue to nasolacrimal duct over each eye when administering drops that may cause systemic effects, avoided pressure against patient's eyeball.   ___ ___ ___ _____

      (7) Asked patient to close eyes gently after instilling drops.   ___ ___ ___ _____

   e. Instilled eye ointment:

      (1) Held applicator above lower lid margin, applied ointment evenly along lower eyelid on conjunctiva.   ___ ___ ___ _____

      (2) Had patient close eye and rub lid lightly if not contraindicated.   ___ ___ ___ _____

      (3) Wiped excess medication from eyelid.   ___ ___ ___ _____

      (4) Applied clean eye patch if needed, completely covered affected eye, taped without applying pressure to eye.   ___ ___ ___ _____

	S	U	NP	Comments

f. Applied intraocular disk:

(1) Opened disk package, positioned convex side of disk on fingertip.

(2) Pulled patient's lower eyelid away from eye, asked patient to look up.

(3) Placed disk properly in the conjunctival sac.

(4) Pulled patient's lower eyelid out and over disk, repeated if you could see the disk.

8. Removed and disposed of gloves and soiled supplies after administering eye medications; performed hand hygiene.

9. Removed intraocular disk:

a. Performed hand hygiene, applied clean gloves, pulled eyelid downward on the lower eyelid.

b. Pinched disk and lifted it out of patient's eye.

c. Removed and disposed of gloves, performed hand hygiene.

10. Instilled eardrops:

a. Performed hand hygiene, applied clean gloves if drainage is present.

b. Warmed medication to room temperature.

c. Positioned patient properly, stabilized patient's head with his or her own hand.

d. Straightened ear canal by pulling pinna appropriately.

e. Wiped away any cerumen or drainage occluding outmost portion of ear canal, did not force cerumen into canal.

f. Instilled prescribed drops holding dropper appropriately above ear canal.

g. Asked patient to remain side-lying for a few minutes, massaged tragus of ear gently.

h. Inserted portion of cotton ball into outermost part of canal if ordered, did not press cotton into canal.

i. Removed cotton after 15 minutes, assisted patient to comfortable position.

12. Disposed of soiled supplies properly, removed and disposed of gloves, performed hand hygiene.

	S	U	NP	Comments

EVALUATION

1. Observed response to medication by assessing vision or hearing changes, asked if symptoms were relieved, noted side effects or discomfort. ___ ___ ___ _____

2. Asked patient to discuss drug's purpose, action, side effects, and technique of administration. ___ ___ ___ _____

3. Had patient or family caregiver demonstrate self-administration of next dose. ___ ___ ___ _____

4. Identified unexpected outcomes. ___ ___ ___ _____

RECORDING AND REPORTING

1. Recorded drug, concentration, dose, drop, site, and time on MAR; included initials or signature, recorded patient teaching and validation of understanding in nurses' notes. ___ ___ ___ _____

2. Recorded objective data related to tissues involved and patient's response to medications, recorded side effects in nurses' notes. ___ ___ ___ _____

3. Reported adverse effects/patient's response/ withheld drugs to nurse in charge or health care provider. ___ ___ ___ _____

Student _____ Date _____

Instructor _____ Date _____

PERFORMANCE CHECKLIST SKILL 21-5 **ADMINISTERING NASAL INSTILLATIONS**

	S	U	NP	Comments
ASSESSMENT				
1. Checked accuracy and completeness of each MAR with medication order, clarified incomplete or unclear orders with health care provider.	___	___	___	_____
2. Reviewed pertinent information related to medication.	___	___	___	_____
3. Assessed patient's history and history of allergies.	___	___	___	_____
4. Performed hand hygiene, used penlight to inspect condition of nose and sinuses, palpated sinuses for tenderness, noted type of any drainage.	___	___	___	_____
5. Assessed patient's knowledge regarding use of nasal instillations, technique for instillation, and willingness to learn self-administration.	___	___	___	_____
PLANNING				
1. Identified expected outcomes.	___	___	___	_____
2. Explained procedure to family and patient regarding positioning and sensations to expect.	___	___	___	_____
IMPLEMENTATION				
1. Prepared medications for instillation, checked label of medication against MAR twice, checked expiration date on container.	___	___	___	_____
2. Took medication(s) to patient at the proper time, applied the six rights of medication.	___	___	___	_____
3. Identified patient using two identifiers.	___	___	___	_____
4. Compared MAR with medication labels at patient's bedside, asked patient if he or she had allergies.	___	___	___	_____
5. Discussed purpose of each medication, action, and possible adverse effects; allowed patient to ask any questions; told patient that he or she may experience burning, stinging, or a choking sensation.	___	___	___	_____
6. Performed hand hygiene, arranged supplies and medications at bedside, applied clean gloves.	___	___	___	_____

	S	U	NP	Comments

7. Shook container, instructed patient to clear or blow nose unless contraindicated. ___ ___ ___ _____

8. Administered nose drops:

   a. Assisted patient to proper position depending on affected nasal passage. ___ ___ ___ _____

   b. Supported patient's head with nondominant hand. ___ ___ ___ _____

   c. Instructed patient to breathe through mouth. ___ ___ ___ _____

   d. Held dropper above nares, instilled prescribed number of drops properly. ___ ___ ___ _____

   e. Had patient remain in supine position for 5 minutes. ___ ___ ___ _____

   f. Offered facial tissue, cautioned patient against blowing nose for several minutes. ___ ___ ___ _____

9. Administered nasal spray:

   a. Helped patient into appropriate position. ___ ___ ___ _____

   b. Helped patient insert tip of spray into nares, occluded other nostril with finger, pointed spray tip properly. ___ ___ ___ _____

   c. Had patient spray medication into nose while inhaling, helped patient remove nozzle, instructed patient to breathe out through mouth. ___ ___ ___ _____

   d. Offered facial tissue, cautioned patient against blowing nose for several minutes. ___ ___ ___ _____

10. Assisted patient to comfortable position until medicine was absorbed. ___ ___ ___ _____

11. Disposed of soiled supplies, removed and disposed of gloves, performed hand hygiene. ___ ___ ___ _____

EVALUATION

1. Observed patient for onset of side effects 15 to 30 minutes after administration. ___ ___ ___ _____

2. Asked if patient was able to breathe through nose, had patient occlude one nostril at a time and breathe deeply if necessary. ___ ___ ___ _____

3. Reinspected condition of nasal passages between instillations. ___ ___ ___ _____

4. Asked patient to describe risks of overuse and methods for administration. ___ ___ ___ _____

5. Had patient demonstrate self-medication. ___ ___ ___ _____

6. Identified unexpected outcomes. ___ ___ ___ _____

	S	U	NP	Comments

RECORDING AND REPORTING

1. Recorded drug, concentration, number of drops, nares, and time on MAR; included initials or signature; recorded patient teaching and validation of understanding in nurses' notes.   ___ ___ ___ _____

2. Reported any unusual systemic effects/adverse effects/patient response/withheld drugs to nurse in charge or health care provider.   ___ ___ ___ _____

PERFORMANCE CHECKLIST SKILL 21-6 **USING METERED-DOSE INHALERS**

	S	U	NP	Comments

ASSESSMENT

1. Checked accuracy and completeness of each MAR against medication order, clarified incomplete or unclear orders with health care provider.

2. Reviewed pertinent information related to medication.

3. Assessed patient's medical history, history of allergies, and medication history.

4. Assessed respiratory pattern, auscultated breath sounds.

5. Assessed patient's ability to hold, manipulate, and depress canister and inhaler.

6. Assessed patient's readiness and ability to learn.

7. Assessed patient's knowledge and understanding of disease and purpose and action of medications.

PLANNING

1. Identified expected outcomes.

2. Explained procedure to patient, explained specifics if patient wished to self-administer drug.

IMPLEMENTATION

1. Prepared medications for inhalation, checked label of medication against MAR twice, checked expiration date.

2. Took medication(s) to patient at correct time, applied the six rights of medication administration.

3. Identified patient using two identifiers.

4. Compared MAR with medication labels at patient's bedside, asked patient if he or she had allergies.

5. Discussed purpose of each medication, action, and possible adverse effects; allowed patient to ask any questions; explained what a metered-dose is and how to administer it, warned about overuse and side effects.

	S	U	NP	Comments

6. Allowed adequate time for patient to manipulate equipment, explained and demonstrated how canister fits into inhaler.   ___ ___ ___ _____

7. Explained steps for administering MDI without spacer:

   a. Removed mouthpiece cover from inhaler after inserting MDI canister into holder.   ___ ___ ___ _____

   b. Shook inhaler well for 2 to 5 seconds.   ___ ___ ___ _____

   c. Held inhaler in dominant hand.   ___ ___ ___ _____

   d. Instructed patient to position inhaler properly.   ___ ___ ___ _____

   e. Had patient take deep breath and exhale completely.   ___ ___ ___ _____

   f. Had patient hold inhaler in three-point or bilateral hand position when positioned properly.   ___ ___ ___ _____

   g. Instructed patient to tilt head back and inhale slowly and deeply through mouth for 3 to 5 seconds while depressing canister fully.   ___ ___ ___ _____

   h. Had patient hold breath for about 10 seconds.   ___ ___ ___ _____

   i. Removed MDI from mouth before exhaling.   ___ ___ ___ _____

8. Explained steps to administer MDI using a spacer.

   a. Removed mouthpiece cover from MDI and mouthpiece of spacer device.   ___ ___ ___ _____

   b. Shook inhaler well for 2 to 5 seconds.   ___ ___ ___ _____

   c. Inserted MDI into end of spacer device.   ___ ___ ___ _____

   d. Instructed patient to place spacer mouthpiece in mouth and close lips, avoided covering exhalation slots with lips.   ___ ___ ___ _____

   e. Had patient breathe normally through mouthpiece.   ___ ___ ___ _____

   f. Instructed patient to spray one puff into spacer device.   ___ ___ ___ _____

   g. Had patient breathe in slowly and fully.   ___ ___ ___ _____

   h. Instructed patient to hold breath for 10 seconds.   ___ ___ ___ _____

9. Instructed patient to wait appropriate length between inhalations.   ___ ___ ___ _____

	S	U	NP	Comments
10. Instructed patient to not repeat inhalation before next scheduled.	___		___	_____
11. Warned patient they may feel gagging sensation.	___		___	_____
12. Instructed patient to rinse and spit with warm water 2 minutes after dose.	___	___	___	_____
13. Instructed patient in daily cleaning of inhaler.	___	___	___	_____
14. Asked if patient had any questions.	___	___	___	_____
15. Assisted patient to comfortable position, performed hand hygiene.	___	___	___	_____

EVALUATION

	S	U	NP	Comments
1. Had patient explain and demonstrate steps in use and cleaning of inhaler.	___	___	___	_____
2. Asked patient to explain drug schedule and dose or medication.	___	___	___	_____
3. Asked patient to describe side effects of medication and criteria for calling health care provider.	___	___	___	_____
4. Assessed patient's respirations, breath sounds, and peak flow measures after medication administration if ordered.	___	___	___	_____
5. Identified unexpected outcomes.	___	___	___	_____

RECORDING AND REPORTING

	S	U	NP	Comments
1. Recorded drug, dose, route, number of inhalations, and time on MAR; included initials or signature; recorded patient teaching and validation of understanding in nurses' notes.	___	___	___	_____
2. Recorded patient's response to MDI, side effects, and patient's ability to use MDI.	___	___	___	_____
3. Reported adverse effects/patient response/ withheld drugs to nurse in charge or health care provider.	___	___	___	_____

Student _____   Date _____

Instructor _____   Date _____

PERFORMANCE CHECKLIST PROCEDURAL GUIDELINE 21-1   **USING DRY POWDER INHALED MEDICATION**

	S	U	NP	Comments
PROCEDURAL GUIDELINE				
1. Checked accuracy and completeness of each MAR with medication order, clarified incomplete or unclear orders with health care provider.	___	___	___	_____
2. Reviewed pertinent information related to medication.	___	___	___	_____
3. Assessed patient's medical history, history of allergies, and medication and diet history.	___	___	___	_____
4. Assessed respiratory pattern, auscultated breath sounds.	___	___	___	_____
5. Assessed patient's knowledge of medication and readiness to learn.	___	___	___	_____
6. Assessed patient's ability to learn.	___	___	___	_____
7. Determined patient's ability to hold, manipulate, and activate DPI.	___	___	___	_____
8. Assessed patient's technique in using a DPI if previously instructed in self-administration.	___	___	___	_____
9. Prepared medication for inhalation, checked label on inhaler against MAR twice, *checked expiration date on container.*	___	___	___	_____
10. Took medication to patient at correct time, applied the six rights of medication administration.	___	___	___	_____
11. Identified patient using two identifiers.	___	___	___	_____
12. Compared MAR with medication labels at patient's bedside, asked patient if he or she had allergies.	___	___	___	_____
13. Discussed purpose of each medication, action, and possible adverse effects; allowed patient to ask any questions; explained about a DPI; warned about overuse and side effects.	___	___	___	_____
14. Noted number of doses remaining if external counter was present.	___	___	___	_____
15. Prepared DPI for administration, performed hand hygiene.	___	___	___	_____

	S	U	NP	Comments

16. Had patient place lips over mouthpiece and inhale quickly and deeply, removed inhaler before exhalation, instructed patient that he or she may not taste the powdered medication. ___ ___ ___ _____

17. Had patient hold breath as long as possible and then exhale. ___ ___ ___ _____

18. Had patient rinse and spit with warm water after using DPI. ___ ___ ___ _____

19. Returned DPI to closed position or removed loaded capsule, noted number if external counter was present. ___ ___ ___ _____

20. Had patient demonstrate use of DPI at next scheduled dose, asked patient to discuss purpose, action, and side effects. ___ ___ ___ _____

21. Auscultated breath sounds, evaluated respiratory rate, asked patient about his or her breathing. ___ ___ ___ _____

22. Recorded drug, dose, route, inhalations, and time on MAR; included initials or signature; recorded patient teaching and validation of understanding in nurses' notes. ___ ___ ___ _____

276

Student _____ Date _____

Instructor _____ Date _____

PERFORMANCE CHECKLIST SKILL 21-7 **USING SMALL-VOLUME NEBULIZERS**

	S	U	NP	Comments
ASSESSMENT				
1. Checked accuracy and completeness of each MAR against medication order, clarified incomplete or unclear orders with health care provider.	___	___	___	_____
2. Reviewed pertinent information related to medication.	___	___	___	_____
3. Assessed patient's medical history, history of allergies, and medication and diet history.	___	___	___	_____
4. Assessed patient's ability to grasp and ability to assemble, hold, and manipulate nebulizer equipment.	___	___	___	_____
5. Assessed pulse, respirations, breath sounds, pulse oximetry, and peak flow measurement if ordered.	___	___	___	_____
6. Assessed patient's knowledge of medication and readiness to learn.	___	___	___	_____
PLANNING				
1. Identified expected outcomes.	___	___	___	_____
2. Explained procedure to patient, explained specifics if patient wished to self-administer drug.	___	___	___	_____
IMPLEMENTATION				
1. Prepared medications for inhalation, checked label of medication against MAR twice, checked expiration date.	___	___	___	_____
2. Took medication(s) to patient at correct time, applied the six rights of medication administration.	___	___	___	_____
3. Performed hand hygiene, arranged equipment needed.	___	___	___	_____
4. Identified patient using two identifiers.	___	___	___	_____
5. Compared MAR with medication labels at patient's bedside, asked patient if he or she had allergies.	___	___	___	_____

	S	U	NP	Comments

6. Discussed purpose of each medication, action, and possible adverse effects; allowed patient to ask any questions; explained how to manipulate nebulizer.

7. Assembled nebulizer equipment properly.

8. Added prescribed medication by pouring medicine into nebulizer cup or using dropper or syringe and diluent to instill medication.

9. Attached top portion of cup and connected mask or mouthpiece.

10. Connected tubing to aerosol compressor and nebulizer cup.

11. Had patient hold mouthpiece between lips or used mask or adapter.

12. Turned on machine, ensured a sufficient mist was formed.

13. Had patient take a deep breath; encouraged brief, end-inspiratory pause; had patient exhale passively:

   a. Encouraged patient to hold every fourth or fifth breath for 5 to 10 seconds.

   b. Reminded patient to repeat breathing pattern until drug was completely nebulized.

   c. Tapped nebulizer cup occasionally.

   d. Monitored patient's pulse during procedure.

14. Turned machine off when medication was completely nebulized, rinsed nebulizer cup per agency policy, dried completely, stored tubing assembly per policy.

15. Instructed patient to rinse and gargle with warm water if steroids were nebulized.

16. Had patient take several breaths and cough after treatment was complete.

17. Assisted patient to comfortable position, performed hand hygiene.

EVALUATION

1. Assessed patient's respirations, breath sounds, cough effort, sputum production, pulse oximetry, and peak flow measures if ordered.

2. Had patient explain and demonstrate steps in use of nebulizer.

	S	U	NP	Comments
3. Asked patient to explain drug schedule.	⎯	⎯	⎯	_____
4. Asked patient to describe side effects of medication and criteria for calling health care provider.	⎯	⎯	⎯	_____
5. Identified unexpected outcomes.	⎯	⎯	⎯	_____

RECORDING AND REPORTING

	S	U	NP	Comments
1. Recorded drug, dose, route, length of treatment, and time on MAR; included initials or signature; recorded patient teaching and validation of understanding in nurses' notes.	⎯	⎯	⎯	_____
2. Recorded patient's response to treatment in nurses' notes.	⎯	⎯	⎯	_____
3. Reported adverse effects/patient response/ withheld drugs to nurse in charge or health care provider.	⎯	⎯	⎯	_____

Student _____ Date _____

Instructor _____ Date _____

PERFORMANCE CHECKLIST SKILL 21-8 **ADMINISTERING VAGINAL INSTILLATIONS**

	S	U	NP	Comments
ASSESSMENT				
1. Checked accuracy and completeness of each MAR against medication order, clarified incomplete and unclear orders with health care provider.	—	—	—	_____
2. Reviewed pertinent information related to medication.	—	—	—	_____
3. Assessed patient's medical history, history of allergies, and medication and diet history.	—	—	—	_____
4. Performed hand hygiene, applied clean gloves, inspected condition of vaginal tissues during perineal care, noted if drainage was present, removed gloves, performed hand hygiene.	—	—	—	_____
5. Asked if patient was experiencing any symptoms of pruritis, burning, or discomfort.	—	—	—	_____
6. Assessed patient's knowledge of medication and readiness to learn.	—	—	—	_____
7. Assessed patient's ability to manipulate applicator, suppository, or irrigation equipment and to properly position self to insert medication.	—	—	—	_____
PLANNING				
1. Identified expected outcomes.	—	—	—	_____
2. Explained procedure to patient, explained specifics if patient wished to self-administer drug.	—	—	—	_____
IMPLEMENTATION				
1. Prepared suppository for administration, checked label of medication against MAR twice, checked expiration date.	—	—	—	_____
2. Took medication(s) to patient at correct time, applied the six rights of medication administration.	—	—	—	_____
3. Identified patient using two identifiers.	—	—	—	_____
4. Compared MAR with medication labels at patient's bedside, asked patient if he or she had allergies.	—	—	—	_____
5. Discussed purpose of each medication, action, and possible adverse effects; allowed patient to ask any questions; explained procedure if patient planned to self-administer medication.	—	—	—	_____

	S	U	NP	Comments

6. Performed hand hygiene, arranged supplies at bedside, applied clean gloves, provided privacy. ___ ___ ___ _____

7. Had patient void, assisted patient to proper position. ___ ___ ___ _____

8. Kept abdomen and lower extremities draped. ___ ___ ___ _____

9. Ensured vaginal orifice was well illuminated, positioned lamp if necessary. ___ ___ ___ _____

10. Inserted vaginal suppository:

  a. Removed suppository from wrapper, applied lubricant to rounded end and gloved index finger, ensured suppository was room temperature. ___ ___ ___ _____

  b. Separated labial folds in front-to-back direction. ___ ___ ___ _____

  c. Inserted rounded end of suppository along posterior wall of vaginal canal. ___ ___ ___ _____

  d. Withdrew finger and wiped remaining lubricant from around labia with tissue. ___ ___ ___ _____

11. Applied cream or foam:

  a. Filled cream or foam applicator following package directions. ___ ___ ___ _____

  b. Separated labial folds with nondominant-gloved hand. ___ ___ ___ _____

  c. Inserted applicator properly with dominant gloved hand, pushed applicator plunger to deposit medication into vagina. ___ ___ ___ _____

  d. Withdrew applicator and placed on paper towel, wiped off residual cream from labia or vaginal orifice with tissue. ___ ___ ___ _____

12. Administered irrigation and douche:

  a. Placed patient on bedpan with absorbent pad underneath. ___ ___ ___ _____

  b. Ensured irrigation or douche fluid was at body temperature, ran fluid through container nozzle. ___ ___ ___ _____

  c. Separated labial folds, directed nozzle toward sacrum. ___ ___ ___ _____

  d. Raised container appropriately above level of vagina, inserted nozzle appropriately, allowed solution to flow while rotating nozzle, administered all irrigating solution. ___ ___ ___ _____

	S	U	NP	Comments

e. Withdrew nozzle, assisted patient to comfortable position. ___ ___ ___ _____

f. Allowed patient to remain on bedpan for a few minutes, cleansed perineum with soap and water. ___ ___ ___ _____

g. Assisted patient off bedpan, dried perineal area. ___ ___ ___ _____

13. Instructed patient who received suppository, cream, or tablet to remain on back for at least 10 minutes. ___ ___ ___ _____

14. Washed applicator with soap and water, rinsed, and stored for future use. ___ ___ ___ _____

15. Offered perineal pad when patient resumes ambulation. ___ ___ ___ _____

16. Discarded gloves and soiled equipment appropriately, performed hand hygiene. ___ ___ ___ _____

EVALUATION

1. Performed hand hygiene, applied clean gloves, inspected condition of vaginal canal and external genitalia between applications, assessed vaginal discharge if present, removed gloves, performed hand hygiene. ___ ___ ___ _____

2. Questioned patient regarding continued pruritis, burning, discomfort, or discharge. ___ ___ ___ _____

3. Asked patient to discuss purpose, action, and side effects of medication. ___ ___ ___ _____

4. Observed patient demonstrate administration of next dose. ___ ___ ___ _____

5. Identified unexpected outcomes. ___ ___ ___ _____

RECORDING AND REPORTING

1. Recorded drug, dose, type of instillation, and time on MAR; included initials or signature; recorded patient teaching, validation of understanding, and ability to self-administer medication in nurses' notes. ___ ___ ___ _____

2. Reported to health care provider if patient stated symptoms persisted or got worse. ___ ___ ___ _____

3. Reported adverse effects/patient response/withheld drugs to nurse in charge of health care provider. ___ ___ ___ _____

Student _____ Date _____

Instructor _____ Date _____

PERFORMANCE CHECKLIST SKILL 21-9 **ADMINISTERING RECTAL SUPPOSITORIES**

	S	U	NP	Comments
ASSESSMENT				
1. Checked accuracy and completeness of each MAR against medication order, clarified incomplete or unclear orders with health care provider.	___	___	___	_____
2. Reviewed pertinent information related to medication.	___	___	___	_____
3. Reviewed patient's medical history for history of rectal surgery or bleeding, cardiac problems, history of allergies, and medication history	___	___	___	_____
4. Reviewed any presenting signs of GI alterations.	___	___	___	_____
5. Assessed patient's ability to hold suppository and position self to insert medication.	___	___	___	_____
6. Reviewed patient's knowledge of purpose of drug therapy and interest in self-administering suppository.	___	___	___	_____
PLANNING				
1. Identified expected outcomes.	___	___	___	_____
2. Explained procedure to patient, explained specifics if patient wished to self-administer drug.	___	___	___	_____
IMPLEMENTATION				
1. Prepared suppository for administration, checked label of medication against MAR twice, checked expiration date on container.	___	___	___	_____
2. Took medication to patient at correct time, applied the six rights of medication administration.	___	___	___	_____
3. Identified patient using two identifiers.	___	___	___	_____
4. Compared MAR with medication labels at patient's bedside, asked patient if he or she had allergies.	___	___	___	_____
5. Discussed purpose of each medication, action, and possible adverse effects; allowed patient to ask any questions; explained procedure if patient plans to self-administer.	___	___	___	_____

	S	U	NP	Comments

6. Performed hand hygiene, arranged supplies at bedside, applied clean gloves, provided privacy.
    _____ _____ _____ _____

7. Assisted patient to proper position.
    _____ _____ _____ _____

8. Assisted to position appropriate for any mobile impairment, obtained assistance if necessary.
    _____ _____ _____ _____

9. Kept patient draped with only anal area exposed.
    _____ _____ _____ _____

10. Examined condition of anus externally, palpated rectal walls as needed, disposed of gloves properly if necessary.
    _____ _____ _____ _____

11. Applied clean gloves if necessary.
    _____ _____ _____ _____

12. Removed suppository from wrapper, lubricated round end of suppository and index finger, handled area gently if patient had hemorrhoids.
    _____ _____ _____ _____

13. Asked patient to take slow, deep breaths through mouth and relax anal sphincter.
    _____ _____ _____ _____

14. Retracted patient's buttocks with nondominant hand, inserted suppository properly.
    _____ _____ _____ _____

15. Gave suppository through colostomy if ordered.
    _____ _____ _____ _____

16. Withdrew finger, wiped patient's anal area.
    _____ _____ _____ _____

17. Asked patient to remain flat for 5 minutes.
    _____ _____ _____ _____

18. Discarded gloves and supplies in appropriate receptacle.
    _____ _____ _____ _____

19. Placed call light within reach if suppository contained laxative or fecal softener.
    _____ _____ _____ _____

20. Reminded patient *not* to flush commode after bowel movement if suppository was given for constipation.
    _____ _____ _____ _____

EVALUATION

1. Returned to bedside within 5 minutes to determine if suppository was expelled.
    _____ _____ _____ _____

2. Asked if patient experienced localized anal or rectal discomfort during insertion.
    _____ _____ _____ _____

3. Evaluated patient for relief of symptoms.
    _____ _____ _____ _____

4. Asked patient to explain purpose of medication.
    _____ _____ _____ _____

5. Had patient demonstrate self-administration of next dose of medication.
    _____ _____ _____ _____

6. Identified unexpected outcomes.
    _____ _____ _____ _____

	S	U	NP	Comments

RECORDING AND REPORTING

1. Recorded drug, dose, route, and time on MAR; included initials or signature; recorded patient teaching, validation of understanding, and self-administration of suppositories in nurses' notes. ⸻ ⸻ ⸻ ⸻⸻⸻⸻⸻

2. Reported adverse effects/patient response/ withheld drugs to nurse in charge or health care provider. ⸻ ⸻ ⸻ ⸻⸻⸻⸻⸻

PERFORMANCE CHECKLIST SKILL 22-1 **PREPARING INJECTIONS: AMPULES AND VIALS**

	S	U	NP	Comments
ASSESSMENT				
1. Checked accuracy and completeness of each MAR with medication order, reprinted any portion of MAR that was difficult to read.	___	___	___	_____
2. Assessed patient's medical and medication history.	___	___	___	_____
3. Assessed patient's history of allergies, knew types of allergies and normal response.	___	___	___	_____
4. Reviewed medication reference information.	___	___	___	_____
5. Assessed patient's body build, muscle size, and weight if giving subcutaneous or IM medication.	___	___	___	_____
PLANNING				
1. Identified expected outcomes.	___	___	___	_____
IMPLEMENTATION				
1. Performed hand hygiene, prepared supplies.	___	___	___	_____
2. Prepared medications.				
a. Moved medication cart outside patient's room if being used.	___	___	___	_____
b. Unlocked medication cart or logged onto computerized dispensing system.	___	___	___	_____
c. Followed "No-Interruption Zone" policy, prepared medication for one patient at a time, kept all pages of MARs for one patient together, looked at only one patient's electronic MAR at a time.	___	___	___	_____
d. Selected correct drug, compared label with MAR.	___	___	___	_____
e. Checked expiration date on each medication.	___	___	___	_____
f. Calculated drug dose as necessary, double-checked calculations, asked another nurse if needed.	___	___	___	_____
g. Checked record for previous drug count and compared with supply if preparing a controlled substance.	___	___	___	_____
h. Did not leave drugs unattended.	___	___	___	_____

	S	U	NP	Comments

3. Prepared ampule.

   a. Tapped top of ampule until fluid moved from neck of ampule. ___ ___ ___ _____

   b. Placed gauze pad around neck of ampule. ___ ___ ___ _____

   c. Snapped neck of ampule properly. ___ ___ ___ _____

   d. Drew up medication quickly, used a long enough filter needle. ___ ___ ___ _____

   e. Held ampule properly, inserted filter needle, did not allow needle to touch rim of ampule. ___ ___ ___ _____

   f. Aspirated medication into syringe. ___ ___ ___ _____

   g. Kept needle tip under surface of liquid, tipped ampule if needed. ___ ___ ___ _____

   h. Did not expel air if air bubbles were aspirated. ___ ___ ___ _____

   i. Expelled air bubble properly outside of ampule, did not eject fluid. ___ ___ ___ _____

   j. Used sink for disposal of excess fluid, rechecked fluid level in syringe properly. ___ ___ ___ _____

   k. Covered needle with safety sheath, replaced filter needle with regular SESIP needle. ___ ___ ___ _____

4. Prepared vial containing solution.

   a. Removed cap covering top of unused vial, wiped surface of rubber seal with alcohol, allowed it to dry. ___ ___ ___ _____

   b. Picked up syringe, removed cap, drew amount of air into syringe equivalent to volume of medication to be aspirated. ___ ___ ___ _____

   c. Inserted needle or needleless device through center of rubber seal, applied pressure to tip of needle during insertion. ___ ___ ___ _____

   d. Injected air into air space of vial, held plunger firmly. ___ ___ ___ _____

   e. Inverted vial, kept hold on syringe and plunger, grasped so as to counteract pressure in vial. ___ ___ ___ _____

   f. Kept tip of needle below fluid level. ___ ___ ___ _____

   g. Allowed air pressure to fill syringe gradually with medication, pulled back on plunger if necessary. ___ ___ ___ _____

	S	U	NP	Comments

h. Positioned needle into air space of vial when desired volume is obtained, dislodged air bubbles, ejected air in top of syringe. ___ ___ ___ _____

i. Removed needle or needleless access device from vial. ___ ___ ___ _____

j. Held syringe properly, ensured correct volume and absence of air bubbles, dislodged any remaining air bubbles, ejected any air, rechecked volume of medication. ___ ___ ___ _____

k. Changed needle to appropriate gauge and length if necessary. ___ ___ ___ _____

l. Labeled vial properly if using multi-dose vial. ___ ___ ___ _____

5. Prepared vial containing a powder.

a. Removed cap covering vials of medication and diluent, swabbed both seals with alcohol, allowed to dry. ___ ___ ___ _____

b. Drew appropriate volume of diluent into syringe. ___ ___ ___ _____

c. Inserted needle or needleless device through rubber seal of vial of powdered medication, injected diluent, removed needle. ___ ___ ___ _____

d. Mixed medication thoroughly, rolled in palms, did not shake. ___ ___ ___ _____

e. Determined appropriate dose after reconstitution. ___ ___ ___ _____

f. Drew medication into syringe, did not add additional air. ___ ___ ___ _____

6. Compared level of medication with MAR. ___ ___ ___ _____

7. Disposed of soiled supplies, placed broken ampule/used vials and used needle or needleless device in puncture- and leak-proof container, cleaned work area, performed hand hygiene. ___ ___ ___ _____

EVALUATION

1. Compared MAR with label of prepared drug, compared dose in syringe with desired dose. ___ ___ ___ _____

2. Identified unexpected outcomes. ___ ___ ___ _____

Student _____ Date _____

Instructor _____ Date _____

PERFORMANCE CHECKLIST PROCEDURAL GUIDELINE 22-1   **MIXING PARENTERAL MEDICATIONS IN ONE SYRINGE**

	S	U	NP	Comments
PROCEDURAL STEPS				
1. Checked accuracy and completeness of MAR with medication order, reprinted/recopied any portion of MAR that was difficult to read.	___	___	___	_____
2. Reviewed pertinent information related to medication.	___	___	___	_____
3. Assessed patient's body build, muscle size, and weight if giving subcutaneous or IM medication.	___	___	___	_____
4. Considered compatibility of medications to be mixed and type of injection.	___	___	___	_____
5. Checked medication's expiration date printed on vial.	___	___	___	_____
6. Performed hand hygiene.	___	___	___	_____
7. Prepared medication for one patient at a time, followed the six rights of medication administration, selected ampule or vial from drawer or system, compared label of each medication with MAR, ensured correct types of insulin were prepared if necessary.	___	___	___	_____
8. Mixed medication from two vials.				
a. Aspirated volume of air equivalent to first medication dose using syringe with needle-less device or filter needle.	___	___	___	_____
b. Injected air into vial A, ensured needle or needleless device did not touch solution.	___	___	___	_____
c. Held plunger, withdrew needle and syringe from vial A, aspirated air equivalent to second medication dose into syringe.	___	___	___	_____
d. Inserted needle or device into vial B, injected volume of air into vial B, withdrew medication into syringe.	___	___	___	_____
e. Withdrew needle and syringe from vial B, ensured proper volume had been obtained.	___	___	___	_____
f. Determined what combined value of medications should measure.	___	___	___	_____

	S	U	NP	Comments
g. Inserted needle or device into vial A, ensured no medication was expelled into vial, inverted vial, withdrew desired amount of medication into syringe.	__	__	__	_____
h. Withdrew needle or device, expelled excess air, checked fluid level in syringe.	__	__	__	_____
i. Changed needle or device for appropriate-sized needle if medication was being injected, kept device capped until administration time.	__	__	__	_____

9. Mixed insulin.

	S	U	NP	Comments
a. Rolled bottle to resuspend insulin preparation if necessary.	__	__	__	_____
b. Wiped off tops of both insulin vials with alcohol.	__	__	__	_____
c. Verified insulin dose against MAR.	__	__	__	_____
d. Prepared insulin in the proper order if relevant.	__	__	__	_____
e. Inserted needle, injected air into first vial, did not let tip of needle touch solution.	__	__	__	_____
f. Removed syringe from vial of insulin without aspirating medication.	__	__	__	_____
g. Injected air equal to dose of second medication into vial, withdrew correct dose into syringe.	__	__	__	_____
h. Removed syringe from vial, removed air bubbles.	__	__	__	_____
i. Verified second dosage with MAR, verified with another nurse, determined and verified combined dosage.	__	__	__	_____
j. Placed needle back in first vial, ensured no insulin was pushed into vial.	__	__	__	_____
k. Inverted vial, withdrew desired amount of insulin into syringe.	__	__	__	_____
l. Withdrew needle, checked fluid level in syringe, kept needle sheathed or capped until administration.	__	__	__	_____

10. Mixed medications from a vial and an ampule.

	S	U	NP	Comments
a. Prepared medication from vial first as in Skill 22-1.	__	__	__	_____
b. Determined what combined volume of medications should measure.	__	__	__	_____

	S	U	NP	Comments
c. Used same syringe to prepare medication from ampule as in Skill 22-1.	___	___	___	_____
d. Withdrew filter needle from ampule, verified fluid level in syringe, changed needle to appropriate SESIP needle, kept device or needle sheathed or capped until administration.	___	___	___	_____
e. Checked syringe for total combined dose of medications.	___	___	___	_____
11. Compared MAR and labels on vials/ampules.	___	___	___	_____
12. Disposed of soiled supplies, placed used ampules/vials and needle or needleless device in puncture- and leak-proof container.	___	___	___	_____
13. Cleaned work area, performed hand hygiene.	___	___	___	_____
14. Checked syringe again for total combined dose.	___	___	___	_____

Student _____ Date _____

Instructor _____ Date _____

PERFORMANCE CHECKLIST SKILL 22-2 **ADMINISTERING INTRADERMAL INJECTIONS**

	S	U	NP	Comments
ASSESSMENT				
1. Checked accuracy and completeness of MAR with medication order, recopied any portion of MAR that was difficult to read.	___	___	___	_____
2. Reviewed medication reference information about expected reaction when testing skin with allergen.	___	___	___	_____
3. Assessed patient's history of allergies, known type of allergens, and normal allergic reaction.	___	___	___	_____
4. Assessed for contraindications to ID injections and history of severe adverse reactions to ID injections.	___	___	___	_____
5. Assessed patient's knowledge of purpose and response to skin testing.	___	___	___	_____
PLANNING				
1. Identified expected outcomes.	___	___	___	_____
IMPLEMENTATION				
1. Prepared medications for one patient at a time, kept all pages of MARs for one patient together, looked at only one patient's electronic MAR at a time, checked label of medication with MAR twice.	___	___	___	_____
2. Took medication(s) to patient at correct time, applied the six rights of medication administration.	___	___	___	_____
3. Provided privacy.	___	___	___	_____
4. Identified patient using two identifiers.	___	___	___	_____
5. Compared MAR with medication labels at bedside, asked patient if he or she had allergies.	___	___	NP	_____
6. Discussed purpose of each medication, action, and possible adverse effects; allowed patient to ask questions; told patient injection would cause a slight burning or stinging sensation.	___	___	___	_____

	S	U	NP	Comments

7. Performed hand hygiene, applied clean gloves, kept sheet draped over body parts not requiring exposure.

8. Selected appropriate site, noted lesions or discoloration of skin.

9. Assisted patient to comfortable position, had patient extend elbow and support forearm on flat surface.

10. Cleansed site with antiseptic swab.

11. Held swab or gauze properly.

12. Removed needle cap.

13. Held syringe properly with bevel of needle pointing up.

14. Administered injection.

    a. Stretched skin over site with nondominant hand.

    b. Inserted needle properly into skin, advanced to appropriate depth.

    c. Injected medication slowly, reinserted needle if necessary.

    d. Noted that small bleb appeared on skin surface.

    e. Withdrew needle, applied alcohol swab or gauze over site.

15. Assisted patient to comfortable position.

16. Discarded needle in puncture- and leak-proof container.

17. Removed gloves, performed hand hygiene.

18. Stayed with patient, observed for allergic reactions.

EVALUATION

1. Returned to room in 15 to 30 minutes; asked if patient felt pain, burning, numbness, or tingling at injection site.

2. Asked patient to discuss implications of skin testing and signs of hypersensitivity.

3. Inspected bleb, drew circle around injection site with skin pencil if necessary.

4. Identified unexpected outcomes.

	S	U	NP	Comments

RECORDING AND REPORTING

1. Recorded drug, dose, route, site, and time on MAR; signed MAR.

2. Recorded area of ID injection and appearance of skin.

3. Reported undesirable effects to health care provider, documented adverse effects properly.

4. Recorded patient teaching, validation of understanding, and patient's response to medication.

Student _____ Date _____

Instructor _____ Date _____

PERFORMANCE CHECKLIST SKILL 22-3 **ADMINSTERING SUBCUTANEOUS INJECTIONS**

	S	U	NP	Comments
ASSESSMENT				
1. Checked accuracy and completeness of MAR with medication order, reprinted/recopied any portion of MAR that was difficult to read.	___	___	___	_____
2. Assessed patient's medical and medication history.	___	___	___	_____
3. Assessed patient's history of allergies.	___	___	___	_____
4. Reviewed all relevant medication information.	___	___	___	_____
5. Observed patient's previous verbal and nonverbal responses to injection.	___	___	___	_____
6. Assessed for contraindication to subcutaneous injections.	___	___	___	_____
7. Assessed patient's symptoms before initiating therapy.	___	___	___	_____
8. Assessed adequacy of patient's adipose tissue.	___	___	___	_____
9. Assessed patient's knowledge of medication.	___	___	___	_____
PLANNING				
1. Identified expected outcomes.	___	___	___	_____
IMPLEMENTATION				
1. Performed hand hygiene, prepared medication using aseptic technique, checked label of medication with MAR twice.	___	___	___	_____
2. Took medication to patient at correct time, applied the six rights of medication administration.	___	___	___	_____
3. Provided privacy.	___	___	___	_____
4. Identified patient using two identifiers.	___	___	___	_____
5. Compared MAR with medication labels at bedside, asked patient if he or she had allergies.	___	___	___	_____
6. Discussed purpose of each medication, action, and possible adverse effects; allowed patient to ask questions; told patient injection would cause a slight burning or stinging sensation.	___	___	___	_____

	S	U	NP	Comments

7. Performed hand hygiene, applied clean gloves, kept sheet draped over body parts not requiring exposure. ___ ___ ___ _____

8. Selected appropriate injection site, inspected skin over site. ___ ___ ___ _____

9. Palpated sites, avoided those with masses or tenderness, ensured needle was correct size by measuring skinfold. ___ ___ ___ _____

10. Assisted patient to comfortable position, had patient relax site. ___ ___ ___ _____

11. Relocated site using anatomic landmarks. ___ ___ ___ _____

12. Cleansed site properly with antiseptic swab. ___ ___ ___ _____

13. Held swab in nondominant hand. ___ ___ ___ _____

14. Removed needle cap or sheath. ___ ___ ___ _____

15. Held syringe properly in dominant hand. ___ ___ ___ _____

16. Administered injection.

   a. Held skin across injection site. ___ ___ ___ _____

   b. Injected needle at appropriate angle quickly and firmly, released skin if pinched. ___ ___ ___ _____

   c. Adjusted injection technique for obese patient if necessary. ___ ___ ___ _____

   d. Stabilized lower end of syringe barrel with nondominant hand, injected medication slowly, avoided moving syringe. ___ ___ ___ _____

   e. Withdrew needle quickly while placing swab or gauze over site. ___ ___ ___ _____

17. Applied pressure to site, *did not massage site.* ___ ___ ___ _____

18. Assisted patient to comfortable position. ___ ___ ___ _____

19. Discarded uncapped needle or needle enclosed in safety shield and attached syringe into puncture- and leak-proof receptacle. ___ ___ ___ _____

20. Removed gloves, performed hand hygiene. ___ ___ ___ _____

21. Stayed with patient for several minutes, observed for any allergic reactions. ___ ___ ___ _____

EVALUATION

1. Returned to room in 15 to 30 minutes; asked if patient felt pain, burning, numbness, or tingling at injection site. ___ ___ ___ _____

2. Inspected site, noted bruising or induration, provided warm compress to site. ___ ___ ___ _____

	S	U	NP	Comments

3. Observed patient's response to medication at time correlating with medication's onset, peak, and duration.

4. Asked patient to explain purpose and effects of medication.

5. Identified unexpected outcomes.

RECORDING AND REPORTING

1. Recorded medication, dose, route, site, and time on MAR immediately after administration; signed MAR properly.

2. Recorded patient teaching, validation of understanding, and patient's response to medication in nurses' notes.

3. Reported any undesirable effects to health care provider, documented adverse effects in record.

Student _____ Date _____

Instructor _____ Date _____

PERFORMANCE CHECKLIST SKILL 22-4 **ADMINISTERING INTRAMUSCULAR INJECTIONS**

	S	U	NP	Comments

ASSESSMENT

1. Checked accuracy and completeness of each MAR with medication order, reprinted/recopied any portion of MAR that was difficult to read. _____ _____ _____ _____

2. Assessed patient's medical and medication history. _____ _____ _____ _____

3. Assessed patient's history of allergies. _____ _____ _____ _____

4. Reviewed medication reference information. _____ _____ _____ _____

5. Observed patient's previous verbal and nonverbal responses toward injection. _____ _____ _____ _____

6. Assessed for contraindications to IM injections. _____ _____ _____ _____

7. Assessed patient's symptoms before initiating therapy. _____ _____ _____ _____

8. Assessed patient's knowledge regarding medication to be received. _____ _____ _____ _____

PLANNING

1. Identified expected outcomes. _____ _____ _____ _____

IMPLEMENTATION

1. Prepared medication for one patient at a time, kept all pages of MAR for one patient together, checked label of medication with MAR twice. _____ _____ _____ _____

2. Took medication to patient at correct time, applied the six rights of medication administration. _____ _____ _____ _____

3. Provided privacy. _____ _____ _____ _____

4. Identified patient using two identifiers. _____ _____ _____ _____

5. Compared MAR with medication labels at bedside, asked patient if he or she had allergies. _____ _____ _____ _____

6. Discussed purpose of each medication, action, and possible adverse effects. _____ _____ _____ _____

7. Performed hand hygiene, applied clean gloves, kept sheet over body parts not requiring exposure. _____ _____ _____ _____

8. Selected appropriate site, noted integrity and size of muscle, palpated for and avoided areas of tenderness or hardness, rotated sites if necessary. _____ _____ _____ _____

	S	U	NP	Comments
9. Assisted patient to comfortable position.	___	___	___	_____
10. Relocated site using anatomic landmarks.	___	___	___	_____
11. Cleansed site with antiseptic swab.	___	___	___	_____
12. Held swab in nondominant hand.	___	___	___	_____
13. Removed needle cap or sheath.	___	___	___	_____
14. Held syringe properly in dominant hand.	___	___	___	_____
15. Administered injection.				
a. Positioned nondominant hand below site and pulled skin, injected needle appropriately into muscle.	___	___	___	_____
b. Grasped body of muscle if necessary.	___	___	___	_____
c. Stabilized end of syringe barrel, moved dominant hand to plunger, avoided moving syringe.	___	___	___	_____
d. Pulled back on plunger, injected medication slowly if no blood appeared.	___	___	___	_____
e. Waited 10 seconds, withdrew needle, released skin, applied gauze over site.	___	___	___	_____
16. Applied pressure to site, did not massage site, applied bandage if needed.	___	___	___	_____
17. Assisted patient to comfortable position.	___	___	___	_____
18. Discarded needle and syringe into a puncture- and leak-proof receptacle.	___	___	___	_____
19. Removed gloves, performed hand hygiene.	___	___	___	_____
20. Stayed with patient, observed for allergic reactions.	___	___	___	_____

EVALUATION

	S	U	NP	Comments
1. Returned to room in 15 to 30 minutes; asked if patient felt any pain, numbness, or tingling at injection site.	___	___	___	_____
2. Inspected site, noted bruising or induration, applied warm compress to site.	___	___	___	_____
3. Observed patient's response to medication at times that correlate with medication's onset, peak, and duration.	___	___	___	_____
4. Asked patient to explain purpose and effects of medication.	___	___	___	_____
5. Identified unexpected outcomes.	___	___	___	_____

	S	U	NP	Comments

RECORDING AND REPORTING

1. Recorded medication, dose, route, site, and time given on MAR immediately after administration; signed MAR properly. ___ ___ ___ _____

2. Recorded patient's teaching, validation of understanding, and patient's response to medication in nurses' notes. ___ ___ ___ _____

3. Reported any undesirable effects to health care provider, documented adverse effects in record. ___ ___ ___ _____

Student _____ Date _____

Instructor _____ Date _____

PERFORMANCE CHECKLIST SKILL 22-5 **ADMINISTERING MEDICATIONS BY INTRAVENOUS BOLUS**

	S	U	NP	Comments
ASSESSMENT				
1. Checked accuracy and completeness of each MAR with medication order, reprinted/recopied any portion of MAR that was difficult to read.	___	___	___	_____
2. Assessed patient's medical and medication history.	___	___	___	_____
3. Reviewed medication reference information.	___	___	___	_____
4. Determined compatibility with IV fluids and additives if necessary.	___	___	___	_____
5. Performed hand hygiene, assessed condition of insertion site for signs of infiltration of phlebitis.	___	___	___	_____
6. Assessed patency of patient's existing IV infusion line or saline lock.	___	___	___	_____
7. Checked patient's history of medication allergies.	___	___	___	_____
8. Assessed patient's symptoms before initiating medication therapy.	___	___	___	_____
9. Assessed patient's understanding of purpose of drug therapy.	___	___	___	_____
PLANNING				
1. Identified expected outcomes.	___	___	___	_____
IMPLEMENTATION				
1. Prepared medications for one patient at a time, kept all pages of MAR for one patient together, checked label of medication with MAR twice.	___	___	___	_____
2. Took medication to patient at correct time, applied the six rights of medication administration.	___	___	___	_____
3. Provided privacy.	___	___	___	_____
4. Identified patient using two identifiers.	___	___	___	_____
5. Compared MAR with medication labels at bedside, asked patient if he or she had allergies.	___	___	___	_____
6. Discussed purpose of each medication, action, and possible adverse effects; allowed patient to ask any questions; explained that medication would be given through existing IV line; encouraged patient to report symptoms of discomfort at IV site.	___	___	___	_____

	S	U	NP	Comments

7. Performed hand hygiene, applied clean gloves. ____ ____ ____ _____

8. Performed IV push using existing line.

   a. Selected injection port of IV closest to patient, used needleless injection port. ____ ____ ____ _____

   b. Cleaned injection port with antiseptic swab, allowed to dry. ____ ____ ____ _____

   c. Connected needleless tip of syringe to IV line. ____ ____ ____ _____

   d. Occluded IV line by pinching tubing, aspirated for blood return. ____ ____ ____ _____

   e. Released tubing, injected medication, timed administration, allowed IV to infuse when not pushing medication. ____ ____ ____ _____

   f. Withdrew syringe, rechecked IV fluid infusion rate. ____ ____ ____ _____

   g. Stopped IV fluids, clamped line, and flushed line if medication was incompatible with fluids; flushed again after administration at *same rate* as medication. ____ ____ ____ _____

   h. Verified agency policy for stopping IV fluids and medications, disconnected IV line and administered IV push or started and new IV site as appropriate. ____ ____ ____ _____

9. Performed IV push using IV lock.

   a. Prepared flush solutions according to agency policy. ____ ____ ____ _____

   b. Administered medication.

     (1) Cleaned injection port with antiseptic swab. ____ ____ ____ _____

     (2) Inserted syringe with normal saline 0.9% through injection port of IV lock. ____ ____ ____ _____

     (3) Pulled back on plunger, checked for blood return. ____ ____ ____ _____

     (4) Flushed IV site. ____ ____ ____ _____

     (5) Removed saline-filled syringe. ____ ____ ____ _____

     (6) Cleaned injection port with antiseptic swab. ____ ____ ____ _____

     (7) Inserted syringe containing prepared medication through injection port. ____ ____ ____ _____

     (8) Injected medication, used a watch to time administration. ____ ____ ____ _____

     (9) Withdrew syringe. ____ ____ ____ _____

	S	U	NP	Comments
(10) Cleaned injection port with antiseptic swab.	___	___	___	_____
(11) Flushed injection port, injected flush at the same rate medication was delivered.	___	___	___	_____
10. Disposed of uncapped needles and syringes in puncture- and leak-proof container.	___	___	___	_____
11. Stayed with patient for several minutes, observed for allergic reactions.	___	___	___	_____
12. Removed clean gloves, performed hand hygiene.	___	___	___	_____

EVALUATION

	S	U	NP	Comments
1. Observed patient for adverse reactions during and after administration.	___	___	___	_____
2. Observed IV site during and after injection for sudden swelling.	___	___	___	_____
3. Assessed patient's status after giving medication to evaluate effectiveness.	___	___	___	_____
4. Asked patient to explain medication's purpose and side effects.	___	___	___	_____
5. Identified unexpected outcomes.	___	___	___	_____

RECORDING AND REPORTING

	S	U	NP	Comments
1. Recorded drug, dose, route, and time on MAR immediately after administration; included initials or signature.	___	___	___	_____
2. Reported any adverse reactions to health care provider.	___	___	___	_____
3. Recorded patient's medication response in nurses' notes.	___	___	___	_____

Student _____ Date _____

Instructor _____ Date _____

PERFORMANCE CHECKLIST SKILL 22-6 ADMINISTERING INTRAVENOUS MEDICATION BY PIGGYBACK, INTERMITTENT INFUSION SETS, AND MINI-INFUSION PUMPS

	S	U	NP	Comments
ASSESSMENT				
1. Checked accuracy and completeness of each MAR with medication order, reprinted/recopied any portion of MAR that was difficult to read.	___	___	___	_____
2. Assessed patient's medical and medication history.	___	___	___	_____
3. Assessed patient's history of allergies.	___	___	___	_____
4. Reviewed medication reference information.	___	___	___	_____
5. Determined compatibility of medication with IV fluids if giving medication through existing IV line.	___	___	___	_____
6. Assessed patency of patient's existing IV infusion line or saline lock.	___	___	___	_____
7. Assessed patient's symptoms before initiating therapy.	___	___	___	_____
8. Assessed patient's knowledge of medication.	___	___	___	_____
PLANNING				
1. Identified expected outcomes.	___	___	___	_____
IMPLEMENTATION				
1. Prepared medications for one patient at a time, kept all pages of MAR for one patient together, checked label of medication with MAR twice.	___	___	___	_____
2. Took medication to patient at correct time, applied the six rights of medication administration.	___	___	___	_____
3. Provided privacy.	___	___	___	_____
4. Identified patient using two identifiers.	___	___	___	_____
5. Compared MAR with medication labels at bedside, asked patient if he or she had allergies.	___	___	___	_____
6. Discussed purpose of each medication, action, and possible adverse effects; allowed patient to ask questions; explained you would give medication through existing IV line; encouraged patient to report discomfort at the site.	___	___	___	_____

	S	U	NP	Comments

7. Administered infusion.

   a. Piggyback infusion:

     (1) Connected infusion tubing to medication bag, filled tubing, closed clamp, capped end of tubing. ____ ____ ____ _____

     (2) Hung piggyback medication bag above level of primary fluid bag. ____ ____ ____ _____

     (3) Connected infusion tubing to appropriate connector on upper Y-port of primary infusion line. ____ ____ ____ _____

     (4) Flushed and prepared saline lock if necessary, wiped port with alcohol, let dry, inserted tip of infusion tubing via needleless access. ____ ____ ____ _____

     (5) Regulated flow rate of medication, referred to medication reference for safe flow rate. ____ ____ ____ _____

     (6) Checked flow rate of primary infusion or disconnected tubing, cleansed port, and flushed IV line after infusion. ____ ____ ____ _____

     (7) Regulated continuous main infusion line to ordered rate. ____ ____ ____ _____

     (8) Left IV piggyback and tubing in place or discarded in puncture- and leak-proof container. ____ ____ ____ _____

   b. Volume-control administration set:

     (1) Filled Volutrol with desired amount of IV fluid. ____ ____ ____ _____

     (2) Closed clamp, ensured clamp on air vent Volutrol chamber was open. ____ ____ ____ _____

     (3) Cleaned injection port with antiseptic swab. ____ ____ ____ _____

     (4) Removed needle cap, inserted needleless syringe or needle through port, injected medication, rotated Volutrol between hands. ____ ____ ____ _____

     (5) Regulated IV infusion rate. ____ ____ ____ _____

     (6) Labeled Volutrol with all pertinent information following ISMP safe medication label format. ____ ____ ____ _____

314

	S	U	NP	Comments

(7) Checked continuous infusion after completion of Volutrol infusion.

(8) Disposed of uncapped needle or needle enclosed in safety shield and syringe in puncture- and leak-proof-container, discarded supplies in appropriate container, performed hand hygiene.

  c. Mini-infusion administration:

    (1) Connected prefilled syringe to mini-infusion tubing, removed end cap.

    (2) Applied pressure to plunger, allowed tubing to fill with medication.

    (3) Placed syringe into mini-infusion pump and hung on IV pole, ensured syringe was secured.

    (4) Connected end of mini-infusion tubing properly to main IV line or saline lock

    (5) Checked flow rate or disconnected tubing, cleansed port with alcohol, and flushed IV line after infusion.

8. Disposed of supplies in puncture- and leak-proof container.

9. Performed hand hygiene.

10. Stayed with patient, observed for allergic reactions.

EVALUATION

1. Observed patient for signs or symptoms of adverse reaction.

2. Checked infusion rate and condition of IV site periodically during infusion.

3. Asked patient to explain purpose and side effects of medication.

4. Identified unexpected outcomes.

RECORDING AND REPORTING

1. Recorded medication, dose, route, rate, and time on MAR immediately; included initials or signature.

2. Recorded volume of fluid in bag or Volutrol on I&O form.

3. Reported any adverse reaction to health care provider.

Student _____ Date _____

Instructor _____ Date _____

PERFORMANCE CHECKLIST SKILL 22-7 **ADMINISTERING CONTINUOUS SUBCUTANEOUS MEDICATIONS**

	S	U	NP	Comments

ASSESSMENT

1. Checked accuracy and completeness of each MAR with medication order, reprinted/recopied any portion of MAR that was difficult to read.

2. Assessed patient's medical and medication history.

3. Assessed patient's history of allergies.

4. Reviewed medication reference information.

5. Assessed patient's previous verbal and nonverbal response to needle insertion.

6. Assessed for contraindications to CSQI.

7. Assessed adequacy of patient's adipose tissue to determine appropriate site.

8. Assessed patient's knowledge of medication and use of medication pump.

9. Assessed patient's symptoms before initiating therapy, determined severity of pain or measured blood glucose level.

PLANNING

1. Identified expected outcomes.

IMPLEMENTATION

1. Reviewed manufacturer's directions for pump.

2. Performed hand hygiene, prepared medication or checked dose on prefilled syringe, connected syringe and prime tubing, compared label of medication with MAR twice.

3. Obtained and programmed medication administration pump, placed syringe in pump.

4. Compared label on prefilled syringe with MAR.

5. Identified patient using two identifiers.

6. Compared MAR with medication labels at bedside, asked if patient had any allergies.

7. Discussed purpose of each medication, action, and possible adverse effects; allowed patient to ask questions; told patient needle insertion would cause slight burning or stinging.

	S	U	NP	Comments

8. Positioned patient, draped, and provided privacy. ___ ___ ___ _____

9. Initiated CSQI.

   a. Assisted patient to comfortable position. ___ ___ ___ _____

   b. Selected appropriate injection site. ___ ___ ___ _____

   c. Performed hand hygiene, applied clean gloves, cleansed injection site with alcohol and antiseptic, allowed both to dry. ___ ___ ___ _____

   d. Held needle in dominant hand, removed needle guard. ___ ___ ___ _____

   e. Pinched or lifted up skin with nondominant hand. ___ ___ ___ _____

   f. Inserted needle per manufacturer's directions. ___ ___ ___ _____

   g. Released skinfold, applied tape over "wings" of needle. ___ ___ ___ _____

   h. Placed occlusive, transparent dressing over insertion site. ___ ___ ___ _____

   i. Attached needle tubing to pump tubing, turned pump on. ___ ___ ___ _____

   j. Disposed of sharps in puncture- and leak-proof container, discarded used supplies, removed gloves, performed hand hygiene. ___ ___ ___ _____

   k. Inspected site before leaving, instructed patient to inform you if site became red or leaked. ___ ___ ___ _____

   l. Stayed with patient, observed for allergic reactions. ___ ___ ___ _____

10. Discontinued CSQL.

   a. Verified order, established alternative method for administration if applicable. ___ ___ ___ _____

   b. Stopped infusion pump. ___ ___ ___ _____

   c. Performed hand hygiene. Applied clean gloves. ___ ___ ___ _____

   d. Removed dressing without dislodging or removing needle. ___ ___ ___ _____

   e. Removed tape from wings of needle, pulled needle out at same angle it was inserted. ___ ___ ___ _____

   f. Applied pressure at site until no fluid leaked out of skin. ___ ___ ___ _____

   g. Applied sterile gauze or adhesive bandage to site. ___ ___ ___ _____

	S	U	NP	Comments
11. Disposed of uncapped needles and syringes in puncture-poof and leak-proof container.	——	——	——	———————
12. Removed and disposed of gloves, performed hand hygiene.	——	——	——	———————

EVALUATION

1. Evaluated patient's response to medication.	——	——	——	———————
2. Assessed site every 4 hours for redness, pain, drainage, or swelling.	——	——	——	———————
3. Asked patient to explain understanding of medication and CSQI therapy.	——	——	——	———————
4. Identified unexpected outcomes.	——	——	——	———————

RECORDING AND REPORTING

1. Recorded drug, dose, route, site, time, and type of pump in patient's medical record immediately after initiating CSQI; used initials or signature.	——	——	——	———————
2. Followed policy for documentation of opioid waste.	——	——	——	———————
3. Recorded patient's response to medication and appearance of site every 4 hours in nurses' notes.	——	——	——	———————
4. Documented and reported adverse side effects from medication or infection at insertion site to patient's health care provider.	——	——	——	———————

Student _____ Date _____

Instructor _____ Date _____

PERFORMANCE CHECKLIST SKILL 23-1 **APPLYING A NASAL CANNULA OR OXYGEN MASK**

	S	U	NP	Comments
ASSESSMENT				
1. Assessed patient's respiratory status.	___	___	___	_____
2. Observed for patent airway, removed airway secretions by having patient cough or by suctioning.	___	___	___	_____
3. Noted patient's most recent ABG results or SpO_2 value.	___	___	___	_____
4. Reviewed patient's medical record for order for oxygen.	___	___	___	_____
PLANNING				
1. Identified expected outcomes.	___	___	___	_____
2. Explained procedure to patient and family.	___	___	___	_____
IMPLEMENTATION				
1. Performed hand hygiene, applied face shield if indicated.	___	___	___	_____
2. Identified patient using two identifiers.	___	___	___	_____
3. Attached oxygen delivery device to oxygen tubing, attached to humidified oxygen source adjusted to prescribed flow rate.	___	___	___	_____
4. Positioned tips of cannula properly in nares, adjusted fit of cannula or face mask to a snug fit.	___	___	___	_____
5. Maintained sufficient slack on oxygen tubing, secured to patient's clothes.	___	___	___	_____
6. Observed for proper function of oxygen delivery device.	___	___	___	_____
7. Verified setting on flowmeter and oxygen source for proper setup and prescribed flow rate.	___	___	___	_____
8. Checked cannula/mask every 8 hours, kept humidification container filled at all times.	___	___	___	_____
9. Posted "Oxygen in Use" signs as needed.	___	___	___	_____
10. Performed hand hygiene.	___	___	___	_____
EVALUATION				
1. Monitored patient's response to changes in flow rate with SpO_2.	___	___	___	_____
2. Observed for improvement in physical signs and symptoms.	___	___	___	_____

	S	U	NP	Comments
3. Assessed adequacy of oxygen flow each shift.	____	____	____	_____
4. Observed patient's ears, nose, nares, and nasal mucous membranes for evidence of skin breakdown.	____	____	____	_____
5. Identified unexpected outcomes.	____	____	____	_____

RECORDING AND REPORTING

	S	U	NP	Comments
1. Recorded all pertinent information in the appropriate log.	____	____	____	_____
2. Reported unexpected outcomes to health care provider or nurse in charge.	____	____	____	_____

Student _____ Date _____

Instructor _____ Date _____

PERFORMANCE CHECKLIST SKILL 23-2 **ADMINISTERING OXYGEN THERAPY TO A PATIENT WITH AN ARTIFICIAL AIRWAY**

	S	U	NP	Comments
ASSESSMENT				
1. Assessed patient's respiratory status.	___	___	___	_____
2. Observed for patent airway, removed airway secretions by having patient cough and by suctioning.	___	___	___	_____
3. Monitored SpO$_2$, noted patient's most recent ABG levels.	___	___	___	_____
4. Reviewed patient's medical record for order for oxygen; noted delivery mother, flow rate, and duration of oxygen therapy.	___	___	___	_____
PLANNING				
1. Identified expected outcomes.	___	___	___	_____
2. Explained purpose of T tube or tracheostomy collar to patient and family.	___	___	___	_____
IMPLEMENTATION				
1. Performed hand hygiene, applied clean gloves and other appropriate PPE.	___	___	___	_____
2. Identified patient using two identifiers.	___	___	___	_____
3. Attached T tube or tracheostomy collar to oxygen tubing and to humidified air or oxygen source if indicated.	___	___	___	_____
4. Adjusted flow rate properly if oxygen was ordered, adjusted nebulizer to proper FiO$_2$ setting, attached T tube or tracheostomy collar to ET or tracheostomy tube.	___	___	___	_____
5. Observed that T tube does not pull on ET or tracheostomy tube.	___	___	___	_____
6. Observed oxygen tubing for accumulation of fluid, drained tube away from patient if necessary, disconnected from collar or T tube, discarded fluid in proper receptacle.	___	___	___	_____
7. Set up suction equipment at patient's bedside.	___	___	___	_____
8. Removed gloves and goggles, performed hand hygiene.	___	___	___	_____

	S	U	NP	Comments

EVALUATION

1. Monitored patient's ABG levels or measured SpO$_2$. ___ ___ ___ _____

2. Observed position of oxygen delivery device, ensured it was not pulling on the artificial airway. ___ ___ ___ _____

3. Monitored patient's vital signs, palpated chest excursion, and observed patient's behavior. ___ ___ ___ _____

4. Identified unexpected outcomes. ___ ___ ___ _____

RECORDING AND REPORTING

1. Recorded all pertinent information in the appropriate log. ___ ___ ___ _____

2. Reported unexpected outcomes to health care provider or nurse in charge. ___ ___ ___ _____

Student _____ Date _____

Instructor _____ Date _____

PERFORMANCE CHECKLIST SKILL 23-3 **USING INCENTIVE SPIROMETRY**

	S	U	NP	Comments
ASSESSMENT				
1. Identified patients who would benefit from incentive spirometry.	___	___	___	_____
2. Assessed patient for confusion, malnutrition, cognitive impairment, and decreased necessary motor skills.	___	___	___	_____
3. Assessed patient's respiratory status.	___	___	___	_____
4. Assessed level of pain.	___	___	___	_____
5. Reviewed health care provider's order for incentive spirometry.	___	___	___	_____
PLANNING				
1. Identified expected outcomes.	___	___	___	_____
2. Explained procedure to patient and family.	___	___	___	_____
3. Indicated to patient where the target volume is on the IS, demonstrated use if possible.	___	___	___	_____
IMPLEMENTATION				
1. Performed hand hygiene.	___	___	___	_____
2. Positioned patient in appropriate position.	___	___	___	_____
3. Instructed patient to exhale completely and place lips tightly around mouthpiece.	___	___	___	_____
4. Instructed patient to take slow, deep breath and maintain a constant flow.	___	___	___	_____
5. Had patient repeat maneuver, encouraged patient to reach prescribed goal.	___	___	___	_____
6. Reminded patient to perform IS exercises 5 to 10 times, followed by controlled coughing every hour, kept IS device within patient's reach.	___	___	___	_____
7. Performed hand hygiene.	___	___	___	_____
EVALUATION				
1. Observed patient's ability to use incentive spirometer by return demonstration.	___	___	___	_____
2. Assessed if patient was able to achieve target volume or frequency.	___	___	___	_____
3. Auscultated chest during respiratory cycle.	___	___	___	_____
4. Identified unexpected outcomes.	___	___	___	_____

	S	U	NP	Comments

RECORDING AND REPORTING

1. Recorded lung sounds before and after incentive spirometry, frequency of use, volumes achieved, and adverse effects. ___ ___ ___ _____

2. Reported changes in respiratory assessment or patient's inability to use IS to health care provider. ___ ___ ___ _____

Student _____ Date _____

Instructor _____ Date _____

PERFORMANCE CHECKLIST SKILL 23-4 **CARE OF A PATIENT RECEIVING NONINVASIVE POSITIVE-PRESSURE VENTILATION**

	S	U	NP	Comments
ASSESSMENT				
1. Assessed patient's respiratory status.	___	___	___	_____
2. Observed patient's skin over bridge of nose, around ears, and back of head.	___	___	___	_____
3. Observed patient's ability to clear and remove airway secretions by coughing.	___	___	___	_____
4. Obtained pulse oximetry results, noted most recent ABG results.	___	___	___	_____
5. Obtained vital signs and pulse oximetry before initiation of therapy.	___	___	___	_____
6. Reviewed patient's medical record for medical order for CPAP/BiPAP and appropriate settings.	___	___	___	_____
PLANNING				
1. Identified expected outcomes.	___	___	___	_____
2. Explained to patient and family purpose and reasons for CPAP/BiPAP.	___	___	___	_____
IMPLEMENTATION				
1. Performed hand hygiene, applied clean gloves and any necessary PPE.	___	___	___	_____
2. Identified patient using two identifiers.	___	___	___	_____
3. Determined correct mask size.	___	___	___	_____
4. Connected CPAP/BiPAP device delivery tubing to pressure generator.	___	___	___	_____
5. Connected patient to pulse oximetry.	___	___	___	_____
6. Set CPAP/BiPAP initial settings properly.	___	___	___	_____
7. Performed frequent skin assessment to determine presence of pressure, skin irritation, or skin breakdown.	___	___	___	_____
8. Disposed of supplies appropriately, removed gloves, performed hand hygiene.	___	___	___	_____

	S	U	NP	Comments

EVALUATION

1. Observed for decreased anxiety, improved LOC and cognitive abilities, and other indicators of response to therapy. ____ ____ ____ _____

2. Monitored pulse oximetry. ____ ____ ____ _____

3. Observed skin integrity over bridge of nose. ____ ____ ____ _____

4. Observed and monitored patient's and family's ability to manipulate device and face mask if NIPPV is planned for use in the home. ____ ____ ____ _____

5. Identified unexpected outcomes. ____ ____ ____ _____

RECORDING AND REPORTING

1. Recorded respiratory findings, CPAP/BiPAP settings, vital signs, pulse oximetry, patient response, and patient teaching outcomes. ____ ____ ____ _____

2. Reported sudden change in respiratory status and decline in ABG levels or pulse oximetry values to nurse in charge or health care provider. ____ ____ ____ _____

Student _____ Date _____

Instructor _____ Date _____

PERFORMANCE CHECKLIST PROCEDURAL GUIDELINE 23-1 **USE OF A PEAK FLOW METER**

	S	U	NP	Comments
PROCEDURAL STEPS				
1. Assessed previous PEFR readings and target set by patient's health care provider.	___	___	___	_____
2. Instructed patient about purpose and rationale.	___	___	___	_____
3. Assisted patient to appropriate position.	___	___	___	_____
4. Slid mouthpiece into base of numbered scale at zero position.	___	___	___	_____
5. Instructed patient to take deep breath.	___	___	___	_____
6. Had patient place meter mouthpiece in mouth and close lips firmly.	___	___	___	_____
7. Had patient blow out hard and fast in one breath.	___	___	___	_____
8. Repeated maneuver twice, recorded highest number in chart.	___	___	___	_____
9. Had patient demonstrate PEFR technique independently, assessed ability to record PEFR accurately on chart.	___	___	___	_____
10. Helped patient implement an appropriate action plan.	___	___	___	_____
11. Instructed patient to clean unit weekly following manufacturer instructions.	___	___	___	_____

Student _____ Date _____

Instructor _____ Date _____

PERFORMANCE CHECKLIST SKILL 23-5 **CARE OF PATIENT ON A MECHANICAL VENTILATOR**

	S	U	NP	Comments
ASSESSMENT				
1. Assessed patient's LOC, ability to cooperate, and need for special positioning.	___	___	___	_____
2. Assessed patient's need for sedation.	___	___	___	_____
3. Assessed patient's respiratory status.	___	___	___	_____
4. Checked ventilator, $EtCO_2$ (if available), SpO_2, and ventilator and cardiac alarms at appropriate times; compared with health care provider's orders.				
5. Applied gloves, verified placement of artificial airway, determined that tube was securely placed.	___	___	___	_____
a. Auscultated over trachea for presence of air leak.	___	___	___	_____
b. Checked inflation of cuff of artificial airway.	___	___	___	_____
6. Observed for patent airway, removed secretions by suctioning if necessary, removed and disposed of gloves, performed hand hygiene.	___	___	___	_____
7. Noted patient's most recent ABG results or SpO_2, determined if any factors changed during mechanical ventilation.	___	___	___	_____
8. Determined method for communication with patient, reviewed previous communication techniques if possible.	___	___	___	_____
9. Reviewed patient's medical record for order for mechanical ventilation; noted mode, rate, oxygen settings, and tidal volume.	___	___	___	_____
PLANNING	S	U	NP	
1. Identified expected outcomes.	___	___	___	_____
2. Explained ventilator system to patient and family, included purpose and reasons for initiation of mechanical ventilation.	___	___	___	_____
3. Positioned patient properly.	___	___	___	_____

	S	U	NP	Comments

IMPLEMENTATION

1. Performed hand hygiene, applied clean gloves and other PPE.

2. Identified patient using two identifiers.

3. Attached mechanical ventilator to ET or tracheostomy tube, observed for proper functioning of mechanical ventilator.

4. Verified that ET or tracheostomy tube was properly positioned during an inspiratory and expiratory cycle.

5. Observed patient for synchronization with mechanical ventilation and response to therapy.

6. Monitored heart rate, blood pressure, respiratory rate, and cardiac rhythm.

7. Reassessed and marked level of ET tube at the lips or nares.

8. Set up suctioning equipment.

9. Repositioned patient to promote best oxygenation and ventilation, monitored SpO_2 levels during and after positioning.

10. Collaborated with health care provider about status of patient, response to therapy, and ongoing monitoring.

11. Performed hourly safety checks on patient and ventilator system.

    a. Ensured patient could reach call light.

    b. Checked security of all ventilator connections, ensured all alarms were turned on.

    c. Verified all settings were correct and corresponded to health care provider's orders.

    d. Checked and refilled humidifier, checked tubing for condensation, drained and appropriately discarded any liquid.

    e. Observed temperature gauges, ensured gas was delivered at correct temperature.

12. Performed mouth care at least four times per 24 hours.

13. Performed nursing activities to prevent hazards of immobility.

14. Kept patient informed on progress and plan for weaning from mechanical ventilator.

15. Removed PPE, performed hand hygiene.

	S	U	NP	Comments

EVALUATION

1. Reassessed and monitored patient's response to mechanical ventilation every 2 to 4 hours. ___ ___ ___ _____

2. Observed pulse oximetry, monitored gas exchange. ___ ___ ___ _____

3. Observed integrity of patient ventilator system. ___ ___ ___ _____

4. Observed and evaluated effectiveness of communication methods. ___ ___ ___ _____

5. Identified unexpected outcomes. ___ ___ ___ _____

RECORDING AND REPORTING

1. Recorded all pertinent information in progress notes. ___ ___ ___ _____

2. Reported sudden change in patient's respiratory status and ventilator-associated problems to nurse in charge or health care provider. ___ ___ ___ _____

Student _____ Date _____

Instructor _____ Date _____

PERFORMANCE CHECKLIST SKILL 24-1 **PERFORMING POSTURAL DRAINAGE**

	S	U	NP	Comments

ASSESSMENT

1. Assessed patient for history of decreased LOC and muscle weakness or disease processes.

2. Reviewed medical record; assessed for signs and symptoms consistent with atelectasis, lobar collapse pneumonia, or bronchiectasis; ineffective coughing; thick, sticky, tenacious, and discolored secretions that are difficult to cough up.

3. Auscultated all lung fields for decreased breath sounds and adventitious lung sounds.

4. Assessed vital signs and pulse oximetry before postural drainage treatment.

5. Determined patient's and caregiver's understanding of and ability to perform home postural drainage.

6. Determined patient's comfort level.

PLANNING

1. Identified expected outcomes.

2. Prepared patient for procedure.

    a. Administered analgesia 20 minutes before CPT maneuvers if necessary.

    b. Explained purpose and rationale for procedure, explained details of procedure.

    c. Encouraged high fluid intake program unless contraindicated and if approved, maintained record of fluid I&O.

    d. Planned treatments so they did not overlap with meals or tube feeding, stopped gastric tube feedings for 30 to 45 minutes before postural drainage, checked for residual feeding in patient's stomach, held treatment if necessary.

    e. Scheduled treatments at appropriate times.

    f. Had patient remove any restrictive clothing.

	S	U	NP	Comments

IMPLEMENTATION

1. Provided privacy, performed hand hygiene, applied gloves. ____ ____ ____ _____

2. Identified patient using two identifiers. ____ ____ ____ _____

3. Used findings from physical assessment and chest x-ray film to select congested areas for drainage. ____ ____ ____ _____

4. Assisted patient to appropriate position, placed pillows for support and comfort, draped patient appropriately. ____ ____ ____ _____

5. Had patient maintain posture for 10 to 15 minutes. ____ ____ ____ _____

6. Performed chest percussion, vibration, and shaking during 15 minutes. ____ ____ ____ _____

7. Had patient sit up and cough, saved secretions if necessary, suctioned if necessary. ____ ____ ____ _____

8. Had patient rest briefly if necessary. ____ ____ ____ _____

9. Had patient take sips of water. ____ ____ ____ _____

10. Repeated steps 4 through 9, ensured each treatment did not exceed 30 to 60 minutes. ____ ____ ____ _____

11. Offered or assisted patient with oral hygiene. ____ ____ ____ _____

12. Performed hand hygiene. ____ ____ ____ _____

EVALUATION

1. Auscultated lung fields. ____ ____ ____ _____

2. Inspected character and amount of sputum. ____ ____ ____ _____

3. Reviewed diagnostic reports. ____ ____ ____ _____

4. Obtained vital signs and pulse oximetry. ____ ____ ____ _____

5. Identified unexpected outcomes. ____ ____ ____ _____

RECORDING AND REPORTING

1. Recorded all pertinent information in the appropriate log. ____ ____ ____ _____

2. Charted all pertinent information about patient and caregiver instruction. ____ ____ ____ _____

Student _____ Date _____

Instructor _____ Date _____

PERFORMANCE CHECKLIST PROCEDURAL 24-1 **USING AN ACAPELLA DEVICE**

	S	U	NP	Comments
PROCEDURAL STEPS				
1. Verified need for a health care provider's order.	___	___	___	_____
2. Identified patient using two identifiers.	___	___	___	_____
3. Assessed respirations, auscultated lung sounds for signs indicating need for this treatment.	___	___	___	_____
4. Assessed patient's and family's understanding of the device and procedure, explained and clarified procedure as needed.	___	___	___	_____
5. Prepared Acapella device properly.	___	___	___	_____
6. Instructed patient to:				
a. Sit comfortably.	___	___	___	_____
b. Take in a breath larger than normal but not full capacity.	___	___	___	_____
c. Place mouthpiece into mouth, maintained a tight seal.	___	___	___	_____
d. Hold breath for 2 to 3 seconds.	___	___	___	_____
e. Try not to cough, exhale slowly for 3 to 4 seconds through device.	___	___	___	_____
f. Repeat cycle for 5 to 10 breaths as tolerated.	___	___	___	_____
g. Remove mouthpieces, perform forced exhalations.	___	___	___	_____
h. Repeat steps a through g if ordered.	___	___	___	_____
7. Auscultated lung fields.	___	___	___	_____
8. Obtained vital sign and pulse oximetry.	___	___	___	_____
9. Inspected color, character, and amount of sputum.	___	___	___	_____
10. Assisted patient with oral hygiene.	___	___	___	_____
11. Reviewed unexpected outcomes for Skill 24-1.	___	___	___	_____
12. Document procedure and patient's tolerance.	___	___	___	_____

Student _____ Date _____

Instructor _____ Date _____

PERFORMANCE CHECKLIST PERFORMED PROCEDURAL GUIDELINE 24-2 **PERFORMING PERCUSSION, VIBRATION, AND SHAKING**

	S	U	NP	Comments
PROCEDURAL STEPS				
1. Identified patient using two identifiers.	___	___	___	_____
2. Assessed breathing pattern.	___	___	___	_____
3. Assessed patient, reviewed medical record for signs, symptoms, and conditions that indicate need to perform these skills.	___	___	___	_____
4. Identified and assessed area of rib cage over affected bronchial segment; determined if percussion, vibration, or shaking were contraindicated.	___	___	___	_____
5. Determined patient's understanding, assessed patient's ability to cooperate with therapy.	___	___	___	_____
6. Explained procedure in detail.	___	___	___	_____
7. Helped patient to relax during procedure, had patient practice exhaling slowly through pursed lips while relaxing chest wall muscles.	___	___	___	_____
8. Performed hand hygiene, applied clean gloves.	___	___	___	_____
9. Elevated bed to working height, stood close to bed with arms in front and knees slightly bent.	___	___	___	_____
10. Positioned patient appropriately, assessed and identified lung region for percussion and vibration.	___	___	___	_____
11. Performed percussion for 3 to 5 minutes in each position as tolerated, began percussion on appropriate part of chest wall, asked if patient experienced any discomfort.				
a. Placed hands properly on chest wall.	___	___	___	_____
b. Clapped with proper motion.	___	___	___	_____
c. Alternately clapped chest with cupped hands, performed clapping at proper speed.	___	___	___	_____

	S	U	NP	Comments

12. Performed chest wall vibration and shaking over each affected area, performed vibrations in sets of three followed by coughing.

    a. Placed flat portion of hand over area; had patient take slow, deep breath through nose.

    b. Resisted chest wall gently as it rose.

    c. Had patient hold breath for 2 to 3 seconds and exhale through pursed lips while contracting abdominal muscles and relaxing chest wall muscles.

    d. Vibrated chest wall properly while patient was exhaling.

    e. Repeated vibration three times, had patient cascade cough, vibrated chest wall as patient coughed, followed natural movement of ribs when applying pressure, allowed patient to sit up and cough as needed.

    f. Monitored patient's tolerance of vibration and ability to relax chest wall and breathe properly as instructed.

13. Performed shaking with vibration.

    a. Placed flat part of hand over area, had patient inhale slowly through nose.

    b. Applied light pressure on ribs and stretched skin during inhalation.

    c. Had patient hold breath for 2 to 3 seconds.

    d. Increased pressure as patient exhaled.

    e. Instructed patient to exhale through pursed lips and relax chest wall muscles.

    f. Repeated shaking three times, had patient inhale deeply, did rib shaking during cascade cough.

14. Performed appropriate number of sets of vibration or shaking with vibration.

15. Used HFCWO device.

    a. Positioned patient comfortably.

    b. Explained procedure and equipment to patient and caregiver.

    c. Placed vest on patient, assessed for proper fit.

    d. Connected tubing to generator and ports of vest, turned power on.

340

	S	U	NP	Comments
e. Adjusted pressure control as ordered.	___	___	___	_____
f. Adjusted frequency.	___	___	___	_____
g. Administered any aerosol therapy as prescribed.	___	___	___	_____
h. Depressed and maintained pressure on control to initiate vest therapy.	___	___	___	_____
i. Released control after 5 to 10 minutes.	___	___	___	_____
16. Instructed patient to cough, suctioned if necessary.	___	___	___	_____
17. Continued with treatment, usually 15 to 30 minutes.	___	___	___	_____
18. Assisted with oral hygiene.	___	___	___	_____
19. Removed gloves, performed hand hygiene.	___	___	___	_____
20. Taught patient and significant others procedure for home use of devices if necessary, referred for outpatient or home care follow-up.	___	___	___	_____
21. Auscultated lung fields.	___	___	___	_____
22. Obtained vital signs and pulse oximetry.	___	___	___	_____
23. Inspected color, character, and amount of sputum.	___	___	___	_____

Student _____ Date _____

Instructor _____ Date _____

PERFORMANCE CHECKLIST SKILL 25-1 **PERFORMING OROPHARYNGEAL SUCTIONING**

	S	U	NP	Comments
ASSESSMENT				
1. Identified risk factors for airway obstruction.	___	___	___	_____
2. Assessed for signs and symptoms of hypoxia, hypoxemia, or hypercapnia.	___	___	___	_____
3. Obtained patient's oxygen saturation level via pulse oximetry, kept oximeter in place.	___	___	___	_____
4. Determined patient's ability to hold or manipulate catheter and knowledge about procedure.	___	___	___	_____
5. Assessed for signs and symptoms of upper airway obstruction.	___	___	___	_____
6. Auscultated for presence of adventitious sounds.	___	___	___	_____
PLANNING				
1. Identified expected outcomes.	___	___	___	_____
2. Explained procedure to patient, encouraged patient to cough out secretions, showed how to splint painful areas during procedure, had patient practice coughing if able.	___	___	___	_____
3. Positioned patient properly, draped patient properly.	___	___	___	_____
IMPLEMENTATION				
1. Identified patient using two identifiers.	___	___	___	_____
2. Performed hand hygiene, applied clean gloves and necessary PPE.	___	___	___	_____
3. Filled cup or basin with appropriate amount of water or saline.	___	___	___	_____
4. Connected one end of tube to suction machine and other to Yankauer suction catheter, turned on suction machine, set vacuum regulator appropriately.	___	___	___	_____
5. Checked that suction machine was functioning properly.	___	___	___	_____
6. Removed patient's oxygen mask if present, kept mask near patient's face.	___	___	___	_____

	S	U	NP	Comments

7. Inserted catheter into mouth along gum line to pharynx, moved catheter around until secretions cleared, encouraged patient to cough, replaced oxygen mask.

8. Rinsed catheter with water until tubing was cleared of secretions, turned off suction, washed face if necessary.

9. Observed respiratory status, repeated procedure if indicated, used standard suction catheter if needed.

10. Removed towel or drape, placed in trash or laundry if soiled, repositioned patient appropriately.

11. Discarded remainder of water into appropriate receptacle; washed basin; dried with paper towels; discarded cup in appropriate receptacle; placed catheter in clean, dry area.

12. Removed gloves and PPE, disposed of in appropriate receptacle, performed hand hygiene.

13. Positioned patient, provided oral hygiene as needed.

EVALUATION

1. Compared assessment findings before and after procedure.

2. Auscultated chest and airways for adventitious sounds.

3. Inspected mouth for any vomitus.

4. Obtained postsuction SpO_2 measure, compared with presuction level.

5. Observed patient or family perform Yankauer suctioning.

6. Identified unexpected outcomes.

RECORDING AND REPORTING

1. Recorded all pertinent information in the appropriate log.

2. Recorded instructions given to caregivers, noted their ability to correctly perform the procedure.

3. Reported any unresolved outcomes to health care provider.

Student _____ Date _____

Instructor _____ Date _____

PERFORMANCE CHECKLIST SKILL 25-2 **AIRWAY SUCTIONING**

	S	U	NP	Comments

ASSESSMENT

1. Assessed for risk factors for upper or lower airway obstruction.

2. Determined presence of symptoms indicating hypoxia, hypothermia, or hypercapnia.

3. Assessed vital signs.

4. Assessed signs and symptoms of upper and lower airway obstruction requiring airway suctioning.

5. Assessed for additional factors that anatomically influence upper or lower airway function.

6. Assessed factors that affect volume and consistency of secretions.

7. Assessed patient's peak inspiratory pressure or tidal volume for endotracheal suctioning.

8. Weighed patient's need for suction, considered contraindications to nasotracheal suctioning.

9. Examined sputum microbiology data.

10. Assessed patient's understanding of procedure.

PLANNING

1. Identified expected outcomes.

2. Explained how procedure would clear airway and relieve breathing; explained that temporary coughing, sneezing, gagging, or shortness of breath was normal.

3. Explained importance of and encouraged coughing to remove secretions during procedure, had patient practice coughing, used splinting if appropriate.

4. Had patient assume appropriate position.

5. Placed pulse oximeter on patient's finger, took reading, left oximeter in place, placed towel across patient's chest if needed.

	S	U	NP	Comments

IMPLEMENTATION

1. Identified patient using two identifiers.

2. Performed hand hygiene, applied PPE if necessary.

3. Connected one end of tubing to suction machine, placed other end near patient, turned device on, set suction pressure as low as possible, occluded end of tubing to check pressure.

4. Prepared suction catheter.

   a. Prepared one-time-use catheter.

     (1) Opened suction kit or catheter using aseptic technique, placed drape across patient's chest or on over-bed table, did not allow suction catheter to touch any nonsterile surface.

     (2) Opened sterile basin, placed on bedside table, did not touch inside of basin, filled properly with sterile saline solution or water.

     (3) Opened lubricant, squeezed small amount onto open sterile catheter package without touching package if necessary.

   b. Prepared closed (in-line) suction following Procedural Guideline 25-1.

5. Applied sterile gloves properly.

6. Picked up suction catheter with dominant hand, picked up connecting tubing with nondominant hand, secured catheter to tubing.

7. Checked that equipment was functioning properly.

8. Suctioned airway.

   a. Performed nasopharyngeal and nasotracheal suctioning.

     (1) Increased oxygen flow rate for face masks as ordered, had patient deep breathe slowly.

     (2) Coated distal end of catheter with lubricant.

     (3) Removed oxygen delivery device if applicable, inserted catheter into nares without applying suction, instructed patient to deep breathe, inserted catheter properly following natural course of the nares, did not force.

	S	U	NP	Comments

(4) Applied continuous suction by placing thumb over vent of catheter and withdrawing catheter while rotating it back and forth between thumb and forefinger, encouraged patient to cough, replaced oxygen device, had patient breathe deeply.

(5) Rinsed catheter and connecting tubing with normal saline or water until cleared.

(6) Assessed need to repeat procedure, did not perform more than two passes with the catheter, observed for alterations in cardiopulmonary status, allowed time between suction passes, encouraged patient to deep breathe with mask and cough.

b. Performed artificial airway suctioning.

(1) Hyperoxygenated patient appropriately before suctioning, did not manually ventilate patient.

(2) Opened swivel adapter or removed delivery device if patient was receiving mechanical ventilation.

(3) Inserted catheter without applying suction until resistance was met or patient coughed, pulled back.

(4) Applied intermittent suction by placing thumb over vent and withdrawing catheter while rotating it between thumb and forefinger, encouraged patient to cough, watched for respiratory distress.

(5) Closed swivel adapter or replaced oxygen delivery device if patient was receiving mechanical ventilation.

(6) Rinsed catheter and connected tubing with normal saline until clear, used continuous suction.

(7) Assessed patient's vital signs, cardiopulmonary status, and ventilatory measures for secretion clearance; repeated steps to clear secretions; allowed adequate times between passes.

(8) Encouraged patient to deep breathe if able, hyperoxygenated for at least 1 minute.

(9) Performed oropharyngeal suctioning to clear mouth after pharynx and trachea were sufficiently cleared, did not suction nose again.

	S	U	NP	Comments

9. Disconnected catheter from tubing, rolled catheter in fingers, pulled glove off inside out so catheter remained in glove, pulled off other glove over first in same way, discarded appropriately, turned off suction device. ____ ____ ____ _____

10. Removed towel, placed in appropriate receptacle, repositioned patient, applied clean gloves to continue personal care. ____ ____ ____ _____

11. Readjusted oxygen to original level if indicated. ____ ____ ____ _____

12. Discarded remainder of saline appropriately, discarded basin appropriately or rinsed and placed in soiled utility room. ____ ____ ____ _____

13. Removed face shield and discarded, performed hand hygiene. ____ ____ ____ _____

14. Placed unopened suction kit on machine table or at head of bed. ____ ____ ____ _____

15. Assisted patient to comfortable position, provided oral hygiene as needed. ____ ____ ____ _____

EVALUATION

1. Compared patient's vital signs, cardiopulmonary assessments, and SpO_2 values before and after suctioning; compared FiO_2 and tidal volumes if on ventilator. ____ ____ ____ _____

2. Asked patient if breathing was easier and if congestion had decreased. ____ ____ ____ _____

3. Observed character of airway secretions. ____ ____ ____ _____

4. Identified unexpected outcomes. ____ ____ ____ _____

RECORDING AND REPORTING

1. Recorded all pertinent information in the appropriate log. ____ ____ ____ _____

2. Documented patient's presuctioning and postsuctioning vital signs, cardiopulmonary status and ventilation measures. ____ ____ ____ _____

Student _____ Date _____

Instructor _____ Date _____

PERFORMANCE CHECKLIST PROCEDURAL GUIDELINE 25-1 CLOSED (IN-LINE) SUCTION

	S	U	NP	Comments

PROCEDURAL GUIDELINE

1. Performed assessment as in Skill 25-2.

2. Identified patient using two identifiers.

3. Explained procedure and importance of coughing during procedure to patient.

4. Assisted patient to appropriate position, placed towel across patient's chest.

5. Performed hand hygiene, applied PPE, attached suction.

   a. Opened catheter package, attached closed suction catheter to ventilator circuit, connected Y on ventilator circuit to catheter with flex tubing.

   b. Connected tubing to suction machine and end of closed-system or in-line suction catheter, turned device on, set regulator to appropriate negative pressure, checked pressure.

6. Hyperoxygenated patient, did not manually ventilate.

7. Picked up suction catheter in plastic sleeve with dominant hand.

8. Waited until patient inhaled to insert catheter, used repeated maneuver of pushing catheter and sliding plastic sleeve back until resistance was felt or patient coughed, pulled back.

9. Encouraged patient to cough, applied suction while withdrawing catheter, applied suction for no longer than 15 seconds, withdrew catheter completely.

10. Reassessed cardiopulmonary status, determined need for subsequent suctioning, repeated steps 5 to 9 one more time to clear secretions, allowed time between suction passes.

11. Withdrew catheter into sheath, ensured colored indicator line was visible in sheath, squeezed vial or pushed syringe while applying suction, rinsed catheter with saline until clear, locked suction mechanism, turned off suction.

	S	U	NP	Comments

12. Hyperoxygenated for at least 1 minute. ___ ___ ___ _____

13. Performed Skill 25-1 or 25-2 with separate suction catheter if patient required it. ___ ___ ___ _____

14. Positioned patient appropriately, removed gloves and PPE and discarded appropriately, performed hand hygiene. ___ ___ ___ _____

15. Compared patient's respiratory assessments before and after suctioning, observed airway secretion, documented findings. ___ ___ ___ _____

Student _____ Date _____

Instructor _____ Date _____

PERFORMANCE CHECKLIST SKILL 25-3 **PERFORMING ENDOTRACHEAL TUBE CARE**

	S	U	NP	Comments
ASSESSMENT				
1. Auscultated lungs, observed respiratory rate and depth.	___	___	___	_____
2. Observed for soiled or loose tape, pressure sores on nares or mouth, patient moving tube with tongue, tube repositioning, or foul-smelling mouth.	___	___	___	_____
3. Observed for factors that increase risk for complications from ET tube.	___	___	___	_____
4. Determined proper ET tube depth.	___	___	___	_____
5. Assessed patient's knowledge of procedure.	___	___	___	_____
PLANNING				
1. Identified expected outcomes.	___	___	___	_____
2. Explained procedure and patient's need to participate.	___	___	___	_____
IMPLEMENTATION				
1. Identified patient using two identifiers.	___	___	___	_____
2. Performed hand hygiene, applied gloves and PPE.	___	___	___	_____
3. Administered endotracheal, nasopharyngeal, or oropharyngeal suction.	___	___	___	_____
4. Connected oral suction catheter to suction source, assisted patient to a comfortable position.	___	___	___	_____
5. Prepared securement option.	___	___	___	_____
a. Prepared tape properly for tape method.	___	___	___	_____
b. Prepared commercial ET tube holder properly.	___	___	___	_____
6. Instructed assistant to apply gloves and hold ET tube at patient's lips or nares, noted number marking on ET tube at gum line or lips.	___	___	___	_____
7. Removed old tape or device.	___	___	___	_____
a. Removed tape properly, moistened if needed, discarded in appropriate receptacle.	___	___	___	_____
b. Removed Velcro strips, removed ET tube holder from patient.	___	___	___	_____

	S	U	NP	Comments

8. Removed any secretions or adhesive from patient's face, used adhesive remover if necessary. ___ ___ ___ _____

9. Removed oral airway or bite block and placed on towel. ___ ___ ___ _____

10. Cleaned mouth, gums, and teeth opposite ET tube appropriately, brushed teeth, rinsed with mouthwash, administered oropharyngeal suctioning. ___ ___ ___ _____

11. Repositioned oral ET tube properly if necessary. ___ ___ ___ _____

12. Repeated oral cleaning on opposite side of mouth. ___ ___ ___ _____

13. Cleaned face and neck with soap, rinsed and dried, shaved male patient if necessary. ___ ___ ___ _____

14. Poured skin protectant or liquid adhesive on gauze, dotted face properly, allowed to dry completely. ___ ___ ___ _____

15. Secured ET tube.

   a. Used tape method.

     (1) Slipped tape properly under patient's head and neck, centered tape. ___ ___ ___ _____

     (2) Secured tape properly on one side of face, tore remaining tape in half, secured each piece properly to face and tube. ___ ___ ___ _____

     (3) Pulled other side of tape, secured to opposite side of face. ___ ___ ___ _____

   b. Used commercially available device.

     (1) Threaded ET tube through opening, ensured pilot balloon was accessible. ___ ___ ___ _____

     (2) Placed strips of ET holder under patient at occipital region of the head. ___ ___ ___ _____

     (3) Verified that ET tube was at established depth. ___ ___ ___ _____

     (4) Attached Velcro at base of patient's head, left slack in strips. ___ ___ ___ _____

     (5) Verified that tube was secure and there were no pressure areas. ___ ___ ___ _____

16. Removed and cleaned oral airway, rinsed well, shook excess water from airway, ensured hydrogen peroxide was rinsed from airway. ___ ___ ___ _____

17. Reinserted oral airway, secured with tape. ___ ___ ___ _____

352

	S	U	NP	Comments

18. Discarded soiled items in appropriate receptacle, removed towel, placed in laundry.

19. Repositioned patient.

20. Removed gloves and PPE, discarded, performed hand hygiene, placed clean items in storage.

EVALUATION

1. Compared respiratory assessments before and after ET tube care.

2. Observed depth and position of ET tube.

3. Assessed security of tape.

4. Assessed skin around mouth and mucous membrane for intactness and pressure sores.

5. Identified unexpected outcomes.

RECORDING AND REPORTING

1. Documented all pertinent information in the appropriate log.

2. Reported unequal breath sounds, accidental extubation, or respiratory distress to health care provider.

Student _____ Date _____

Instructor _____ Date _____

PERFORMANCE CHECKLIST SKILL 25-4   **PERFORMING TRACHEOSTOMY CARE**

	S	U	NP	Comments
ASSESSMENT				
1. Observed for need for tracheostomy care due to secretions at stoma site or in tube.	___	___	___	_____
2. Assessed patient's hydration status, humidity delivered to airway, status of existing infection, patient's nutritional status, and ability to cough.	___	___	___	_____
3. Assessed vital signs, oxygen saturation, lung sounds, and patient's ability to clear airway.	___	___	___	_____
4. Assessed patient's understanding of and ability to perform tracheostomy care.	___	___	___	_____
5. Checked when tracheostomy care was last performed.	___	___	___	_____
PLANNING				
1. Identified expected outcomes.	___	___	___	_____
2. Obtained nurse or NAP to assist.	___	___	___	_____
3. Explained procedure and patient's participation.	___	___	___	_____
4. Assisted patient to appropriate position.	___	___	___	_____
5. Placed towel across patient's chest.	___	___	___	_____
IMPLEMENTATION				
1. Identified patient using two identifiers.	___	___	___	_____
2. Performed hand hygiene, applied gloves and PPE if applicable.	___	___	___	_____
3. Applied pulse oximeter sensor.	___	___	___	_____
4. Suctioned tracheostomy, removed soiled dressing, discarded in glove with coiled catheter.	___	___	___	_____
5. Performed hand hygiene, prepared equipment on bedside table.	___	___	___	_____
a. Opened sterile kit and two gauze packages, poured saline on one, opened cotton swab packages, poured saline on one, did not recap saline.	___	___	___	_____
b. Opened sterile tracheostomy dressing package.	___	___	___	_____
c. Unwrapped sterile basin, poured proper amount of saline into it.	___	___	___	_____

	S	U	NP	Comments

d. Opened sterile brush package, placed in basin. ___ ___ ___ _____

e. Prepared length of twill tape, cut ends diagonally, laid aside to dry. ___ ___ ___ _____

f. Opened commercially prepared package according to manufacturer's direction if appropriate. ___ ___ ___ _____

6. Hyperoxygenated patient appropriately. ___ ___ ___ _____

7. Applied sterile gloves, kept dominant hand sterile throughout. ___ ___ ___ _____

8. Provided care of tracheostomy with inner cannula. ___ ___ ___ _____

a. Unlocked and removed inner cannula while touching only outer aspect of the tube, dropped inner cannula into normal saline basin. ___ ___ ___ _____

b. Replaced tracheostomy collar, T tube, or ventilator oxygen source over outer cannula. ___ ___ ___ _____

c. Used small brush to remove secretions inside and outside inner cannula. ___ ___ ___ _____

d. Held inner cannula over basin, rinsed with saline, used nondominant hand to pour. ___ ___ ___ _____

e. Replaced inner cannula, secured locking mechanism, reapplied ventilator after hyperoxygenating if needed. ___ ___ ___ _____

9. Provided care of tracheostomy with disposable inner cannula. ___ ___ ___ _____

a. Removed new cannula from packaging. ___ ___ ___ _____

b. Withdrew inner cannula while touching only the outer aspect of the tube, replaced and locked new cannula. ___ ___ ___ _____

c. Disposed of contaminated cannula in appropriate receptacle, reconnected ventilator or oxygen supply. ___ ___ ___ _____

10. Cleaned exposed outer cannula surfaces and stoma under faceplate properly with wet cotton and gauze. ___ ___ ___ _____

11. Used dry gauze to pat skin and cannula surfaces dry. ___ ___ ___ _____

12. Secured tracheostomy.

a. Used tracheostomy tie method.

(1) Instructed assistant to apply clean gloves and hold tube in place, cut old ties. ___ ___ ___ _____

	S	U	NP	Comments

(2) Inserted one end of tie through faceplate eyelet, pulled ends even.

(3) Slid ends of tie behind head, inserted ties through proper eyelets.

(4) Pulled snugly.

(5) Tied ends properly, allowed proper amount of space within tie.

(6) Inserted fresh dressing under clean ties and faceplate.

b. Used tracheostomy tube holder method.

(1) Maintained hold on tracheostomy tube, left old tube holder in place until new device was secure.

(2) Aligned strap under patient's neck, ensured Velcro attachments were properly placed.

(3) Placed narrow end of tie under and through faceplate eyelets, pulled ends even, secured with Velcro.

(4) Verified space under neck strap.

13. Positioned patient comfortably, assessed respiratory status.

14. Ensured oxygen or humidification delivery sources were in place and set at correct levels.

15. Removed gloves and PPE, discarded appropriately.

16. Replaced cap on normal saline bottles, stored reusable liquids, dated container, stored unused supplies appropriately.

17. Performed hand hygiene.

EVALUATION

1. Compared assessments before and after tracheostomy care.

2. Assessed fit of new tracheostomy ties, asked patient if tube felt comfortable.

3. Inspected inner and outer cannulas for secretions.

4. Assessed stoma for inflammation, edema, or discolored secretions.

5. Identified unexpected outcomes.

	S	U	NP	Comments

RECORDING AND REPORTING

1. Recorded all pertinent information in the appropriate log. _____ _____ _____ _____

2. Reported accidental decannulation or respiratory distress to health care provider. _____ _____ _____ _____

Student _____ Date _____

Instructor _____ Date _____

PERFORMANCE CHECKLIST SKILL 25-5 **INFLATING THE CUFF ON AN ENDOTRACHEAL OR TRACHEOSTOMY TUBE**

	S	U	NP	Comments
ASSESSMENT				
1. Observed for signs and symptoms of gurgling on expiration, decreased exhaled tidal volume, spasmodic coughing, tense test balloon on tube, flaccid test balloon on tube, and unexpected phonation.	___	___	___	_____
2. Assessed vital signs, respiratory effort, and tidal volume if appropriate.	___	___	___	_____
3. Determined family caregiver's understanding of and ability to perform procedure if necessary.	___	___	___	_____
PLANNING				
1. Identified expected outcomes.	___	___	___	_____
2. Explained procedure and how patient could participate, explained that coughing during procedure was normal.	___	___	___	_____
IMPLEMENTATION				
1. Identified patient using two identifiers.	___	___	___	_____
2. Performed hand hygiene, applied gloves and face shield if indicated.	___	___	___	_____
3. Assisted patient to comfortable position.	___	___	___	_____
4. Suctioned secretions through ET or tracheostomy tube and mouth.	___	___	___	_____
5. Connected syringe to pilot balloon.	___	___	___	_____
6. Placed stethoscope in sternal notch or above tracheostomy tube, listened for minimal amount of air leak at end of inspiration.	___	___	___	_____
7. Removed all air from cuff if air leak was not heard.	___	___	___	_____
8. Reinflated cuff according to agency policy.	___	___	___	_____
9. Slowly added air if excessive leak was heard.	___	___	___	_____
10. Removed stethoscope, wiped diaphragm with alcohol wipe.	___	___	___	_____
11. Removed syringe, discarded appropriately.	___	___	___	_____
12. Repositioned patient appropriately.	___	___	___	_____
13. Removed gloves and PPE, discarded appropriately, performed hand hygiene.	___	___	___	_____

	S	U	NP	Comments

EVALUATION

1. Compared respiratory assessments before and after cuff care.

2. Observed exhaled tidal volume from mechanical ventilator.

3. Auscultated for audible air leak.

4. Observed for excessive phonation, presence of gastric secretions in airway secretions, or tracheoesophageal fistula.

5. Identified unexpected outcomes.

RECORDING AND REPORTING

1. Documented all pertinent information in the appropriate log.

Student _____ Date _____

Instructor _____ Date _____

PERFORMANCE CHECKLIST SKILL 26-1 **MANAGING CLOSED CHEST DRAINAGE SYSTEM**

	S	U	NP	Comments
ASSESSMENT				
1. Measured vital signs and pulse oximetry.	___	___	___	_____
2. Performed a complete respiratory assessment.	___	___	___	_____
3. Assessed patient for known allergies; asked patient if he or she has had a problem with medications, latex, or anything applied to skin.	___	___	___	_____
4. Reviewed patient's medication record for anticoagulant therapy.	___	___	___	_____
5. Reviewed patient's hemoglobin and hematocrit levels.	___	___	___	_____
6. Observed dressing and insertion site, tubing, and system orientation for patient who has chest tubes.	___	___	___	_____
7. Assessed patient's knowledge of procedure.	___	___	___	_____
PLANNING				
1. Identified expected outcomes.	___	___	___	_____
IMPLEMENTATION				
1. Identified patient using two identifiers.	___	___	___	_____
2. Determined whether informed consent was needed.	___	___	___	_____
3. Reviewed health care provider's order for chest tube placement.	___	___	___	_____
4. Performed hand hygiene.	___	___	___	_____
5. Set up water-seal system.				
a. Obtained chest drainage system, removed wrappers, prepared to set up.	___	___	___	_____
b. Maintained sterility of drainage system, stood system upright, added sterile water or saline to appropriate compartments.	___	___	___	_____
6. Set up waterless system.				
a. Removed sterile wrappers, prepared to set up.	___	___	___	_____
b. Connected tubing from suction control chamber to suction source for three-chamber system.	___	___	___	_____
c. Instilled water or saline into diagnostic indicator injection port.	___	___	___	_____

	S	U	NP	Comments

7. Secured all tubing connections with tape or zip ties, checked system for patency.   ____   ____   ____   _____

8. Turned off suction source and unclamped drainage tubing before connecting patient to system, ensured drainage tubing was not excessively long, turned suction source on after patient was connected.   ____   ____   ____   _____

9. Administered premedication as ordered.   ____   ____   ____   _____

10. Provided psychological support to patient, included reinforcement of preprocedural explanation and coaching and support.   ____   ____   ____   _____

11. Performed hand hygiene, applied clean gloves, positioned patient properly for tube insertion.   ____   ____   ____   _____

12. Assisted health care provider with chest tube insertion.   ____   ____   ____   _____

13. Helped health care provider attach drainage tube to chest tube, removed clamp, turned on suction to prescribed level.   ____   ____   ____   _____

14. Taped or zip- tied all connections between chest tube and drainage tube.   ____   ____   ____   _____

15. Checked systems for proper functioning.   ____   ____   ____   _____

16. Positioned patient appropriately after tube placement.   ____   ____   ____   _____

17. Checked patency of air vents in systems.   ____   ____   ____   _____

18. Positioned excess tubing horizontally on mattress next to patient, secured with clamp.   ____   ____   ____   _____

19. Adjusted tubing to hang straight from chest tube to drainage chamber.   ____   ____   ____   _____

20. Placed two rubber-tipped hemostats in an easily accessible position.   ____   ____   ____   _____

21. Disposed of sharps and used supplies properly, performed hand hygiene.   ____   ____   ____   _____

22. Provided care for patient after chest tube insertion.

   a. Performed hand hygiene; applied clean gloves; assessed vital signs, oxygen saturation, skin color, breath sounds, character of respirations, and insertion site at appropriate times.   ____   ____   ____   _____

   b. Monitored color, consistency, and amount of chest tube drainage; indicated level of drainage, date, and time on chamber's surface.   ____   ____   ____   _____

   c. Observed chest dressing for drainage.   ____   ____   ____   _____

	S	U	NP	Comments

d. Palpated around tube for swelling and crepitus. ___ ___ ___ _____

e. Ensured tubing was free of kinks and dependent loops. ___ ___ ___ _____

f. Observed for fluctuation of drainage in tubing and water-seal chamber, observed for clots or debris in tubing. ___ ___ ___ _____

g. Kept drainage system upright and below level of patient's chest. ___ ___ ___ _____

h. Checked for air leaks by monitoring bubbling in water-seal chamber. ___ ___ ___ _____

i. Removed gloves, disposed of equipment in appropriate biohazard container, performed hand hygiene. ___ ___ ___ _____

EVALUATION

1. Assessed patient for decreased respiratory distress and chest pain, auscultated patient's lungs and observed chest expansion. ___ ___ ___ _____

2. Monitored vital signs and pulse oximetry. ___ ___ ___ _____

3. Reassessed patient's level of comfort. ___ ___ ___ _____

4. Evaluated patient's ability to use deep-breathing exercises while maintaining comfort. ___ ___ ___ _____

5. Monitored continued functioning of system. ___ ___ ___ _____

6. Identified unexpected outcomes. ___ ___ ___ _____

RECORDING AND REPORTING

1. Recorded respiratory assessment, amount of suction, amount of drainage in chamber, and presence of an air leak, included initials; recorded patient teaching and validation of understanding. ___ ___ ___ _____

2. Recorded patient comfort and baseline vital signs appropriately. ___ ___ ___ _____

3. Recorded integrity of dressing and presence of drainage on dressing. ___ ___ ___ _____

Student _____ Date _____

Instructor _____ Date _____

PERFORMANCE CHECKLIST SKILL 26-2 **ASSISTING WITH REMOVAL OF CHEST TUBES**

	S	U	NP	Comments
ASSESSMENT				
1. Assessed status of patient's lung reexpansion.	___	___	___	_____
2. Assessed patient's level of comfort, determined when last analgesic medication was given.	___	___	___	_____
3. Determined patient's understanding of chest tube removal procedure.	___	___	___	_____
4. Did not clamp chest tube before removal; assessed changes in vital signs, oxygen saturation, chest pain, apprehension, and symptoms of tension pneumothorax.	___	___	___	_____
PLANNING				
1. Identified expected outcomes.	___	___	___	_____
2. Explained procedure to patient.	___	___	___	_____
IMPLEMENTATION				
1. Identified patient using two identifiers.	___	___	___	_____
2. Administered prescribed medication for pain relief 30 minutes before procedure.	___	___	___	_____
3. Performed hand hygiene, applied PPE if needed.	___	___	___	_____
4. Assisted patient to appropriate position, placed pad under chest tube site.	___	___	___	_____
5. Supported patient physically and emotionally while health care provider removed dressing and clips sutures.	___	___	___	_____
6. Assisted with application of sterile occlusive dressing over wound and secured with tape.	___	___	___	_____
7. Assisted patient to appropriate position.	___	___	___	_____
8. Removed used equipment from bedside, placed in appropriate receptacle.	___	___	___	_____
9. Removed gloves, performed hand hygiene.	___	___	___	_____

	S	U	NP	Comments

EVALUATION

1. Auscultated lung sounds, palpated over lung, observed patient for subcutaneous emphysema, evaluated for respiratory distress. ___ ___ ___ _____

2. Evaluated patient's vital signs, oxygen saturation, pulmonary status, and psychological status. ___ ___ ___ _____

3. Reviewed chest x-ray film. ___ ___ ___ _____

4. Asked about patient's level of pain, observed for nonverbal cues. ___ ___ ___ _____

5. Checked chest dressing for drainage and patency, noted wound for signs of healing. ___ ___ ___ _____

6. Identified unexpected outcomes. ___ ___ ___ _____

RECORDING AND REPORTING

1. Recorded all pertinent information in appropriate log. ___ ___ ___ _____

Student _____ Date _____

Instructor _____ Date _____

PERFORMANCE CHECKLIST SKILL 26-3 **AUTOTRANSFUSION OF CHEST TUBE DRAINAGE**

	S	U	NP	Comments
ASSESSMENT				
1. Performed assessment outline in Skill 26-1.	___	___	___	_____
2. Determined presence of active bleeding through chest tube.	___	___	___	_____
3. Assessed IV site, noted size of IV catheter.	___	___	___	_____
4. Obtained baseline laboratory data.	___	___	___	_____
PLANNING				
1. Identified expected outcomes.	___	___	___	_____
2. Explained procedure to patient.	___	___	___	_____
IMPLEMENTATION				
1. Set up system.				
a. Set up ATS according to instructions and to maintain sterility of unit.	___	___	___	_____
b. Ensured all connections were tight and all clamps were open.	___	___	___	_____
2. Identified patient using two identifiers.	___	___	___	_____
3. Performed hand hygiene, applied gloves.	___	___	___	_____
4. Prepared chest drainage for reinfusion.				
a. Opened replacement bag following directions, closed the two white clamps.	___	___	___	_____
b. Used high-negativity relief valve to reduce excessive negativity.	___	___	___	_____
c. Performed bag transfer.				
(1) Closed clamp on chest drainage tubing.	___	___	___	_____
(2) Closed clamps on top of initial ATS collection bag.	___	___	___	_____
(3) Connected chest drainage tube to new bag.	___	___	___	_____
(4) Ensured all connections were tight.	___	___	___	_____
(5) Opened all clamps on chest drainage tube and replacement bag.	___	___	___	_____
d. Connected connectors of initial bag, removed appropriately.	___	___	___	_____

	S	U	NP	Comments

e. Secured replacements bag, secured frame onto the hook.

f. Placed thumbs on metal frame, pushed up to slide bag out, removed replacement bag.

5. Reinfused chest drainage.

   a. Used a new microaggregate filter to reinfuse each autotransfusion bag.

   b. Accessed bag by inverting bag and spiking it and twisting.

   c. Squeezed bag upside down to remove air, primed filler with blood.

   d. Hung bag on IV pole; primed until all air was gone; clamped tubing, attached to patient's IV access, and adjusted clamp to deliver reinfusion at appropriate rate.

   e. Added anticoagulants properly if ordered.

   f. Monitored patient's vital signs and SpO_2 properly.

6. Discontinued autotransfusion.

   a. Clamped chest drainage tube briefly, connected directly to chest drainage unit with red and blue connectors.

   b. Opened chest drainage tube clamp.

7. Discarded used supplies and performed hand hygiene.

EVALUATION

1. Monitored vital signs, hematocrit, and hemoglobin.

2. Monitored chest drainage system and patient's lung sounds.

3. Evaluated IV infusion site for infiltration and phlebitis.

4. Identified unexpected outcomes.

RECORDING AND REPORTING

1. Recorded all pertinent information in the appropriate log.

Student _____ Date _____

Instructor _____ Date _____

PERFORMANCE CHECKLIST SKILL 27-1 **INSERTING AN OROPHARYNGEAL AIRWAY**

	S	U	NP	Comments

ASSESSMENT

1. Identified need to insert oral airway.

2. Determined factors that may contribute to upper airway obstruction.

3. Assessed for presence of gag reflex.

4. Ensured patient did not have dentures in place.

PLANNING

1. Identified expected outcomes.

IMPLEMENTATION

1. Positioned unconscious patient appropriately.

2. Performed hand hygiene, applied clean gloves and PPE.

3. Used padded tongue blade to open patient's mouth, used thumb and forefingers as necessary.

4. Inserted oral airway.

   a. Held oral airway properly until back of throat was found, turned airway over and followed natural curve of tongue.

5. Suctioned secretions as needed.

6. Reassessed patient's respiratory status, auscultated lungs.

7. Cleaned patient's face with tissue or washcloth.

8. Discarded tissue into appropriate receptacle, placed washcloth in soiled linen bag, removed and discarded gloves and PPE, performed hand hygiene.

9. Administered mouth care frequently.

EVALUATION

1. Observed patient's respiratory status and compared respiratory assessments before and after insertion.

2. Assessed that airway was patent and that patient's tongue did not obstruct airway.

	S	U	NP	Comments

3. Reassessed need for oral airway if patient pushed airway out with tongue or coughed.   ____ ____ ____ _____

4. Identified unexpected outcomes.   ____ ____ ____ _____

RECORDING AND REPORTING

1. Recorded all pertinent information in the appropriate log.   ____ ____ ____ _____

Student _____ Date _____

Instructor _____ Date _____

PERFORMANCE CHECKLIST SKILL 27-2   **USE OF AN AUTOMATED EXTERNAL DEFIBRILLATOR**

	S	U	NP	Comments
ASSESSMENT				
1. Established a person's unresponsiveness, called for help.	___	___	___	_____
2. Established absence of respirations and lack of circulation.	___	___	___	_____
PLANNING				
1. Identified expected outcomes.	___	___	___	_____
IMPLEMENTATION				
1. Assessed patient for unresponsiveness, not breathing, and pulselessness.	___	___	___	_____
2. Activated code team in accordance with policy and procedure.	___	___	___	_____
3. Started chest compressions, continued until AED was attached to patient and device advised you to not touch the patient.	___	___	___	_____
4. Placed AED next to patient near chest or head.	___	___	___	_____
5. Turned power on.	___	___	___	_____
6. Attached the device properly, ensured cables were connected to the AED.	___	___	___	_____
7. Did *not* touch the patient when the AED prompted you, announced "Clear," allowed AED to analyze rhythm, pressed button if required.	___	___	___	_____
8. Announced "clear," performed a visual check to ensure no one was in contact with the victim.	___	___	___	_____
9. Began chest compressions after the shock, continued for 2 minutes, did *not* remove the pads.	___	___	___	_____
10. Delivered two breaths using mouth-to-mouth with a barrier device or mask, delivered 10 to 12 breaths per minute.	___	___	___	_____
11. Cleared patient when AED prompted you, continued until patient regained pulse or a health care provider determined death.	___	___	___	_____

	S	U	NP	Comments

EVALUATION

1. Inspected pad adhesion to chest wall, applied new set of pads if necessary. ____ ____ ____ _____

2. Continued efforts until patient regained pulse or health care provider determined death. ____ ____ ____ _____

3. Identified unexpected outcomes. ____ ____ ____ _____

RECORDING AND REPORTING

1. Reported arrest via hospital-wide communication system immediately, included exact location. ____ ____ ____ _____

2. Documented arrest properly. ____ ____ ____ _____

3. Recorded all pertinent information in the appropriate log. ____ ____ ____ _____

372

Student _____ Date _____

Instructor _____ Date _____

PERFORMANCE CHECKLIST SKILL 27-3 **CODE MANAGEMENT**

	S	U	NP	Comments
ASSESSMENT				
1. Determined if patient was unconscious by shaking the patient and shouting, assessed patient unresponsiveness.	——	——	——	_____
PLANNING				
1. Identified expected outcomes.	——	——	——	_____
2. Activated hospital's code team or EMS immediately, told co-workers to bring AED and crash cart to bedside.	——	——	——	_____
IMPLEMENTATION: PRIMARY SURVEY				
1. Checked carotid pulse properly.	——	——	——	_____
2. Placed patient on a hard surface, ensured patient was flat, logrolled patient if trauma was suspected.	——	——	——	_____
3. Applied clean gloves and face shield.	——	——	——	_____
4. Opened airway by head tilt–chin lift or jaw thrust.	——	——	——	_____
5. Attempted to ventilate patients with slow breaths using appropriate method.	——	——	——	_____
6. Inserted oral airway if available.	——	——	——	_____
7. Suctioned secretions if necessary or turned patient's head to one side if appropriate.	——	——	——	_____
8. Applied AED immediately if appropriate and available in absence of patient's pulse.	——	——	——	_____
9. Initiated chest compressions if AED was unavailable, used correct hand position and compression ratio.	——	——	——	_____
IMPLEMENTATION: SECONDARY SURVEY				
1. Gave leader verbal report of events performed before code team's arrival.	——	——	——	_____
2. Delegated tasks appropriately while core group continued resuscitation efforts.	——	——	——	_____
a. Assisted victim's roommates or visitors away from code scene.	——	——	——	_____
b. Delegated someone to removed excess equipment from the room.	——	——	——	_____
c. Had someone bring patient's chart or access patient's electronic medical record.	——	——	——	_____

	S	U	NP	Comments

d. Assigned a nurse as recorder of events. ____ ____ ____ _____

e. Assigned a nurse to get medications and supplies to hand off to code team members. ____ ____ ____ _____

3. Attached manual defibrillator/monitor to patient appropriately. ____ ____ ____ _____

4. Continued CPR and defibrillation if cardiac rhythm was "shockable." ____ ____ ____ _____

   a. Turned on defibrillator, selected proper energy level. ____ ____ ____ _____

   b. Applied conductive gel or gel pads to patient's chest. ____ ____ ____ _____

   c. Placed paddles or pads on patient's chest wall. ____ ____ ____ _____

   d. Verified that everyone had cleared the patient, called, "Clear." ____ ____ ____ _____

5. Established IV access with large-bore IV needle, began infusion of 0.9% NS. ____ ____ ____ _____

6. Assisted with procedure as needed. ____ ____ ____ _____

7. Continued CPR until appropriate point. ____ ____ ____ _____

8. Assisted code team with ET intubation if respirations were absent, had appropriate equipment available, ensured light source on laryngoscope was functional. ____ ____ ____ _____

9. Assisted in confirmation of ET tube placement or advanced airway support. ____ ____ ____ _____

10. Ventilated bag device upon intubation. ____ ____ ____ _____

11. Assisted health care provider in obtaining laboratory and diagnostic studies. ____ ____ ____ _____

EVALUATION

1. Reassessed the primary and secondary surveys throughout the code event. ____ ____ ____ _____

2. Palpated carotid pulse at least every 5 minutes after first minute of CPR. ____ ____ ____ _____

3. Observed for spontaneous return of respirations or heart rate every 2 minutes. ____ ____ ____ _____

4. Ensured that interruptions in CPR were minimized. ____ ____ ____ _____

5. Identified unexpected outcomes. ____ ____ ____ _____

RECORDING AND REPORTING

1. Reported arrest immediately, included exact location. ____ ____ ____ _____

2. Recorded all pertinent information in the appropriate log. ____ ____ ____ _____

Student _____ Date _____

Instructor _____ Date _____

PERFORMANCE CHECKLIST SKILL 28-1 **INITIATING INTRAVENOUS THERAPY**

	S	U	NP	Comments

ASSESSMENT

1. Reviewed accuracy and completeness of the order for type and amount of IV fluid, medication additives, infusion rate, and length of therapy; followed six rights of medication administration.

2. Assessed patient's knowledge of procedure and reason for prescribed therapy.

3. Assessed for clinical factors that would respond to or be affected by administration of solutions.

4. Determined if patient was going to undergo any surgeries or operations.

5. Assessed laboratory data.

6. Assessed patient's history of allergies, especially to iodine, adhesive, or latex.

PLANNING

1. Identified expected outcomes.

IMPLEMENTATION

1. Identified patient using two identifiers, compared identifiers in MAR and on patient's ID bracelet.

2. Instructed patient about rationale for infusion, medications ordered, procedure, and signs and symptoms of complications.

3. Assisted patient to comfortable position, provided adequate lighting.

4. Performed hand hygiene, organized equipment on bedside stand or over-bed table.

5. Changed patient's gown to more easily removable gown if available.

6. Opened sterile packages using sterile aseptic technique.

7. Prepared tubing and solution for continuous infusion.

   a. Checked IV solution using six rights of administration, ensured additives had been added, checked solution and bag.

	S	U	NP	Comments

b. Opened infusion set, maintained sterility at both tubing ends. ___ ___ ___ _____

c. Placed roller clamp below drip chamber, moved roller clamp to *off* position. ___ ___ ___ _____

d. Removed protective sheath over IV tubing port on bag or bottle. ___ ___ ___ _____

e. Removed protective cap from insertion spike, inserted spike into port of IV bag, cleansed rubber stopper, inserted spike into rubber stopper. ___ ___ ___ _____

f. Filled drip chamber one-third to one-half full. ___ ___ ___ _____

g. Primed infusion tubing by filling with IV solution, removed protective cape on tubing, opened roller clamp, inverted Y connector to displace air, returned roller clamp to *off* position, replaced protective cap on end of tubing. ___ ___ ___ _____

h. Ensured tubing was clear of air and bubbles, checked entire length of tubing. ___ ___ ___ _____

i. If optional long extension tubing was used, removed protective cap, attached to distal end of IV tubing, primed extension tubing. ___ ___ ___ _____

8. Performed hand hygiene, applied clean gloves, wore PPE if necessary. ___ ___ ___ _____

9. Applied tourniquet around arm above antecubital fossa, checked for presence of radial pulse. ___ ___ ___ _____

10. Selected appropriate vein for VAD insertion. ___ ___ ___ _____

a. Used most distal site in nondominant arm if possible. ___ ___ ___ _____

b. Selected a well-dilated vein. ___ ___ ___ _____

c. Palpated vein; noted resilience, soft feeling while releasing pressure; avoided veins that felt hard. ___ ___ ___ _____

d. Avoided areas with tenderness, redness, rash, pain, or infection; extremity affected by previous CVA, paralysis, dialysis shunt, or mastectomy; sites distal to previous venipuncture site; sclerosed or hardened veins; infiltrate site; areas of venous valves or phlebotic vessels; and fragile dorsal veins in older patients. ___ ___ ___ _____

e. Chose site that did not interfere with ADL. ___ ___ ___ _____

	S	U	NP	Comments

11. Released tourniquet temporarily and carefully, clipped arm hair if necessary, applied topical anesthetic if needed.

12. Applied clean gloves if necessary.

13. Placed adapter end of tubing or extension/injection cap for saline lock nearby in the sterile package.

14. Cleansed insertion area if necessary, allowed to dry completely, refrained from touching cleansed site.

15. Reapplied tourniquet properly, checked presence of radial pulse.

16. Performed venipuncture, anchored vein below site, instructed patient to relax hand, warned patient of a sharp stick, inserted needle appropriately.

17. Observed for blood return through flashback chamber, lowered and advanced catheter appropriately, loosened stylet over the needle catheter, held skin taught while stabilizing needle, advanced catheter off needle, threaded catheter into vein properly.

18. Stabilized catheter with nondominant hand, released cuff or tourniquet with the other, applied pressure above insertion site, kept catheter stable with index finger.

19. Connected Luer-Lok end of set to end of catheter, did not touch point of entry of connection, secured connection.

20. Flushed primed extension set with saline from attached prefilled syringe or began infusion by opening clamp or adjusting roller clamp of IV tubing.

21. Secured catheter according to agency policy.

22. Applied appropriate sterile dressing over site properly.

23. Looped set tubing alongside arm, placed tape over tubing and secured.

24. Rechecked flow rate and drops per minute for IV fluid administration, connected to EID as per agency policy.

25. Labeled dressing properly.

	S	U	NP	Comments

26. Disposed of sharps in the appropriate container, discarded supplies, removed gloves, performed hand hygiene.

27. Instructed patient in how to move without dislodging VAD.

EVALUATION

1. Observed patient at established intervals.

   a. Checked correct type/amount of IV solution infused.

   b. Checked drip rate or rate on infusion pump.

   c. Checked patency of VAD.

   d. Observed patient for signs of discomfort during palpation of vessel.

   e. Inspected color of insertion site, inspected for signs of inflammation and phlebitis.

2. Observed patient to determine response to therapy.

3. Identified unexpected outcomes.

RECORDING AND REPORTING

1. Recorded all pertinent information in the appropriate log.

2. Documented type and rate of infusion and device ID number if using an EID.

3. Recorded patient's status, IV fluid, amount infused, and integrity and patency of system according to policy.

4. Reported pertinent information to oncoming nursing staff.

5. Reported signs and symptoms of IV-related complications to health care provider.

Student _____ Date _____

Instructor _____ Date _____

PERFORMANCE CHECKLIST SKILL 28-2 **REGULATING INTRAVENOUS FLOW RATE**

	S	U	NP	Comments
ASSESSMENT				
1. Reviewed accuracy and completeness of health care provider order, followed six rights of drug administration.	___	___	___	_____
2. Assessed patient's knowledge of how positioning of IV site affects flow rate.	___	___	___	_____
3. Inspected IV site for signs and symptoms of IV-related complications.	___	___	___	_____
4. Observed for patency of IV tubing and VAD.	___	___	___	_____
5. Identified patient risk for fluid imbalance.	___	___	___	_____
PLANNING				
1. Identified expected outcomes.	___	___	___	_____
IMPLEMENTATION				
1. Identified patient using two identifiers, compared identifiers in MAR and on patient's ID bracelet.	___	___	___	_____
2. Used paper and pencil or calculator to calculate flow.	___	___	___	_____
3. Verified calibration in drops per milliliter of infusion set used.	___	___	___	_____
4. Determined how long each liter of fluid should run.	___	___	___	_____
5. Selected appropriate formula to calculate minute flow rate based on drop factor of the infusion set.	___	___	___	_____
6. Confirmed hourly and minute rate if using gravity infusion set.	___	___	___	_____
7. Followed manufacturer guidelines for setup if using EID.	___	___	___	_____
8. Followed manufacturer guidelines if using volume-control device.	___	___	___	_____
9. Instructed patient in purpose of alarms, to avoid raising hand or arm that affects flow rate, and to avoid touching control clamp.	___	___	___	_____

	S	U	NP	Comments

EVALUATION

1. Monitored IV infusion at least every hour, noted volume of fluid infused and rate. ___ ___ ___ _____

2. Observed patient for signs of fluid volume excess or deficit and signs of fluid and electrolyte balance. ___ ___ ___ _____

3. Evaluated signs of IV-related complications. ___ ___ ___ _____

4. Identified unexpected outcomes. ___ ___ ___ _____

RECORDING AND REPORTING

1. Recorded rate of infusion in the appropriate log. ___ ___ ___ _____

2. Documented use of EID or control device and ID number of device. ___ ___ ___ _____

3. Reported rate of and volume left in infusion to nurse in charge or oncoming nurse. ___ ___ ___ _____

Student _____ Date _____

Instructor _____ Date _____

PERFORMANCE CHECKLIST SKILL 28-3   **CHANGING INTRAVENOUS SOLUTIONS**

	S	U	NP	Comments

ASSESSMENT

1. Reviewed health care provider's order, followed six rights of drug administration.

2. Noted date and time when IV tubing and solution were last changed.

3. Determined compatibility of all IV fluids and additives.

4. Determined patient's understanding of need for continued IV therapy.

5. Assessed patency of current VAD site, observed for signs of complications.

6. Assessed IV tubing for puncture, contamination, or occlusions.

PLANNING

1. Identified expected outcomes.

IMPLEMENTATION

1. Collected equipment; had solution prepared at least 1 hour before needed, ensured it had been delivered, allowed solution to warm to room temperature if necessary, checked that solution was correct and labeled, checked expiration date, ensured light sensitivity restrictions were followed.

2. Identified patient using two identifiers, compared identifiers in MAR and on patient's ID bracelet.

3. Changed solution at the appropriate time.

4. Prepared patient and caregiver by explaining procedure, its purpose, and what was expected of patient.

5. Performed hand hygiene.

6. Prepared new solution for changing, removed cover from IV tubing port or metal cap and disks.

	S	U	NP	Comments

7. Closed roller clamp on existing solution, removed tubing from EID, removed old fluid container from IV pole, held container with tubing port pointing upward. ____ ____ ____ _____

8. Removed spike from new solution container, inserted into new container. ____ ____ ____ _____

9. Hung new container of solution on IV pole. ____ ____ ____ _____

10. Checked for air in tubing, removed properly if necessary. ____ ____ ____ _____

11. Ensured drip chamber was one-third to one-half full, adjusted level appropriately if necessary. ____ ____ ____ _____

12. Regulated flow to ordered rate using either roller clamp or EID. ____ ____ ____ _____

13. Placed time label on side of container, labeled appropriately. ____ ____ ____ _____

EVALUATION

1. Observed functioning, intactness, and patency of IV systems and flow rate. ____ ____ ____ _____

2. Observed patient for signs of FVD or FVE to determine response to IV therapy. ____ ____ ____ _____

3. Assessed patient for signs of IV-related complications. ____ ____ ____ _____

4. Identified unexpected outcomes. ____ ____ ____ _____

RECORDING AND REPORTING

1. Recorded amount and type of solution started and flow rate in the appropriate log. ____ ____ ____ _____

2. Recorded solution and tubing change in the appropriate log. ____ ____ ____ _____

Student _____ Date _____

Instructor _____ Date _____

PERFORMANCE CHECKLIST SKILL 28-4   **CHANGING INFUSION TUBING**

	S	U	NP	Comments
ASSESSMENT				
1. Noted date and time when IV tubing was last changed.	___	___	___	_____
2. Assessed tubing for puncture, contamination, or occlusion that required immediate change.	___	___	___	_____
3. Determined patient's understanding of need for continued IV therapy.	___	___	___	_____
PLANNING				
1. Identified expected outcomes.	___	___	___	_____
IMPLEMENTATION				
1. Identified patient with two identifiers, compared identifiers in MAR and on patient's ID bracelet.	___	___	___	_____
2. Prepared patient by explaining procedure, purpose, and what was expected of the patient.	___	___	___	_____
3. Coordinated tubing changes with solution changes when possible.	___	___	___	_____
4. Performed hand hygiene.	___	___	___	_____
5. Opened new infusion set, connected add-on pieces, kept protective coverings over spike and distal adapter, secured all connections.	___	___	___	_____
6. Applied clean gloves, removed IV dressing if necessary, did not remove tape securing cannula.	___	___	___	_____
7. Prepared infusion tubing with new bag.	___	___	___	_____
8. Prepared infusion tubing with existing continuous IV infusion.				
a. Moved roller clamp on new IV tubing to off position.	___	___	___	_____
b. Slowed rate of infusion to existing IV.	___	___	___	_____
c. Compressed and filled drip chamber of old tubing.	___	___	___	_____
d. Inverted container, removed old tubing, kept spike sterile and upright, taped old drip chamber to IV pole if necessary.	___	___	___	_____

	S	U	NP	Comments

e. Placed insertion spike of new tubing into solution container, hung solution bag on IV pole, compressed and released drip chamber on new tubing, filled drip chamber appropriately.

____ ____ ____ _____

f. Opened roller clamp, removed protective cap from adapter, primed new tubing with solution, stopped infusion, replaced cap, placed end of adapter near patient's IV site.

____ ____ ____ _____

g. Stopped EID of turned roller clamp on old tubing to *off* position.

____ ____ ____ _____

9. Prepared tubing with extension set.

a. Connected new injection cap to new extension tubing if needed.

____ ____ ____ _____

b. Swabbed injection cap with antiseptic swab, inserted syringe and injected with saline solution.

____ ____ ____ _____

10. Reestablished infusion.

a. Disconnected old tubing from extension set, inserted adapter of new tubing or saline lock into connection.

____ ____ ____ _____

b. Opened roller clamp on new tubing for continuous infusion, regulated drip using roller clamp of EID.

____ ____ ____ _____

c. Attached tape or label with date and time of change onto tubing below drip chamber.

____ ____ ____ _____

d. Formed a loop of tubing, secured to patient's arm with tape.

____ ____ ____ _____

11. Removed and discarded old IV tubing, applied new dressing if necessary, removed and disposed of gloves, performed hand hygiene.

____ ____ ____ _____

EVALUATION

1. Evaluated flow rate hourly, observed connection site for leaking.

____ ____ ____ _____

2. Observed patient for signs of FVD or FVE to determine response to IV therapy.

____ ____ ____ _____

3. Checked system for patency starting with solution bag and working down system to insertion site.

____ ____ ____ _____

4. Identified unexpected outcomes.

____ ____ ____ _____

RECORDING AND REPORTING

1. Recorded tubing change, type of solution, volume, and rate in appropriate record; recorded parenteral fluids appropriately.

____ ____ ____ _____

Student _____ Date _____

Instructor _____ Date _____

PERFORMANCE CHECKLIST SKILL 28-5 **CHANGING A SHORT PERIPHERAL INTRAVENOUS DRESSING**

	S	U	NP	Comments
ASSESSMENT				
1. Determined when dressing was last changed, labeled dressing properly.	___	___	___	_____
2. Performed hand hygiene, observed dressing for moisture and intactness, determined source of any moisture.	___	___	___	_____
3. Observed IV system for proper functioning or complications; palpated catheter site through dressing for complaints of tenderness, pain, or burning.	___	___	___	_____
4. Monitored body temperature.	___	___	___	_____
5. Assessed patient's understanding of need for continued IV infusion.	___	___	___	_____
PLANNING				
1. Identified expected outcomes.	___	___	___	_____
IMPLEMENTATION				
1. Explained procedure and purpose to patient and family caregiver, explained that patient would hold affected extremity still, explained how long procedure would take.	___	___	___	_____
2. Performed hand hygiene, collected equipment, applied clean gloves.	___	___	___	_____
3. Identified patient using two identifiers, compared with information on patient's ID bracelet.	___	___	___	_____
4. Removed tape and transparent semipermeable dressing properly, stabilized catheter hub and tubing properly.	___	___	___	_____
5. Observed insertion site for signs and symptoms of IV related complications, discontinued infusion if necessary.	___	___	___	_____
6. Prepared new tape strips for use, removed tape or stabilization device if IV was infusing properly, stabilized VAD with one finger, used adhesive remover to cleanse skin if needed.	___	___	___	_____
7. Cleansed insertion site with antiseptic swab, allowed to dry completely.	___	___	___	_____

	S	U	NP	Comments
8. Applied skin protectant solution if necessary, allowed to dry.	——	——	——	_____
9. Applied appropriate sterile dressing over site while securing catheter.	——	——	——	_____
10. Removed and discarded gloves.	——	——	——	_____
11. Applied site protection device if necessary.	——	——	——	_____
12. Anchored IV tubing with additional tape if necessary, avoided placing tape over dressing.	——	——	——	_____
13. Labeled dressing appropriately.	——	——	——	_____
14. Discarded equipment, performed hand hygiene.	——	——	——	_____

EVALUATION

1. Observed function, patency of IV system, and flow rate after changing dressing.	——	——	——	_____
2. Inspected condition of short peripheral site for signs and symptoms of IV-related complications.	——	——	——	_____
3. Monitored patient's body temperature.	——	——	——	_____
4. Identified unexpected outcomes.	——	——	——	_____

RECORDING AND REPORTING

1. Recorded all pertinent dressings in the appropriate log.	——	——	——	_____
2. Reported dressing change and significant information to nurse in charge or oncoming shift nurse.	——	——	——	_____
3. Reported to health care provider, documented any complications.	——	——	——	_____

Student _____ Date _____

Instructor _____ Date _____

PERFORMANCE CHECKLIST PROCEDURAL GUIDELINE 28-1 **DISCONTINUING SHORT PERIPHERAL INTRAVENOUS ACCESS**

	S	U	NP	Comments
PROCEDURAL STEPS				
1. Observed existing IV site for signs of IV-related complications.	___	___	___	_____
2. Reviewed accuracy and completeness of order for discontinuation of IV therapy.	___	___	___	_____
3. Assessed patient's understanding of need for IV to be discontinued.	___	___	___	_____
4. Identified patient using two identifiers, compared identifiers with information on patient's ID bracelet.	___	___	___	_____
5. Explained procedure to patient before you removed catheter, explained that patient needs to hold affected extremity still.	___	___	___	_____
6. Turned IV tubing roller clamp to *off* position, turned EID off first if necessary.	___	___	___	_____
7. Performed hand hygiene, applied clean gloves.	___	___	___	_____
8. Removed IV site dressing and stabilizing IV device, removed tape securing catheter.	___	___	___	_____
9. Placed clean sterile gauze above site, withdrew catheter properly, kept hub parallel to skin.	___	___	___	_____
10. Applied pressure to site for appropriate length of time.	___	___	___	_____
11. Inspected catheter for intactness after removal, noted tip integrity and length.	___	___	___	_____
12. Observed site for evidence of any complications.	___	___	___	_____
13. Applied clean gauze dressing over insertion site, secured with tape.	___	___	___	_____
14. Discarded used supplies, removed gloves, performed hand hygiene.	___	___	___	_____
15. Documented procedure in patient's medical record.	___	___	___	_____

Student _____ Date _____

Instructor _____ Date _____

PERFORMANCE CHECKLIST SKILL 28 6 **CARING FOR CENTRAL VASCULAR ACCESS DEVICES**

	S	U	NP	Comments

ASSESSMENT

1. Reviewed accuracy and completeness of order for insertion of CVAD for size and type, assessed treatment schedule, followed six rights of medication administration.

2. Assessed patient's hydration status.

3. Assessed patient for any surgical procedures of the upper chest or anatomic irregularities of the proposed insertion site.

4. Assessed CVAD placement site for skin integrity and signs of infection.

5. Assessed patient for allergy to iodine, lidocaine, latex, or chlorhexidine.

6. Assessed type of CVAD intended for placement, reviewed manufacturer's directions.

7. Assessed for proper function of CVAD before therapy.

8. Assessed if lumens require flushing or site needs dressing change.

9. Assessed patient's understanding of CVAD and knowledge of purpose, care, and maintenance; asked patient to discuss steps in care and perform procedure.

PLANNING

1. Identified expected outcomes.

IMPLEMENTATION

1. Explained procedure and purpose to patient and family caregiver, instructed patient not to move during procedure.

2. Identified patient using two identifiers, compared identifiers in MAR and on patient's ID bracelet.

3. Catheter insertion for nontunneled device:

   a. Assisted physician in positioning patient properly.

   b. Performed hand hygiene.

	S	U	NP	Comments

c. Used scissors or electric clippers to remove hair around insertion site.

d. Positioned drape underneath area to be cannulated.

e. Applied PPE.

f. Prepared site with chlorhexidine, allowed to air dry.

g. Performed hand hygiene, changed into new sterile gloves.

h. Set up IV bag, filled tubing, covered end of tubing with sterile cap.

i. Wiped off top of lidocaine bottle with alcohol, held bottle upside down, applied transdermal anesthetic agents before insertion if necessary.

j. Adjusted IV infusion to prescribed rate, connected to electronic infusion pump once chest x-ray study was obtained.

4. Performed insertion site care and dressing change.

  a. Positioned patient properly.

  b. Prepared dressing materials.

  c. Performed hand hygiene, applied mask.

  d. Applied clean gloves, removed old dressing properly, discarded appropriately.

  e. Removed catheter stabilization device properly if used.

  f. Inspected catheter, insertion site, and surrounding skin.

  g. Removed and discarded gloves, performed hand hygiene, opened CVAD dressing kit using sterile technique, applied sterile gloves.

  h. Cleansed site appropriately.

  i. Applied skin protectant to entire area, allowed to dry completely.

  j. Used chlorhexidine-impregnated dressing if appropriate.

  k. Applied new catheter stabilization device appropriately if needed.

  l. Applied proper dressing over insertion site.

	S	U	NP	Comments

m. Applied appropriate label. ___ ___ ___ _____

n. Disposed of supplies and used equipment appropriately, removed gloves, performed hand hygiene. ___ ___ ___ _____

5. Took blood sample properly. ___ ___ ___ _____

  a. Performed hand hygiene, applied clean gloves. ___ ___ ___ _____

  b. Turned off all infusions for at least 1 minute before drawing blood, drew blood from a peripheral vein if necessary. ___ ___ ___ _____

  c. Used appropriate lumen of a multilumen catheter. ___ ___ ___ _____

  d. Cleansed injection cap with antiseptic, allowed to dry, flushed with sodium chloride. ___ ___ ___ _____

  e. Performed syringe method properly, checked agency policy for use of Vacutainer with CVADs. ___ ___ ___ _____

    (1) Removed end of IV tubing or injection cap from the catheter hub, kept end of tubing sterile. ___ ___ ___ _____

    (2) Disinfected catheter hub with antiseptic solution. ___ ___ ___ _____

    (3) Attached an empty syringe, unclamped catheter, and withdrew blood; filled volume of catheter for discard sample. ___ ___ ___ _____

    (4) Reclamped catheter, removed syringe with blood, discarded in appropriate biohazard container. ___ ___ ___ _____

    (5) Cleansed hub with another antiseptic solution. ___ ___ ___ _____

    (6) Attached second syringe(s) to obtain required volume of blood for specimen. ___ ___ ___ _____

    (7) Unclamped catheter to withdraw blood if necessary. ___ ___ ___ _____

    (8) Reclamped catheter after obtaining specimen, removed syringe. ___ ___ ___ _____

    (9) Cleansed catheter hub with antiseptic solution. ___ ___ ___ _____

    (10) Attached prefilled injection cap to syringe of sodium chloride to catheter, unclamped if necessary, flushed, reclamped catheter if needed. ___ ___ ___ _____

    (11) Removed syringe, discarded in appropriate container. ___ ___ ___ _____

	S	U	NP	Comments

f. Transferred blood using transfer vacuum device. _____ _____ _____ _____

g. Flushed catheter with heparin solution. _____ _____ _____ _____

h. Removed syringe, attached IV tubing, resumed infusion as ordered or clamped catheter if needed. _____ _____ _____ _____

i. Disposed of soiled equipment and used supplies, removed gloves, performed hand hygiene. _____ _____ _____ _____

6. Changed injection cap properly.

a. Determined if injection caps should be changed. _____ _____ _____ _____

b. Prepared new injection cap(s) properly. _____ _____ _____ _____

c. Clamped catheter lumens one at a time if needed. _____ _____ _____ _____

d. Removed old caps using aseptic technique. _____ _____ _____ _____

e. Applied clean gloves, cleansed catheter hub with antiseptic, connected new injection cap(s) on catheter hub. _____ _____ _____ _____

f. Flushed catheter with sodium chloride followed by heparin solution. _____ _____ _____ _____

g. Disposed of all soiled supplies and used equipment, removed gloves, performed hand hygiene. _____ _____ _____ _____

7. Flushed positive-pressure device properly.

a. Performed hand hygiene, applied clean gloves. _____ _____ _____ _____

b. Attached prefilled saline syringe, primed device, left syringe attached. _____ _____ _____ _____

c. Clamped catheter if necessary, removed injection cap and discarded. _____ _____ _____ _____

d. Connected positive-pressure device, unclamped catheter, flushed through with saline as ordered. _____ _____ _____ _____

e. Reclamped after syringe had been removed. _____ _____ _____ _____

f. Disposed of all soiled supplies and used equipment, removed gloves, performed hand hygiene. _____ _____ _____ _____

8. Discontinued nontunneled catheters or PICCs properly.

a. Verified order to discontinue line, checked agency policy for the person who should discontinue CVAD. _____ _____ _____ _____

	S	U	NP	Comments
b. Prepared to convert IV fluids or medications to a short peripheral or middle before CVAD continuation.	___	___	___	_____
c. Positioned patient in 10-degree Trendelendburg's position.	___	___	___	_____
d. Performed hand hygiene.	___	___	___	_____
e. Turned off IV fluids infusing through central line.	___	___	___	_____
f. Placed moisture-proof pad under site.	___	___	___	_____
g. Applied PPE.	___	___	___	_____
h. Removed CVAD dressing appropriately, discarded in biohazard container, inspected catheter and insertion site.	___	___	___	_____
i. Removed gloves, performed hand hygiene, opened CVAD dressing change kit and suture removal kit, added additional items to sterile fields, applied sterile gloves.	___	___	___	_____
j. Cleaned CVAD site properly with chlorhexidine swabs, allowed to dry completely.	___	___	___	_____
k. Removed catheter from securement device with alcohol if necessary.	___	___	___	_____
l. Removed sutures with nondominant hand, avoided damaging skin or catheter, discarded sutures appropriately.	___	___	___	_____
m. Applied sterile gauze to site, instructed patient to take a deep breath and hold it.	___	___	___	_____
n. Removed catheter smoothly and properly, noted any resistance, inspected catheter for intactness, applied pressure to site until bleeding stopped.	___	___	___	_____
o. Applied petroleum-based ointment to exit site, applied sterile occlusive dressing to site, changed dressing every 24 hours until healed.	___	___	___	_____
p. Labeled dressing properly.	___	___	___	_____
q. Inspected catheter integrity, discarded in biohazard container.	___	___	___	_____
r. Returned patient to comfortable position, ensured short peripheral IV or midline was infusing at correct rate.	___	___	___	_____
s. Disposed of soiled supplies, removed gloves and PPE, performed hand hygiene.	___	___	___	_____

	S	U	NP	Comments

EVALUATION

1. Observed patient for shortness of breath and pain in chest or shoulders after CVAD insertion, auscultated for breath sounds. ___ ___ ___ _____

2. Observed patient for bleeding or swelling at insertion site or neck and occlusiveness of dressing. ___ ___ ___ _____

3. Monitored I&O as directed for fluid balance, monitored laboratory values for electrolyte balance. ___ ___ ___ _____

4. Assessed vital signs of patient routinely, noted changes symptomatic of infection. ___ ___ ___ _____

5. Observed catheter insertion site and exit for signs of inflammation or infection. ___ ___ ___ _____

6. Observed all catheter connection points. ___ ___ ___ _____

7. Inspected condition of catheter and connection tubing for breaks in integrity. ___ ___ ___ _____

8. Observed for clot formation in catheter, air embolism, and infiltration/extravasation. ___ ___ ___ _____

9. Consulted x-ray examination reports for catheter placement. ___ ___ ___ _____

10. Evaluated ability of patient and family caregiver to provide care and maintain catheter or infusion port, determined need for restrictions on daily activities. ___ ___ ___ _____

11. Identified unexpected outcomes. ___ ___ ___ _____

RECORDING AND REPORTING

1. Notified health care provider of signs and symptoms of any complications. ___ ___ ___ _____

2. Documented catheter site care in nurses' notes. ___ ___ ___ _____

3. Documented in nurses' notes condition of site or port insertion site. ___ ___ ___ _____

4. Documented in nurses' notes catheter removal. ___ ___ ___ _____

5. Documented in nurses' notes blood draw. ___ ___ ___ _____

6. Documented in nurses' notes unexpected outcomes, health care provider notification, interventions, and patient response to treatment. ___ ___ ___ _____

Student _____ Date _____

Instructor _____ Date _____

PERFORMANCE CHECKLIST SKILL 29-1 **INITIATING BLOOD THERAPY**

	S	U	NP	Comments
ASSESSMENT				
1. Verified health care provider's order for specific blood or blood product and all pertinent information.	___	___	___	_____
2. Obtained patient's transfusion history, noted known allergies and previous transfusion reactions, verified that type and crossmatch had been completed appropriately.	___	___	___	_____
3. Verified that IV cannula was patent and without complications, administered blood or components using appropriate peripheral catheter.	___	___	___	_____
4. Assessed laboratory values such as hematocrit, coagulation values, and platelet count.	___	___	___	_____
5. Checked that patient had completed and signed transfusion consent before retrieving blood.	___	___	___	_____
6. Knew indications or reasons for a transfusion, packed RBCs if necessary.	___	___	___	_____
7. Obtained and recorded pretransfusion baseline vital signs, notified health care provider if patient was febrile.	___	___	___	_____
8. Assessed patient's need for IV fluids or medications while transfusion was infusing.	___	___	___	_____
9. Assessed patient's understanding of procedure and rationale.	___	___	___	_____
PLANNING				
1. Identified expected outcomes.	___	___	___	_____
2. Explained procedure to patient and caregiver.	___	___	___	_____
IMPLEMENTATION				
1. Performed preadministration protocol.				
a. Obtained blood component following agency protocol.	___	___	___	_____
b. Checked blood bag for signs of contamination and presence of leaks.	___	___	___	_____
c. Compared verbally; correctly verified patient, blood product, and type with another qualified person before initiating transfusion.	___	___	___	_____

	S	U	NP	Comments

d. Reviewed purpose of transfusion, asked patient to report any changes he or she may feel during the transfusion. ___ ___ ___ _____

e. Emptied urine drainage collection container, or had patient void. ___ ___ ___ _____

2. Administered transfusion.

a. Performed hand hygiene, applied gloves. ___ ___ ___ _____

b. Opened Y-tubing blood administration set, used multiset if needed. ___ ___ ___ _____

c. Set all clamps to *off* position. ___ ___ ___ _____

d. Spiked normal saline IV bag with spike, hung bag on pole, primed tubing, opened upper clamp on saline side of tubing, squeezed drip chamber until fluid covered filter and appropriate amount of drip chamber. ___ ___ ___ _____

e. Maintained clamp on blood product side of tubing in *off* position, opened common tubing clamp, closed clamp when tubing was filled with saline, maintained protective sterile cap on tubing connector. ___ ___ ___ _____

f. Prepared blood component for administration, agitated blood unit bag, removed covering from access port, spiked unit with other Y connection, closed saline clamp, opened blood unit clamp, primed tubing with blood, ensured residual air was removed. ___ ___ ___ _____

g. Maintained asepsis, attached primed tubing to patient's VAD, opened tubing clamp, regulated blood flow properly. ___ ___ ___ _____

h. Remained with patient for first 15 minutes. ___ ___ ___ _____

i. Monitored patient's vitals at the appropriate times. ___ ___ ___ _____

j. Regulated rate appropriately if there was no transfusion reaction, checked drop factor for the blood tubing. ___ ___ ___ _____

k. Cleared IV line with saline, discarded blood bag appropriately, maintained patency when consecutive units were ordered. ___ ___ ___ _____

l. Disposed of all supplies appropriately, removed gloves, performed hand hygiene. ___ ___ ___ _____

	S	U	NP	Comments

EVALUATION

1. Observed IV site and status of infusion each time vitals were taken.
2. Observed for change in vital signs and signs of transfusion reactions.
3. Observed patient, assessed laboratory values to determine response.
4. Identified unexpected outcomes.

RECORDING AND REPORTING

1. Recorded pretransfusion medication, vital signs, location and condition of IV site, and patient education.
2. Recorded all pertinent transfusion information in the appropriate log.
3. Recorded volume of saline and blood component infused.
4. Reported signs and symptoms of a transfusion reaction immediately.
5. Recorded amount of blood received by autotransfusion. and patient's response to therapy.
6. Reported any intratransfusion/posttransfusion deterioration in cardiac, pulmonary, or renal status.
7. Recorded vital signs before, during, and after transfusion.

Student _____ Date _____

Instructor _____ Date _____

PERFORMANCE CHECKLIST SKILL 29-2 **MONITORING FOR ADVERSE TRANSFUSION REACTIONS**

	S	U	NP	Comments
ASSESSMENT				
1. Observed patient for fever with or without chills in conjunction with initiation of transfusion.	___	___	___	_____
2. Assessed patient for tachycardia/tachypnea and dyspnea.	___	___	___	_____
3. Observed patient for drop in blood pressure.	___	___	___	_____
4. Observed patient for hives or skin rash.	___	___	___	_____
5. Observed patient for flushing.	___	___	___	_____
6. Observed patient for gastrointestinal symptoms.	___	___	___	_____
7. Observed patient for wheezing, chest pain, and possible cardiac arrest.	___	___	___	_____
8. Remained alert to patient complaints of headache or muscle pain in presence of a fever.	___	___	___	_____
9. Monitored patient for DIC, renal failure, anemia, and hemoglobinemia/hemoglobinuria by reviewing laboratory test results.	___	___	___	_____
10. Auscultated patient's lungs, monitored CVP if possible.	___	___	___	_____
11. Observed patient for signs of liver damage and bone marrow suppression.	___	___	___	_____
12. Observed for mild hypothermia, cardiac dysrhythmias, hypotension, hypocalcemia, and hemochromatosis in patients receiving massive transfusions.	___	___	___	_____
PLANNING				
1. Identified expected outcomes.	___	___	___	_____
2. Explained treatment of reaction to patient and family caregiver.	___	___	___	_____

	S	U	NP	Comments

IMPLEMENTATION

1. Responded to suspected transfusion reaction.

    a. Stopped transfusion immediately.

    b. Removed blood component and tubing containing blood product, replaced with normal saline and new tubing, connected tubing to hub of IV catheter, administered antihistamine instead if appropriate.

    c. If mild allergic reaction suspected, administered antihistamine, followed health care providers orders on whether or not to restart transfusion.

    d. Maintained patent IV line using normal saline.

    e. Obtained vital signs, did not leave patient alone.

    f. Notified health care provider.

    g. Notified blood bank.

    h. Obtained blood samples from extremity not receiving transfusion if needed.

    i. Returned remainder of blood component, attached blood tubing to blood bank according to policy.

    j. Monitored patient's vitals as frequently as needed.

    k. Administered prescribed medication according to type and severity of transfusion reaction.

    l. Initiated cardiac resuscitation if necessary.

    m. Obtained first voided urine sample, sent to laboratory, inserted catheter if necessary.

EVALUATION

1. Continued monitoring patient for signs and symptoms of transfusion reactions.

2. Identified unexpected outcomes.

RECORDING AND REPORTING

1. Documented all pertinent information in the appropriate record, completed transfusion reaction report.

2. Reported presence of transfusion reaction and patient's physical assessment findings to nurse in charge and health care provider.

Student _____ Date _____

Instructor _____ Date _____

PERFORMANCE CHECKLIST SKILL 30-1 **PERFORMING A NUTRITIONAL ASSESSMENT**

	S	U	NP	Comments
ASSESSMENT				
1. Assessed patient's knowledge of procedure.				
2. Asked patient to report usual body weight, noted recent changes in weight, asked if any weight loss was intentional.	___	___	___	_____
3. Obtained complete nursing history, determined patient's current nutritional habits.	___	___	___	_____
4. Performed physical assessment, noted any mental changes.	___	___	___	_____
5. Reviewed results of relevant laboratory tests.	___	___	___	_____
6. Determined medications and other dietary supplements patient was taking, was aware of common drug-drug and drug-nutrition interactions.	___	___	___	_____
7. Measured ABW properly.	___	___	___	_____
8. Measured actual height properly.	___	___	___	_____
9. Calculated IBW properly.	___	___	___	_____
10. Calculated BMI properly.	___	___	___	_____
11. Assessed patient's diet history.	___	___	___	_____
12. Had patient provide 24-hour diet recall.	___	___	___	_____
13. Determined patient's ability to manipulate eating utensils and self-feed.	___	___	___	_____
14. Explained to patient that nutritional assessment was complete.	___	___	___	_____
15. Reported diet restrictions and food preferences to nutrition department.	___	___	___	_____
EVALUATION				
1. Reviewed history and physical findings, noted abnormal findings or areas of concern.	___	___	___	_____
2. Compared patient's weight for height with IBW, compared BMI with recommended BMI.	___	___	___	_____
3. Compared normal laboratory test levels with patient's levels.	___	___	___	_____
4. Identified unexpected outcomes.	___	___	___	_____

	S	U	NP	Comments

RECORDING AND REPORTING

1. Recorded assessment finding results on nutritional screening form, notified health care provider of abnormal findings.

	___	___	___	_____

2. Made referral to the RD.

	___	___	___	_____

Student _____ Date _____

Instructor _____ Date _____

PERFORMANCE CHECKLIST SKILL 30-2 **ASSISTING AN ADULT PATIENT WITH ORAL NUTRITION**

	S	U	NP	Comments
ASSESSMENT				
1. Assessed patient's knowledge of procedure.	___	___	___	_____
2. Assessed if patient passed flatus and was without nausea, auscultated bowel sounds.	___	___	___	_____
3. Reviewed diet order.	___	___	___	_____
4. Assessed presence and condition of teeth, determined if dentures were poorly fitted.	___	___	___	_____
5. Assessed neurologic patient's cranial nerve function; assessed cranial nerves V, VII, IX, and X.	___	___	___	_____
6. Determined to what extent patient as able to self-feed; assessed physical motor skills; evaluated LOC, visual acuity, peripheral vision, and mood.	___	___	___	_____
7. Assessed patient's appetite, tolerance of foods, recent fluid intake, cultural and religious preferences, and food likes and dislikes.	___	___	___	_____
8. Assessed patient's ability to swallow.	___	___	___	_____
PLANNING				
1. Identified expected outcomes.	___	___	___	_____
IMPLEMENTATION				
1. Prepared patient's room for mealtime.				
a. Performed hand hygiene, cleared over-bed table.	___	___	___	_____
2. Prepared patient for meal.				
a. Assisted patient with elimination needs, helped patient perform hand hygiene before meals.	___	___	___	_____
b. Helped patient to apply dentures, eyeglasses, or contact lenses if necessary.	___	___	___	_____
c. Helped patient to comfortable position.	___	___	___	_____
3. Asked in what order patient would like to eat his or her meal, asked about seasonings, assisted patient to cut food if necessary.	___	___	___	_____
4. Used adaptive eating and drinking aids as needed.	___	___	___	_____

	S	U	NP	Comments

5. Identified food placement as if plate were a clock for disoriented, visually impaired, or easily fatigued patients. ___ ___ ___ _____

6. Fed patient in an appropriate manner that facilitated chewing and swallowing. ___ ___ ___ _____

7. Provided fluids as requested, encouraged patients not to drink all liquid at the beginning of the meal. ___ ___ ___ _____

8. Talked with patient during the meal. ___ ___ ___ _____

9. Used the meal as an opportunity to educate patient. ___ ___ ___ _____

10. Assisted patient with hand hygiene and mouth care. ___ ___ ___ _____

11. Helped patient to appropriate position. ___ ___ ___ _____

12. Returned patient's trays to appropriate place, performed hand hygiene. ___ ___ ___ _____

EVALUATION

1. Monitored body weight appropriately. ___ ___ ___ _____

2. Monitored laboratory values as indicated. ___ ___ ___ _____

3. Monitored I&O and percentage of food on tray after meal. ___ ___ ___ _____

4. Observed patient's ability to self-feed. ___ ___ ___ _____

5. Observed patient for choking, coughing, gagging, or food left in mouth during eating. ___ ___ ___ _____

6. Identified unexpected outcomes. ___ ___ ___ _____

RECORDING AND REPORTING

1. Documented patient's tolerance of diet and amount of food eaten in the appropriate log. ___ ___ ___ _____

2. Recorded caloric intake and fluid intake in appropriate log if necessary. ___ ___ ___ _____

3. Recorded amount of oral nutritional supplements taken and communicated patient tolerance to health care team if necessary. ___ ___ ___ _____

4. Reported any swallowing difficulties, food dislikes, or refusal to eat. ___ ___ ___ _____

Student _____ Date _____

Instructor _____ Date _____

PERFORMANCE CHECKLIST SKILL 30-3 **ASPIRATION PRECAUTIONS**

	S	U	NP	Comments
ASSESSMENT				
1. Assessed patient's knowledge of aspiration risks.	___	___	___	_____
2. Performed nutritional assessment.	___	___	___	_____
3. Assessed mental status.	___	___	___	_____
4. Determined if patient was at increased risk for aspiration, assessed for signs of dysphagia, used dysphagia screening tool if available.	___	___	___	_____
5. Assessed patient's oral health; checked level of dental hygiene, missing teeth, or poorly fitting dentures; applied clean gloves if needed.	___	___	___	_____
6. Observed patient during mealtime for signs of dysphagia, noted if patient was fatigued.	___	___	___	_____
PLANNING				
1. Identified expected outcomes.	___	___	___	_____
IMPLEMENTATION				
1. Performed hand hygiene.	___	___	___	_____
2. Indicated presence of dysphagia/aspiration risk on chart.	___	___	___	_____
3. Applied pulse oximeter to patient's finger.	___	___	___	_____
4. Positioned patient properly.	___	___	___	_____
5. Used penlight and tongue blade to inspect for pockets of food.	___	___	___	_____
6. Had patient assume chin-tuck position, had patient swallow, monitored for respiratory difficulty.	___	___	___	_____
7. Added thickener to thin liquids if necessary.	___	___	___	_____
8. Encouraged patient to self-feed.	___	___	___	_____
9. Told patient not to tilt head backward while eating or drinking.	___	___	___	_____
10. Placed appropriate amount of food on unaffected side of patient's mouth if patient was unable to self-feed, allowed utensils to touch mouth.	___	___	___	_____

	S	U	NP	Comments

11. Provided verbal cueing while feeding, reminded patient to chew and think about swallowing. ___ ___ ___ _____

12. Avoided mixing food of different textures, alternated liquid and bites of food. ___ ___ ___ _____

13. Minimized distractions, did not rush patient, allowed adequate time for chewing. ___ ___ ___ _____

14. Used sauces to facilitate cohesive food bolus formation. ___ ___ ___ _____

15. Reported signs of dysphagia or aspiration to health care provider. ___ ___ ___ _____

16. Asked patient to sit upright after meal. ___ ___ ___ _____

17. Provided oral hygiene after meals. ___ ___ ___ _____

18. Performed hand hygiene. ___ ___ ___ _____

EVALUATION

1. Evaluated patient ability to cough and manage oral secretions continually, monitored ability to swallow foods and fluids without choking. ___ ___ ___ _____

2. Weighed patient with appropriate frequency. ___ ___ ___ _____

3. Monitored patient's I&O, calorie count, and food intake. ___ ___ ___ _____

4. Monitored pulse oximetry readings for high-risk patients when eating. ___ ___ ___ _____

5. Identified unexpected outcomes. ___ ___ ___ _____

RECORDING AND REPORTING

1. Documented all pertinent information in the appropriate log. ___ ___ ___ _____

2. Reported coughing, gagging, choking, or swallowing difficulties to health care provider. ___ ___ ___ _____

Student _____ Date _____

Instructor _____ Date _____

	S	U	NP	Comments

ASSESSMENT

1. Verified order for type of tube and feeding schedule.

2. Assessed patient's knowledge of procedure.

3. Had patient close each nostril alternately and breathe, examined each naris for patency and skin breakdown.

4. Reviewed patient's medical history.

5. Assessed patient's mental status.

6. Performed physical assessment of the abdomen.

PLANNING

1. Identified expected outcomes.

2. Explained procedure to patient, included sensations he or she would feel.

3. Explained how to communicate during intubation.

IMPLEMENTATION

1. Identified patient using two identifiers.

2. Performed hand hygiene.

3. Positioned patient appropriately, obtained assistance if necessary.

4. Applied pulse oximeter, measured vital signs.

5. Determined length of tube to be inserted, marked location properly.

6. Prepared NG or nasoenteric tube for intubation.

   a. Injected water from catheter-tip syringe into the tube.

   b. Ensured stylet was securely positioned within the tube.

7. Cut hypoallergenic tape or prepared other securing device.

	S	U	NP	Comments
8. Applied clean gloves.	___	___	___	_____
9. Dipped tube with surface lubricant into room-temperature water or applied lubricant.	___	___	___	_____
10. Explained the step, inserted tube through nostril to back of throat, aimed appropriately.	___	___	___	_____
11. Had patient flex head toward chest at appropriate time.	___	___	___	_____
12. Encouraged patient to swallow with ice chips or small sips of water, advanced tube as patient swallowed.	___	___	___	_____
13. Reemphasized mouth breathing and swallowing.	___	___	___	_____
14. Listened for air exchange from distal portion of tube when tip of tube reached carina.	___	___	___	_____
15. Advanced tube each time patient swallowed, until desired length had been passed.	___	___	___	_____
16. Checked for position of tube in back of throat.	___	___	___	_____
17. Anchored tube to nose temporarily.	___	___	___	_____
18. Checked placement of tube by aspirating stomach contents.	___	___	___	_____
19. Anchored tube to patient's nose, marked exit site on tube, selected appropriate option for anchoring.				
a. Applied tape properly.	___	___	___	_____
b. Applied membrane dressing or tube fixation device properly.	___	___	___	_____
21. Fastened end of NG tube properly to patient's gown.	___	___	___	_____
22. Assisted patient to a comfortable position.	___	___	___	_____
23. Obtained x-ray film of chest/abdomen.	___	___	___	_____
24. Applied clean gloves, administered oral hygiene, cleansed tubing at nostril properly.	___	___	___	_____
25. Removed gloves, disposed of equipment, performed hand hygiene.	___	___	___	_____

TUBE REMOVAL

	S	U	NP	Comments
1. Verified order for type of tube and feeding schedule.	___	___	___	_____
2. Gathered equipment.	___	___	___	_____
3. Explained procedure to patient.	___	___	___	_____
4. Performed hand hygiene, applied gloves.	___	___	___	_____

	S	U	NP	Comments
5. Positioned patient appropriately.	___	___	___	_____
6. Placed disposable pad over patient's chest.	___	___	___	_____
7. Disconnected tube from feeding administration set.	___	___	___	_____
8. Removed securement device from the patient's nose	___	___	___	_____
9. Instructed patient to take a deep breath and hold.	___	___	___	_____
10. Kinked the tube by folding it over on itself.	___	___	___	_____
11. Withdrew tube in one motion, disposed of tube appropriately.	___	___	___	_____
12. Offered tissues to patient.	___	___	___	_____
13. Removed gloves, performed hand hygiene.	___	___	___	_____
14. Offered mouth care.	___	___	___	_____

EVALUATION

1. Identified unexpected outcomes.	___	___	___	_____

RECORDING AND REPORTING

1. Recorded and reported all pertinent information in the appropriate log.	___	___	___	_____
2. Recorded removal of tube and patient's tolerance.	___	___	___	_____
3. Reported any type of unexpected outcome and interventions performed.	___	___	___	_____

Student _____ Date _____

Instructor _____ Date _____

PERFORMANCE CHECKLIST SKILL 31-2 **VERIFYING FEEDING TUBE PLACEMENT**

	S	U	NP	Comments
ASSESSMENT				
1. Maintained awareness of agency policy and procedures for checking tube placement, did not insufflate air into tube.	___	___	___	_____
2. Identified signs of inadvertent respiratory distress during feeding.	___	___	___	_____
3. Identified conditions that increase the risk for spontaneous tube dislocation.	___	___	___	_____
4. Observed external portion of tube for movement of ink mark.	___	___	___	_____
5. Reviewed patient's medication record for orders for continuous feeding or gastric acid inhibitor or a proton pump inhibitor.	___	___	___	_____
6. Reviewed patient's record for history of prior tube displacement.	___	___	___	_____
PLANNING				
1. Identified expected outcomes.	___	___	___	_____
2. Explained procedure to patient.	___	___	___	_____
IMPLEMENTATION				
1. Identified patient using two identifiers.	___	___	___	_____
2. Prepared equipment at patient's bedside, performed hand hygiene, applied clean gloves.	___	___	___	_____
3. Verified tube placement at the appropriate times.	___	___	___	_____
4. Drew up appropriate amount of air into syringe, attached to end of feeding tube, flushed tube with air before attempting to aspirate, repositioned patient if needed.	___	___	___	_____
5. Drew back on syringe slowly, obtained proper amount of gastric aspirate, observed appearance of aspirate.	___	___	___	_____
6. Mixed aspirate in syringe, expelled a few drops into a clean medicine cup, measured pH of aspirated GI contents, compared color of strip with color on the chart.	___	___	___	_____

	S	U	NP	Comments
7. Monitored external length of tube, observed patient for evidence of respiratory distress if fluids could not be aspirated.	___	___	___	_____
8. Irrigated tube.	___	___	___	_____
9. Removed and disposed of gloves and supplies, performed hand hygiene.	___	___	___	_____

EVALUATION

1. Observed patient for respiratory distress.	___	___	___	_____
2. Verified that external length of tube, pH, and appearance of aspirate were consistent with initial tube placement.	___	___	___	_____
3. Identified unexpected outcomes.	___	___	___	_____

RECORDING AND REPORTING

1. Recorded and reported pH and appearance of aspirate.	___	___	___	_____

Student _____ Date _____

Instructor _____ Date _____

PERFORMANCE CHECKLIST SKILL 31-3 **IRRIGATING A FEEDING TUBE**

	S	U	NP	Comments

ASSESSMENT

1. Inspected volume, color, and character of gastric aspirates. ___ ___ ___ _____

2. Assessed bowel sounds. ___ ___ ___ _____

3. Noted ease with which tube feeding infused through tubing. ___ ___ ___ _____

4. Monitored volume of enteral formula administered during a shift, compared with ordered amount. ___ ___ ___ _____

5. Referred to agency policies regarding routine irrigation. ___ ___ ___ _____

PLANNING

1. Identified expected outcomes. ___ ___ ___ _____

2. Explained procedure to patient. ___ ___ ___ _____

3. Positioned patient properly. ___ ___ ___ _____

IMPLEMENTATION

1. Identified patient using two identifiers. ___ ___ ___ _____

2. Performed hand hygiene, prepared equipment at bedside, applied clean gloves. ___ ___ ___ _____

3. Verified tube placement if fluid could be aspirated for pH testing. ___ ___ ___ _____

4. Irrigated routinely and before, between, and after final medication; irrigated before intermittent feeding was administered. ___ ___ ___ _____

5. Drew up water into syringe, ensured patient had individual bottle of solution. ___ ___ ___ _____

6. Changed irrigation bottle every 24 hours. ___ ___ ___ _____

7. Kinked feeding tube while disconnecting from administration tubing or while removing plug at end of tube. ___ ___ ___ _____

8. Inserted tip of syringe into feeding tube, released kink, slowly instilled irrigation solution. ___ ___ ___ _____

9. Repositioned patient on left side and tried again if unable to instill fluid. ___ ___ ___ _____

10. Removed and discarded gloves, disposed of supplies, performed hand hygiene. ___ ___ ___ _____

	S	U	NP	Comments

EVALUATION

1. Observed ease with which tube feeding instilled.   ___ ___ ___ _____

2. Monitored patient's caloric intake.   ___ ___ ___ _____

3. Identified unexpected outcomes.   ___ ___ ___ _____

RECORDING AND REPORTING

1. Recorded time of irrigation, amount and type of fluid instilled.   ___ ___ ___ _____

2. Reported if tubing had become clogged.   ___ ___ ___ _____

Student _____ Date _____

Instructor _____ Date _____

PERFORMANCE CHECKLIST SKILL 31-4 **ADMINISTERING ENTERAL NUTRITION: NASOENTERIC, GASTROSTOMY, OR JEJUNOSTOMY TUBE**

	S	U	NP	Comments
ASSESSMENT				
1. Assessed patient's clinical status to determine potential need for tube feedings, consulted with nutrition support team or health care provider.	___	___	___	_____
2. Assessed patient for food allergies.	___	___	___	_____
3. Performed physical assessment of abdomen.	___	___	___	_____
4. Obtained baseline weight; reviewed serum electrolytes and blood glucose measurement; assessed patient for fluid volume excess or deficit, electrolyte abnormalities, and metabolic abnormalities.	___	___	___	_____
5. Verified health care provider's order for type of formula, rate, route, and frequency.	___	___	___	_____
PLANNING				
1. Identified expected outcomes.	___	___	___	_____
2. Explained procedure to patient.	___	___	___	_____
IMPLEMENTATION				
1. Identified patient using two identifiers.	___	___	___	_____
2. Performed hand hygiene, applied clean gloves.	___	___	___	_____
3. Obtained formula to administer:				
a. Verified correct formula, checked expiration date, noted condition of container.	___	___	___	_____
b. Provided formula at proper temperature.	___	___	___	_____
4. Prepared formula for administration.				
a. Used aseptic technique when manipulating components of feeding system.	___	___	___	_____
b. Shook formula container well, cleaned top of can with alcohol swab.	___	___	___	_____
c. Connected tubing to container for closed system, poured formula from brick pack or can into administration bag.	___	___	___	_____

	S	U	NP	Comments

5. Opened roller clamp, allowed administration tubing to fill, clamped off tubing, hung container on IV pole.

6. Placed patient in appropriate position.

7. Verified tube placement, observed appearance of aspirate, noted pH measure.

8. Checked GRV properly before each feeding and appropriately thereafter, did not administer feeding if GRV measurements were too high.

9. Traced tube to point of origin before attaching feeding administration set to tube, labeled administration set properly.

10. Intermittent gravity drip:

   a. Pinched proximal end of feeding tube, removed cap.

   b. Set rate properly, allowed bag to empty gradually, labeled bag properly.

   c. Changed bag every 24 hours.

11. Continuous drip method:

   a. Connected distal end of administration set tubing to feeding tube properly.

   b. Threaded tubing through feeding pump, set rate and turned pump on.

12. Advanced rate of tube feeding as ordered.

13. Flushed tubing with water at appropriate times, had registered dietitian recommend total free water requirement per day, obtained health care provider's order.

14. Rinsed bag and tubing with warm water whenever feedings were interrupted, used new administration set every 24 hours.

15. Disposed of supplies, performed hand hygiene.

EVALUATION

1. Measured GRV per policy, asked if nausea or abdominal cramping was present.

2. Monitored I&O at least every 8 hours, calculated daily totals.

3. Weighed patient daily or three times per week as appropriate.

4. Monitored laboratory values.

5. Observed patient's respiratory status.

416

	S	U	NP	Comments
6. Auscultated bowel sounds.	___	___	___	_____
7. Inspected site for impaired skin integrity for tubes placed through abdominal wall.	___	___	___	_____
8. Identified unexpected outcomes.	___	___	___	_____

RECORDING AND REPORTING

	S	U	NP	Comments
1. Recorded and reported all pertinent information in the appropriate log.	___	___	___	_____
2. Recorded volume of formula and additional water on I&O form.	___	___	___	_____
3. Reported type of feeding, status of tube, patient's tolerance, and adverse outcomes.	___	___	___	_____

Student _____ Date _____

Instructor _____ Date _____

PERFORMANCE CHECKLIST PROCEDURAL GUIDELINE 31-1 **CARE OF A GASTROSTOMY OR JEJUNOSTOMY TUBE**

	S	U	NP	Comments
PROCEDURAL STEPS				
1. Determined whether exit site was left to open air or if dressing was indicated, checked order.	___	___	___	_____
2. Identified patient using two identifiers.	___	___	___	_____
3. Performed hand hygiene, applied clean gloves.	___	___	___	_____
4. Removed old dressing, folded appropriately, removed gloves inside out over dressing, discarded appropriately.	___	___	___	_____
5. Assessed exit site for evidence of excoriation, drainage, infection, or bleeding.	___	___	___	_____
6. Cleansed skin around site with water and soap using gauze.	___	___	___	_____
7. Dried site completely.	___	___	___	_____
8. Applied thin layer of protective skin barrier to exit site if indicated.	___	___	___	_____
9. Placed drain-gauze over external bar or disc if dressing was ordered.	___	___	___	_____
10. Secured dressing with tape.	___	___	___	_____
11. Placed date, time, and initials on new dressing.	___	___	___	_____
12. Removed gloves, disposed of supplies, performed hand hygiene.	___	___	___	_____
13. Documented in nurses' note appearance of exit site, drainage noted, and dressing application.	___	___	___	_____
14. Reported any exit site complications to health care provider.	___	___	___	_____

Student _____ Date _____

Instructor _____ Date _____

PERFORMANCE CHECKLIST SKILL 32-1 **ADMINISTERING PARENTERAL NUTRITION THROUGH A CENTRAL LINE**

	S	U	NP	Comments
ASSESSMENT				
1. Assessed indications of and risks for protein/caloric malnutrition.	___	___	___	_____
2. Inspected condition of central vein access site for presence of inflammation, edema, and tenderness; inspected tubing of access device for patency and kinking.	___	___	___	_____
3. Assessed level of serum albumin, total protein, transferrin, prealbumin, and triglycerides; checked blood glucose levels.	___	___	___	_____
4. Assessed patient's medical history for factors influenced by PCN administration and for history of allergies.	___	___	___	_____
5. Assessed vital signs, auscultated lung sounds, measured weight.	___	___	___	_____
6. Consulted with health care provider and dietitian on calculation of calorie, protein, and fluid requirements for patient.	___	___	___	_____
7. Verified order for nutrients, minerals, vitamins, trace elements, added medications, and flow rate; checked for compatibility of added medications.	___	___	___	_____
PLANNING				
1. Identified expected outcomes.	___	___	___	_____
2. Explained purpose of CPN to a patient.	___	___	___	_____
3. Removed from refrigeration 1 hour before infusion if necessary.	___	___	___	_____
IMPLEMENTATION				
1. Performed hand hygiene.	___	___	___	_____
2. Compared label of CPN bag with MAR and patient's name, checked for correct additives and solution expiration date.	___	___	___	_____
3. Inspected 2:1 solution for particulate matter, inspected 3:1 CPN solution for separation of solution.	___	___	___	_____

	S	U	NP	Comments

4. Identified patient using two identifiers.   ___ ___ ___ _____

5. Applied clean gloves.   ___ ___ ___ _____

6. Attached appropriate filter to IV tubing, primed tubing with solution, ensured no air bubbles remained, turned off flow with roller clamp, connected end of tubing to appropriate port of central catheter, labeled port, opened roller clamp to appropriate rate.   ___ ___ ___ _____

7. Placed IV tubing into infusion pump, opened clamp completely, regulated flow rate as ordered.   ___ ___ ___ _____

8. Infused all IV medications or blood through alternative IV line, did not obtain blood samples or CVP readings through same port.   ___ ___ ___ _____

9. Did not interrupt PN infusion, ensured rate did not exceed ordered rate.   ___ ___ ___ _____

10. Changed infusing tubing and filter using aseptic technique, changed administration sets every 24 hours and upon suspected contamination.   ___ ___ ___ _____

11. Discarded used supplies, performed hand hygiene.   ___ ___ ___ _____

EVALUATION

1. Monitored flow rate routinely.   ___ ___ ___ _____

2. Monitored I&O every 8 hours.   ___ ___ ___ _____

3. Obtained weights daily or as ordered.   ___ ___ ___ _____

4. Assessed for fluid retention, palpated skin of extremities, auscultated lung sounds.   ___ ___ ___ _____

5. Monitored patient's glucose levels as ordered, monitored other laboratory parameters daily or as ordered.   ___ ___ ___ _____

6. Inspected central venous access site.   ___ ___ ___ _____

7. Monitored for signs of systemic infection.   ___ ___ ___ _____

8. Identified unexpected outcomes.   ___ ___ ___ _____

RECORDING AND REPORTING

1. Recorded all pertinent information in the appropriate log.   ___ ___ ___ _____

2. Notified health care provider if signs of infection, occlusion, fluid retention, or infiltration occurred.   ___ ___ ___ _____

Student _____ Date _____

Instructor _____ Date _____

PERFORMANCE CHECKLIST SKILL 32-2 **ADMINISTERING PARENTERAL NUTRITION THROUGH A PERIPHERAL LINE**

	S	U	NP	Comments
ASSESSMENT				
1. Assessed patient for potential hypertriglyceridemia, obtained a serum triglyceride level before initiation of PPN and weekly thereafter.	___	___	___	_____
2. Selected or initiated appropriate functional IV site, assessed its patency and function.	___	___	___	_____
3. Checked health care provider's order against MAR for volume of fat emulsion, PPN solution, and administration time for fat emulsion.	___	___	___	_____
4. Read label of fat emulsion solution.	___	___	___	_____
5. Assessed blood glucose level.	___	___	___	_____
6. Assessed patient's fluid status.	___	___	___	_____
7. Obtained patient's weight and vital signs prior to beginning infusion.	___	___	___	_____
PLANNING				
1. Identified expected outcomes.	___	___	___	_____
2. Explained purposes of PPN and fat emulsion.	___	___	___	_____
3. Placed patient in comfortable position.	___	___	___	_____
4. Removed solution from refrigerator 1 hour before infusion.	___	___	___	_____
IMPLEMENTATION				
1. Performed hand hygiene.	___	___	___	_____
2. Compared label of bag and bottle with MAR and patient's name, checked for correct additives and expiration date.	___	___	___	_____
3. Examined lipid solution for separation of emulsion or presence of froth.	___	___	___	_____
4. Identified patient using two identifiers.	___	___	___	_____
5. Measured patient's vital signs.	___	___	___	_____
6. Applied clean gloves. Prepared IV tubing for PPN solution, ran solution through tubing to remove excess air, added sterile capped needle or placed sterile cap on tubing, turned roller clamp off, followed same procedure with set for lipid infusion.	___	___	___	_____

	S	U	NP	Comments

7. Connected PPN solution to functional peripheral IV, disconnected old tubing from site, inserted adapter of new PPN tubing, opened clamp on new tubing, ensured tubing was patent, regulated IV drip rate. ___ ___ ___ _____

8. Cleaned needleless peripheral line tubing injection port with antimicrobial swab. ___ ___ ___ _____

9. Inserted needleless valve at end of fat emulsion tubing appropriately into injection port of main IV, labeled tubing. ___ ___ ___ _____

10. Opened roller clamp completely on fat emulsion infusion, checked flow rate on infusion pump. ___ ___ ___ _____

11. Infused lipids at appropriate rate, increased rate as ordered. ___ ___ ___ _____

12. Began PPN at ordered rate, infused for appropriate length of time. ___ ___ ___ _____

13. Discarded supplies, performed hand hygiene. ___ ___ ___ _____

EVALUATION

1. Monitored flow rate routinely as necessary. ___ ___ ___ _____

2. Measured vital signs and patient comfort every 10 minutes for first 30 minutes. ___ ___ ___ _____

3. Monitored patient's laboratory values daily, performed blood glucose monitoring as ordered, measured serum lipids 4 hours after discontinuing infusion. ___ ___ ___ _____

4. Monitored temperature every 4 hours, inspected venipuncture site for signs of phlebitis or infiltration. ___ ___ ___ _____

5. Assessed patient's weight, I&O, condition of peripheral extremities, and breath sounds. ___ ___ ___ _____

6. Identified unexpected outcomes. ___ ___ ___ _____

RECORDING AND REPORTING

1. Recorded pertinent information in the appropriate log. ___ ___ ___ _____

2. Recorded adverse reactions in nurses' notes. ___ ___ ___ _____

3. Notified health care provider of signs of fat intolerance, infection, occlusion, fluid retention, or infiltration. ___ ___ ___ _____

424

Student _____ Date _____

Instructor _____ Date _____

PERFORMANCE CHECKLIST PROCEDURAL GUIDELINE 33-1 **ASSISTING WITH USE OF A URINAL**

	S	U	NP	Comments
PROCEDURAL STEPS				
1. Assessed patient's normal urinary elimination habits.	___	___	___	_____
2. Determined how much assistance was needed to place and remove urinal.	___	___	___	_____
3. Determined if a urine specimen was to be collected.	___	___	___	_____
4. Explained procedure to patient.	___	___	___	_____
5. Provided privacy.	___	___	___	_____
6. Assessed for distended bladder.	___	___	___	_____
7. Performed hand hygiene, applied gloves.	___	___	___	_____
8. Assisted patient into appropriate position.	___	___	___	_____
9. Assisted male patient in holding urinal or positioning penis if necessary.	___	___	___	_____
10. Assisted female patient in positioning urinal if necessary.	___	___	___	_____
11. Covered patient with bed linens, placed call light within reach, provided privacy.	___	___	___	_____
12. Removed urinal and assessed characteristics of urine, assisted patient with washing and drying genitalia.	___	___	___	_____
13. Measured urine, recorded output on I&O if needed.	___	___	___	_____
14. Emptied and cleansed urinal, returned urinal to patient for future use.	___	___	___	_____
15. Assisted patient to perform hand hygiene.	___	___	___	_____
16. Removed and disposed of gloves, performed hand hygiene.	___	___	___	_____

Student _____ Date _____

Instructor _____ Date _____

INSERTION OF A STRAIGHT OR INDWELLING URINARY CATHETER

	S	U	NP	Comments
ASSESSMENT				
1. Reviewed patient's medical record, noted previous catheterization.	___	___	___	_____
2. Reviewed medical record for any pathologic condition that may impair passage of catheter.	___	___	___	_____
3. Asked patient and checked chart for allergies.	___	___	___	_____
4. Assessed patient's weight, LOC, developmental level, ability to cooperate, and mobility.	___	___	___	_____
5. Assessed patient's gender and age.	___	___	___	_____
6. Assessed patient's knowledge, prior experience with catheterization, and feelings about procedure.	___	___	___	_____
7. Assessed for pain and bladder fullness.	___	___	___	_____
8. Performed hand hygiene, applied gloves, inspected perineal region, removed gloves, performed hand hygiene.	___	___	___	_____
PLANNING				
1. Identified expected outcomes.	___	___	___	_____
2. Explained procedure to patient.	___	___	___	_____
3. Arranged for extra personnel to assist as necessary.	___	___	___	_____
IMPLEMENTATION				
1. Identified patient using two identifiers.	___	___	___	_____
2. Checked patient's plan for care for size and type of catheter, used smallest size possible, collected all required equipment.	___	___	___	_____
3. Performed hand hygiene.	___	___	___	_____
4. Provided privacy.	___	___	___	_____
5. Raised bed to appropriate height, raised side rail on opposite side, lowered side rail on working side.	___	___	___	_____
6. Placed waterproof pad under patient.	___	___	___	_____

	S	U	NP	Comments

7. Assisted patient to appropriate position, asked patient to relax thighs, draped patient properly so that only perineum was exposed. ___ ___ ___ _____

8. Applied gloves; washed, rinsed, and dried perineal area; used gloves to examine patient and identified urinary meatus; removed and discarded gloves. ___ ___ ___ _____

9. Positioned light to illuminate genitals or had assistant hold light. ___ ___ ___ _____

10. Performed hand hygiene. ___ ___ ___ _____

11. Opened outer wrapping of catheterization kit, placed inner wrapped kit on appropriate clean surface. ___ ___ ___ _____

12. Opened inner sterile wrap using sterile technique. ___ ___ ___ _____

13. Put on sterile gloves. ___ ___ ___ _____

14. Draped perineum, kept gloves sterile.

   a. Female patient:

     (1) Unfolded square drape without touching unsterile surfaces, allowed top edge to form cuff over both hands, placed drape shiny side down between patient's thighs, asked patient to lift hips, slipped cuffed edge just under buttocks. ___ ___ ___ _____

     (2) Unfolded fenestrated sterile drape without touching unsterile surfaces, allowed top edge to form cuff over both hands, draped over perineum, exposed labia. ___ ___ ___ _____

   b. Male patient:

     (1) Unfolded square drape without touching unsterile surfaces, placed over thighs just below penis, placed fenestrated drape with opening centered over penis. ___ ___ ___ _____

15. Arranged supplies on sterile field, maintained sterility of gloves, placed loaded sterile tray on sterile drape.

   a. Poured antiseptic solution over cotton balls if necessary. ___ ___ ___ _____

   b. Opened sterile specimen container if specimen was to be obtained. ___ ___ ___ _____

	S	U	NP	Comments

c. Opened inner sterile wrapper of catheter, attached drainage bag if part of a closed system, ensured clamp on drainage port of bag was closed, attached catheter to drainage tubing if part of sterile tray.

d. Opened lubricant, squeezed onto sterile field, lubricated catheter in gel appropriately.

16. Cleansed urethral meatus.

   a. Female patient:

   (1) Separated labia with fingers of nondominant hand.

   (2) Maintained position of nondominant hand throughout procedure.

   (3) Cleansed labia with one cotton ball using forceps, cleaned labia and urinary meatus appropriately.

   b. Male patient:

   (1) Retracted foreskin if present with nondominant hand, held penis appropriately.

   (2) Used uncontaminated hand to appropriately cleanse meatus.

17. Held catheter properly away from catheter tip with catheter coiled in hand, positioned urine tray appropriately if necessary.

18. Inserted catheter.

   a. Female patient:

   (1) Asked patient to bear down, inserted catheter slowly through urethral meatus.

   (2) Advanced catheter appropriately or until urine flows out end.

   b. Male patient:

   (1) Applied upward traction to penis as it was held at 90-degree angle from body.

   (2) Asked patient to bear down, slowly inserted catheter through urethral meatus.

   (3) Advanced catheter appropriately or until urine flows out end.

   (4) Lowered penis, held catheter securely.

	S	U	NP	Comments

19. Allowed bladder to empty fully unless volume was restricted.

20. Collected urine specimen as needed, labeled and bagged specimen in front of patient according to agency policy, sent to laboratory as soon as possible.

21. If straight catheterization, withdrew catheter slowly until removed.

22. Inflated catheter balloon with designated amount of fluid.

   a. Continued to hold catheter with nondominant hand.

   b. Connected prefilled syringe to injection port with free dominant hand.

   c. Injected total amount of solution.

   d. Released catheter after inflating balloon, pulled catheter gently until resistance was felt, advanced catheter slightly.

   e. Connected drainage tubing to catheter if not preconnected.

23. Secured indwelling catheter with securement device, left enough slack to allow leg movement, attached device just at the catheter bifurcation.

   a. For female patient, secured tubing to inner thigh, allowed enough slack.

   b. For male patient, secured catheter tubing to upper thigh or lower abdomen, allowed enough slack, replaced foreskin if retracted.

24. Clipped drainage tubing to edge of mattress, positioned bag lower than bladder, did not attach side rails of bed.

25. Ensured there was no obstruction to urine flow, coiled excess tubing on bed, fastened to bottom sheet with securement device.

26. Provided hygiene as needed, assisted patient to comfortable position.

27. Disposed of supplies in appropriate receptacles.

28. Measured urine and recorded amount.

29. Removed gloves, performed hand hygiene.

	S	U	NP	Comments

EVALUATION

1. Palpated bladder for distention or used bladder scan. ___ ___ ___ _____

2. Asked patient to describe level of comfort. ___ ___ ___ _____

3. Observed character and amount of urine in drainage system for indwelling catheter. ___ ___ ___ _____

4. Ensured there was no urine leaking from catheter or tubing connections for indwelling catheter. ___ ___ ___ _____

5. Identified unexpected outcomes. ___ ___ ___ _____

RECORDING AND REPORTING

1. Recorded and reported all pertinent information in the appropriate log. ___ ___ ___ _____

2. Recorded amount of urine on I&O flow sheet record. ___ ___ ___ _____

3. Reported persistent catheter-related pain, inadequate urine output, and discomfort to health care provider. ___ ___ ___ _____

Student _____ Date _____

Instructor _____ Date _____

	S	U	NP	Comments

ASSESSMENT

1. Catheter care:

   a. Observed urinary output and urine characteristics.

   _____ _____ _____ _____

   b. Assessed for history or presence of bowel incontinence.

   _____ _____ _____ _____

   c. Observed for any discharge, redness, bleeding, or presence of tissue trauma around urethral meatus.

   _____ _____ _____ _____

   d. Assessed patient's knowledge of catheter care.

   _____ _____ _____ _____

2. Catheter removal:

   a. Reviewed patient's medical record, noted length of time catheter was in place.

   _____ _____ _____ _____

   b. Assessed patient's knowledge and prior experience with catheter removal.

   _____ _____ _____ _____

   c. Assessed urine color, clarity, odor, and amount; noted any urethral discharge, irritation, or trauma.

   _____ _____ _____ _____

   d. Determined size of catheter inflation balloon by looking at valve.

   _____ _____ _____ _____

PLANNING

1. Identified expected outcomes.

   _____ _____ _____ _____

2. Explained procedure to patient, discussed signs and symptoms of UTI, taught patient how to perform catheter hygiene.

   _____ _____ _____ _____

IMPLEMENTATION

1. Identified patient using two identifiers.

   _____ _____ _____ _____

2. Provided privacy.

   _____ _____ _____ _____

3. Performed hand hygiene.

   _____ _____ _____ _____

4. Raised bed to appropriate working height, lowered side rails on working side.

   _____ _____ _____ _____

5. Organized equipment for perineal care and/or removal of catheter.

   _____ _____ _____ _____

	S	U	NP	Comments

6. Positioned patient with waterproof pad under buttocks, covered with bath blanket, exposed genital area and catheter only. ___ ___ ___ _____

7. Applied gloves. ___ ___ ___ _____

8. Removed catheter securement device while maintaining connection with drainage tubing. ___ ___ ___ _____

9. Catheter care:

   a. Separated labia or retracted foreskin to expose meatus, maintained position throughout procedure. ___ ___ ___ _____

   b. Grasped catheter with two fingers to stabilize it. ___ ___ ___ _____

   c. Assessed urethral meatus and surrounding tissues for inflammation, swelling, discharge, or tissue trauma; asked patient if burning or discomfort was present. ___ ___ ___ _____

   d. Provided perineal hygiene with soap and water. ___ ___ ___ _____

   e. Cleaned catheter properly with clean washcloth. ___ ___ ___ _____

10. Checked drainage tubing and bag routinely for proper securement and positioning. ___ ___ ___ _____

11. Catheter removal:

   a. Loosened syringe, withdrew plunger, inserted hub of syringe into inflation valve, allowed balloon fluid to drain into syringe, ensured entire amount of fluid was removed. ___ ___ ___ _____

   b. Pulled catheter appropriately, ensured catheter was whole, did not use force. ___ ___ ___ _____

   c. Wrapped contaminated catheter in waterproof pad, unhooked bag and drainage tubing from bed. ___ ___ ___ _____

   d. Repositioned patient as necessary, provided hygiene, lowered bed and raised side rails. ___ ___ ___ _____

   e. Emptied, measured, and recorded urine present in drainage bag. ___ ___ ___ _____

   f. Encouraged patient to maintain or increase fluid intake. ___ ___ ___ _____

   g. Initiated voiding record or bladder diary, instructed patient to tell you when need to empty bladder occurred and that all urine was measured, ensured patient knew how to use collection container. ___ ___ ___ _____

	S	U	NP	Comments

h. Explained that many patients experience mild burning, discomfort, or small-volume voiding which will subside.

i. Informed patient to report signs of UTI.

j. Ensured easy access to toilet or bedpan, placed urine "hat" on toilet seat, placed call bell within easy reach.

12. Disposed of all contaminated supplies in appropriate receptacle, performed hand hygiene.

EVALUATION

1. Inspected catheter and genital area for soiling irritation, and skin breakdown; asked patient about discomfort.

2. Observed time and measured amount of first voiding after catheter removal.

3. Evaluated patient for signs and symptoms of UTI.

4. Identified unexpected outcomes.

RECORDING AND REPORTING

1. Recorded time for catheter care and appearance of urine, described condition of meatus and catheter.

2. Recorded and reported time of catheter removal; amount of water removed from balloon; condition of urethral meatus and catheter; and time, amount, and characteristics of first voided urine.

3. Recorded teaching related to catheter care, catheter removal, and fluid intake.

4. Reported hematuria, dysuria, inability or difficulty voiding, or any new incontinence after catheter removal.

Student _____ Date _____

Instructor _____ Date _____

	S	U	NP	Comments
PROCEDURAL STEPS				
1. Identified patient using two identifiers.	___	___	___	_____
2. Assessed I&O record to determine urine output trends, verified correct timing of the bladder scan measurement.	___	___	___	_____
3. Performed hand hygiene, applied clean gloves.	___	___	___	_____
4. Provided privacy.	___	___	___	_____
5. Discussed procedure with patient, asked patient to void, measured voided urine value if measurement was for PVR.	___	___	___	_____
6. Measured PVR with bladder scan.				
a. Assisted patient to appropriate position, raised bed to working height, lowered side rail on working side.	___	___	___	_____
b. Exposed patient's lower abdomen.	___	___	___	_____
c. Turned on scanner per manufacturer's guidelines.	___	___	___	_____
d. Set gender designation per manufacturer's guidelines.	___	___	___	_____
e. Wiped scanner head with cleanser, allowed to air dry.	___	___	___	_____
f. Palpated patient's symphysis pubis, applied ultrasound gel to midline abdomen.	___	___	___	_____
g. Placed scanner head on gel, ensured scanner head was oriented properly.	___	___	___	_____
h. Applied light pressure, kept head steady, pointed scanner head toward bladder, pressed and released scan button.	___	___	___	_____
i. Verified accurate aim, completed scan, printed image.	___	___	___	_____
j. Removed ultrasound gel from abdomen with paper towel.	___	___	___	_____

	S	U	NP	Comments

k. Removed ultrasound gel from scanner head, wiped with cleanser, let air dry. ___ ___ ___ _____

l. Assisted patient to comfortable position, lowered bed, replaced side rails accordingly. ___ ___ ___ _____

m. Removed gloves, performed hand hygiene. ___ ___ ___ _____

7. Measured PVR using straight/intermittent catheterization. ___ ___ ___ _____

8. Reviewed prescriber's order to determine how often to assess residual urine. ___ ___ ___ _____

9. Reviewed I&O record to determine urine output trends. ___ ___ ___ _____

Student _____ Date _____

Instructor _____ Date _____

PERFORMANCE CHECKLIST SKILL 33-3 **PERFORMING CATHETER IRRIGATION**

	S	U	NP	Comments
ASSESSMENT				
1. Verified order for irrigation method, type, and amount of irrigant, as well as type of catheter in place.	___	___	___	_____
2. Palpated bladder for distention and tenderness.	___	___	___	_____
3. Assessed patient for abdominal pain or spasms, sensation of bladder fullness, or catheter bypassing.	___	___	___	_____
4. Observed urine for color, amount, clarity, and presence of mucus, clots, or sediment.	___	___	___	_____
5. Monitored I&O.	___	___	___	_____
6. Assessed patient's knowledge regarding purpose of performing catheter irrigation.	___	___	___	_____
PLANNING				
1. Identified expected outcomes.	___	___	___	_____
2. Explained procedure to patient.	___	___	___	_____
IMPLEMENTATION				
1. Identified patient using two identifiers.	___	___	___	_____
2. Performed hand hygiene.	___	___	___	_____
3. Provided privacy.	___	___	___	_____
4. Raised bed to working height, lowered side rail on working side.	___	___	___	_____
5. Positioned patient properly, exposed catheter junctions.	___	___	___	_____
6. Removed old catheter securement device.	___	___	___	_____
7. Organized supplies according to type of irrigation prescribed, applied gloves.	___	___	___	_____
8. Closed continuous irrigation:				
a. Closed clamp on irrigation tubing, hung bag of irrigation solution on IV pole, inserted tip of sterile irrigation tubing into port of solution bag.	___	___	___	_____

	S	U	NP	Comments

b. Filled drip chamber half full, allowed solution to flow through tubing, closed clamp and recapped end of tubing once fluid had completely filled tubing.   ___ ___ ___ _____

c. Connected tubing securely to drainage port of Y-connector on double-/triple-lumen catheter using aseptic technique.   ___ ___ ___ _____

d. Adjusted clamp on tubing to begin flow of solution into bladder, calculated drip rate and adjusted at roller clamp, increased irrigation rate if necessary.   ___ ___ ___ _____

e. Observed for outflow of fluid into drainage bag, emptied catheter drainage bag as needed.   ___ ___ ___ _____

9. Closed intermittent irrigation:

a. Poured prescribed irrigation solution into sterile container.   ___ ___ ___ _____

b. Drew prescribed volume of irrigant into syringe using aseptic technique, placed sterile cap on tip of needleless syringe.   ___ ___ ___ _____

c. Clamped catheter tubing appropriately with screw clamp.   ___ ___ ___ _____

d. Cleaned catheter port with antiseptic swab.   ___ ___ ___ _____

e. Inserted tip of needleless syringe properly into port.   ___ ___ ___ _____

f. Injected solution properly.   ___ ___ ___ _____

g. Removed syringe, removed clamp to allow solution to drain into bag.   ___ ___ ___ _____

10. Open intermittent irrigation:

a. Applied sterile gloves if necessary.   ___ ___ ___ _____

b. Opened sterile irrigation tray, arranged sterile field properly.   ___ ___ ___ _____

c. Positioned sterile drape under catheter.   ___ ___ ___ _____

d. Aspirated prescribed volume of solution into syringe, placed syringe in sterile container until ready to use.   ___ ___ ___ _____

e. Moved sterile collection close to patient's thigh.   ___ ___ ___ _____

f. Wiped connection point between catheter and drainage tubing with antiseptic.   ___ ___ ___ _____

	S	U	NP	Comments

g. Disconnected catheter from drainage tubing, allowed any urine to flow into basin, covered open end of tubing with cap, positioned tubing appropriately.

    ___ ___ ___   _____

h. Inserted top of syringe into lumen of catheter, instilled solution.

    ___ ___ ___   _____

i. Removed syringe, lowered catheter, allowed solution to drain into basin, repeated sequence if ordered.

    ___ ___ ___   _____

j. Removed protector cap from tubing end, cleansed end tubing with antiseptic, reinserted lumen of catheter.

    ___ ___ ___   _____

11. Anchored catheter with catheter securement device.

    ___ ___ ___   _____

12. Assisted patient to safe and comfortable position, lowered bed, placed side rail appropriately.

    ___ ___ ___   _____

13. Disposed of all contaminated supplies appropriately, removed gloves, performed hand hygiene.

    ___ ___ ___   _____

EVALUATION

1. Measured actual urine output properly.

    ___ ___ ___   _____

2. Reviewed I&O flow sheet to verify appropriate hourly output.

    ___ ___ ___   _____

3. Inspected urine for blood clots and sediment, ensured tubing was not kinked or occluded.

    ___ ___ ___   _____

4. Assessed patient comfort.

    ___ ___ ___   _____

5. Assessed for signs of infection.

    ___ ___ ___   _____

6. Identified unexpected outcomes.

    ___ ___ ___   _____

RECORDING AND REPORTING

1. Recorded all pertinent information in the appropriate log.

    ___ ___ ___   _____

2. Reported catheter occlusion, sudden bleeding, infection, or increased pain to health care provider.

    ___ ___ ___   _____

3. Recorded I&O on appropriate flow sheet.

    ___ ___ ___   _____

Student _____ Date _____

Instructor _____ Date _____

PERFORMANCE CHECKLIST SKILL 33-4 **APPLYING A CONDOM-TYPE EXTERNAL CATHETER**

	S	U	NP	Comments

ASSESSMENT

1. Assessed urinary pattern, ability to empty bladder effectively, and degree of urinary continence.

2. Assessed skin of penis for rashes, erythema, and/or open areas.

3. Assessed patient's mental status, knowledge of purpose for use of condom-type catheter, and ability to apply the device; included family members if appropriate.

4. Verified patient's size and type of catheter properly.

PLANNING

1. Identified expected outcomes.

2. Explained procedure to patient.

IMPLEMENTATION

1. Identified patient using two identifiers.

2. Performed hand hygiene.

3. Provided privacy.

4. Raised bed to working height, lowered side rail on working side.

5. Prepared drainage collection bag and tubing, clamped off drainage bag port, placed nearby ready to attach.

6. Assisted patient to appropriate position, placed bath blanket over upper torso, folded sheets so only penis was exposed.

7. Applied gloves, provided perineal care, dried thoroughly, ensured foreskin was in normal position, did not apply barrier cream.

8. Clipped hair at base of penis as necessary, applied hair guard or paper towel if appropriate.

9. Applied condom catheter properly.

10. Applied appropriate securement device as indicated in manufacturer's guidelines.

	S	U	NP	Comments

11. Connected drainage tubing to end of condom catheter, ensured condom was not twisted, placed excess tubing on bed and secured.   ____ ____ ____ _____

12. Assisted patient to appropriate position, lowered bed, placed side rail accordingly.   ____ ____ ____ _____

13. Disposed of contaminated supplies, removed gloves, performed hand hygiene.   ____ ____ ____ _____

14. Removed and reapplied daily unless extended-wear device was used, removed condom properly when appropriate.   ____ ____ ____ _____

EVALUATION

1. Observed urinary drainage.   ____ ____ ____ _____

2. Inspected penis with condom catheter in place after application, assessed for swelling and discoloration, asked patient if there was any discomfort.   ____ ____ ____ _____

3. Inspected skin on shaft for signs of breakdown or irritation appropriately.   ____ ____ ____ _____

4. Identified unexpected outcomes.   ____ ____ ____ _____

RECORDING AND REPORTING

1. Recorded condom application; condition of penis, skin, and scrotum; urinary output; and voiding pattern in nurses' notes.   ____ ____ ____ _____

2. Reported penile erythema, rashes, and/or skin breakdown.   ____ ____ ____ _____

Student _____ Date _____

Instructor _____ Date _____

PERFORMANCE CHECKLIST SKILL 33-5   **SUPRAPUBIC CATHETER CARE**

	S	U	NP	Comments

ASSESSMENT

1. Assessed urine in drainage bag for amount, clarity, color, odor, and sediment.   ___ ___ ___ _____

2. Observed dressing for drainage and intactness.   ___ ___ ___ _____

3. Assessed catheter insertion site for signs of inflammation, asked patient if there was any pain at site.   ___ ___ ___ _____

4. Assessed for elevated temperature and chills.   ___ ___ ___ _____

5. Assessed patient's knowledge of purpose of catheter and its care.   ___ ___ ___ _____

6. Checked for allergies.   ___ ___ ___ _____

PLANNING

1. Identified expected outcomes.   ___ ___ ___ _____

2. Explained procedure to patient.   ___ ___ ___ _____

IMPLEMENTATION

1. Performed hand hygiene.   ___ ___ ___ _____

2. Provided privacy.   ___ ___ ___ _____

3. Raised bed to working height, lowered side rail on working side.   ___ ___ ___ _____

4. Prepared supplies properly.   ___ ___ ___ _____

5. Applied gloves, removed existing dressing, noted type and presence of drainage, removed gloves, performed hand hygiene.   ___ ___ ___ _____

6. Cleansed using sterile technique for newly established catheter:

   a. Applied sterile gloves.   ___ ___ ___ _____

   b. Held catheter with nondominant hand, used gauze and saline to cleanse skin appropriately.   ___ ___ ___ _____

   c. Cleansed base of catheter properly with fresh, moistened gauze.   ___ ___ ___ _____

   d. Applied drain dressing with sterile gloved hand around catheter, taped in place.   ___ ___ ___ _____

	S	U	NP	Comments

7. Cleansed using aseptic technique for new or established catheter.

   a. Applied clean gloves. ___ ___ ___ _____

   b. Held catheter with nondominant hand, cleansed properly with soap and water. ___ ___ ___ _____

   c. Cleansed base of catheter properly with fresh washcloth or gauze. ___ ___ ___ _____

   d. Applied drain dressing around catheter if necessary, taped in place. ___ ___ ___ _____

8. Secured catheter to lateral abdomen with tape or Velcro. ___ ___ ___ _____

9. Coiled excess tubing on bed, kept drainage bag below level of bladder. ___ ___ ___ _____

10. Disposed of all contaminated supplies properly, removed gloves, performed hand hygiene. ___ ___ ___ _____

EVALUATION

1. Asked patient to rate pain or discomfort. ___ ___ ___ _____

2. Monitored for signs of infection. ___ ___ ___ _____

3. Observed catheter insertion site for erythema, edema, discharge, and tenderness; checked dressing at least every 8 hours. ___ ___ ___ _____

4. Identified unexpected outcomes. ___ ___ ___ _____

RECORDING AND REPORTING

1. Recorded and reported character of urine, type of dressing, and patient's comfort level. ___ ___ ___ _____

2. Recorded urine output on I&O flow sheet properly. ___ ___ ___ _____

Student _____ Date _____

Instructor _____ Date _____

PERFORMANCE CHECKLIST SKILL 34-1 **ASSISTING A PATIENT IN USING A BEDPAN**

	S	U	NP	Comments

ASSESSMENT

1. Assessed patient's normal bowel elimination habits.

2. Auscultated abdomen for bowel sounds, palpated lower abdomen for distention.

3. Assessed patient's level of mobility.

4. Assessed patient's level of comfort; noted rectal or abdominal pain, presence of hemorrhoids, or irritation of skin surrounding anus.

5. Determined need for stool specimen.

PLANNING

1. Identified expected outcomes.

2. Explained procedure to patient.

3. Obtained assistance from additional nursing personnel as warranted.

IMPLEMENTATION

1. Performed hand hygiene.

2. Provided privacy.

3. Raised bed on opposite side.

4. Raised bed horizontally according to nurses' height.

5. Had patient assume supine position.

6. Placed patient who can assist on bedpan.

   a. Applied clean gloves, raised head of patient's bed appropriately.

   b. Removed upper bed linens, did not expose patient.

   c. Instructed patient in how to flex knees and lift hips upward.

   d. Placed hand under patient' sacrum to assist lifting, asked patient to bend knees and raise hips, slipped bedpan under patient with other hand, ensured open rim faced foot of bed, did not force.

	S	U	NP	Comments

7. Placed patient with mobility restrictions on bedpan.

   a. Applied clean gloves, lowered head of bed appropriately.   ___ ___ ___ _____

   b. Removed top linens as necessary.   ___ ___ ___ _____

   c. Assisted patient with rolling onto side, placed bedpan on buttocks and down into mattress, ensured open rim faced foot of bed.   ___ ___ ___ _____

   d. Kept one hand against bedpan and other around patient's far hip, asked patient to roll onto bedpan, did not force the pan under the patient.   ___ ___ ___ _____

   e. Raised patient's head properly.   ___ ___ ___ _____

   f. Had patient bend knees or raised knee gatch.   ___ ___ ___ _____

8. Maintained patient's comfort and safety, covered patient for warmth, placed pillow or towel under lumbar curve of back.   ___ ___ ___ _____

9. Had call bell and toilet tissue within reach of patient.   ___ ___ ___ _____

10. Ensured that bed was in lowest position, raised upper side rails.   ___ ___ ___ _____

11. Removed and discarded gloves, performed hand hygiene.   ___ ___ ___ _____

12. Allowed patient to be alone, monitored status and responded promptly.   ___ ___ ___ _____

13. Performed hand hygiene, applied clean gloves.   ___ ___ ___ _____

14. Removed bedpan.

   a. Placed patient's bedside chair close to working side of bed.   ___ ___ ___ _____

   b. Maintained privacy, determined if patient is able to wipe own perineal area, used toilet tissue or washcloths if nurse is needed to cleanse perineal area, cleansed patient properly.   ___ ___ ___ _____

   c. Deposited contaminated tissue in bedpan if appropriate, allowed patient to perform hand hygiene.   ___ ___ ___ _____

   d. For mobile patient, asked patient to flex knees and lift buttocks up, placed hand properly for support, had patient lift and remove bedpan, placed bedpan on draped chair, covered bedpan.   ___ ___ ___ _____

   e. For immobile patient, lowered head of bed, assisted patient with rolling off bedpan, held bedpan flat while patient rolled, placed bedpan on bedside chair, covered bedpan.   ___ ___ ___ _____

	S	U	NP	Comments
15. Assisted patient with hand hygiene. Changed soiled linens, removed gloves, and returned patient to comfortable position.	___	___	___	_____
16. Placed bed in its lowest position; ensured call bell, phone, water, and personal items are within reach.	___	___	___	_____
17. Obtained stool specimen as ordered, wore gloves when emptying bedpan, used spray faucet to rinse bedpan, used disinfectant if required.	___	___	___	_____
18. Removed and discarded gloves, performed hand hygiene.	___	___	___	_____

EVALUATION

	S	U	NP	Comments
1. Assessed characteristics of stool and urine.	___	___	___	_____
2. Evaluated patient's ability to use bedpan.	___	___	___	_____
3. Inspected patient's perineal area and surrounding skin while removing bedpan.	___	___	___	_____
4. Evaluated patient's overall activity tolerance and comfort.	___	___	___	_____
5. Identified unexpected outcomes.	___	___	___	_____

RECORDING AND REPORTING

	S	U	NP	Comments
1. Recorded type of assistance needed, patient's tolerance, character and amount of stool, and urine output.	___	___	___	_____
2. Completed laboratory requisition, sent specimen to lab, recorded type of specimen sent.	___	___	___	_____

Student _____   Date _____

Instructor _____   Date _____

PERFORMANCE CHECKLIST SKILL 34-2   **REMOVING FECAL IMPACTION DIGITALLY**

	S	U	NP	Comments
ASSESSMENT				
1. Assessed patient.				
a. Asked patient about normal and current bowel elimination patterns.	___	___	___	_____
b. Inspected patient's abdomen for distention.	___	___	___	_____
c. Auscultated all four quadrants for presence of bowel sounds.	___	___	___	_____
d. Palpated patient's abdomen for distention, discomfort, and masses.	___	___	___	_____
e. Measured patient's current vital signs and comfort level.	___	___	___	_____
f. Performed hand hygiene, applied clean gloves, observed consistency of stool, observed anal area for signs of irritation or hemorrhoids, removed gloves, performed hand hygiene.	___	___	___	_____
g. Determined if patient is receiving anticoagulant therapy.	___	___	___	_____
2. Checked patient's record for order for digital removal of impaction and use of anesthetic anesthetic lubricant.	___	___	___	_____
PLANNING				
1. Identified expected outcomes.	___	___	___	_____
2. Explained procedure to patient.	___	___	___	_____
IMPLEMENTATION				
1. Identified patient using two identifiers.	___	___	___	_____
2. Obtained assistance to help change patient's position if necessary, raised bed to working height.	___	___	___	_____
3. Provided privacy.	___	___	___	_____
4. Lowered side rail on patient's right side, assisted patient to appropriate position.	___	___	___	_____
5. Draped patient's trunk and lower extremities with bath blanket, placed waterproof pad under patient's buttocks.	___	___	___	_____

	S	U	NP	Comments
6. Placed bedpan next to patient.	___	___	___	_____
7. Performed hand hygiene, applied gloves, lubricated gloved fingers of dominant hand.	___	___	___	_____
8. Instructed patient to take slow deep breaths, inserted index finger properly, inserted middle finger when appropriate.	___	___	___	_____
9. Advanced fingers slowly along rectal wall toward umbilicus.	___	___	___	_____
10. Loosened fecal mass appropriately, worked fingers into hardened mass.	___	___	___	_____
11. Worked stool downward, removed small sections of feces, discarded in bedpan.	___	___	___	_____
12. Observed patient's response, assessed heart rate, looked for signs of fatigue.	___	___	___	_____
13. Continued to clear rectum, allowed patient to rest at intervals.	___	___	___	_____
14. Performed perineal hygiene after removal of impaction.	___	___	___	_____
15. Removed bedpan, inspected feces for color and consistency, disposed of feces, cleaned bed pan, removed and disposed of gloves properly.	___	___	___	_____
16. Assisted patient to toilet if needed.	___	___	___	_____
17. Performed hand hygiene.	___	___	___	_____

EVALUATION

	S	U	NP	Comments
1. Applied clean gloves. Performed rectal examination, observed anal and perianal area for irritation or breakdown.	___	___	___	_____
2. Reassessed vital signs, compared to baseline values, monitored patient for bradycardia for 1 hour.	___	___	___	_____
3. Auscultated bowel sounds.	___	___	___	_____
4. Palpated abdomen to determine if it is soft and nontender.	___	___	___	_____
5. Asked patient to rate comfort level.	___	___	___	_____
6. Identified unexpected outcomes.	___	___	___	_____

RECORDING AND REPORTING

	S	U	NP	Comments
1. Recorded all pertinent information on the appropriate log.	___	___	___	_____
2. Reported any changes in vital signs and adverse affects to health care provider.	___	___	___	_____

Student _____ Date _____

Instructor _____ Date _____

PERFORMANCE CHECKLIST SKILL 34-3 **ADMINISTERING AN ENEMA**

	S	U	NP	Comments

ASSESSMENT

1. Reviewed health care provider's order for enema, clarified reason for administration.

2. Assessed last bowel movement, normal versus most recent bowel pattern, presence of hemorrhoids, mobility, and presence of abdominal pain or cramping.

3. Inspected abdomen for presence of distention, auscultated for bowel sounds.

4. Determined patient's level of understanding of purpose of enema.

PLANNING

1. Identified expected outcomes.

IMPLEMENTATION

1. Checked accuracy and completeness of each MAR with written order, compared MAR with label of solution.

2. Identified patient using two identifiers.

3. Provided privacy.

4. Raised bed to working height, raised side rail on patient's left.

5. Assisted patient to appropriate position, encouraged patient to remain in position until procedure is complete.

6. Performed hand hygiene, applied clean gloves, placed waterproof pad under hips and buttocks.

7. Covered patient with bath blanket, exposed only rectal area.

8. Separated buttocks, examined perianal region for abnormalities.

9. Placed bedpan in easily accessible position, ensured toilet is available and slippers and bathrobe are accessible if necessary.

10. Administered enema.

  a. Administered prepackaged disposable enema.

    (1) Removed cap from container, applied more water-soluble lubricant as needed.

	S	U	NP	Comments

(2) Gently separated buttocks, instructed patient to relax by breathing out through the mouth. ____ ____ ____ _____

(3) Expelled any air from enema container. ____ ____ ____ _____

(4) Inserted lubricated tip of container properly into anal canal. ____ ____ ____ _____

(5) Rolled bottle until all of solution entered rectum, instructed patient to retain solution until urge to defecate occurs. ____ ____ ____ _____

b. Administered enema in standard enema bag.

(1) Added warmed solution to enema bag properly, checked temperature of solution on inner wrist. ____ ____ ____ _____

(2) Added castile soap if SSE is ordered. ____ ____ ____ _____

(3) Raised container, released clamp, allowed solution to flow until tubing was filled. ____ ____ ____ _____

(4) Reclamped tubing. ____ ____ ____ _____

(5) Lubricated tip of rectal tube. ____ ____ ____ _____

(6) Separated buttocks, instructed patient to relax by breathing out through the mouth, touched patient's skin next to anus with tip of tube. ____ ____ ____ _____

(7) Inserted tip of rectal tube appropriately. ____ ____ ____ _____

(8) Held tubing constantly until end of fluid instillation. ____ ____ ____ _____

(9) Opened regulating clamp, allowed solution to enter properly. ____ ____ ____ _____

(10) Raised height of enema container to appropriate level above anus. ____ ____ ____ _____

(11) Instilled all solution, clamped tubing, told patient that procedure is complete and you will be removing tubing. ____ ____ ____ _____

11. Placed layers of toilet tissue around anus, withdrew rectal tube and tip. ____ ____ ____ _____

12. Explained to patient that distention and abdominal cramping is normal, asked patient to retain solution as long as possible, stayed at beside, had patient lie quietly in bed if possible. ____ ____ ____ _____

13. Discarded enema container and tubing in proper receptacle. ____ ____ ____ _____

14. Assisted patient to bathroom or with bedpan if possible. ____ ____ ____ _____

	S	U	NP	Comments

15. Observed character of stool and solution, cautioned patient against flushing toilet before inspection.

16. Assisted patient as needed with washing anal area with soap and water.

17. Removed and discarded gloves, performed hand hygiene.

EVALUATION

1. Inspected color, consistency, and amount of stool, odor, and fluid passed.

2. Assessed for abdominal distention.

3. Identified unexpected outcomes.

RECORDING AND REPORTING

1. Recorded all pertinent information in the appropriate log.

2. Reported failure of patient to defecate and any adverse effects to health care provider.

Student _____ Date _____

Instructor _____ Date _____

PERFORMANCE CHECKLIST SKILL 34-4 **INSERTION, MAINTENANCE, AND REMOVAL OF A NASOGASTRIC TUBE FOR GASTRIC DECOMPRESSION**

	S	U	NP	Comments
ASSESSMENT				
1. Inspected condition of patient's nasal and oral cavity.	___	___	___	_____
2. Asked if patient has history of nasal surgery or congestion and allergies, noted if deviated nasal septum is present.	___	___	___	_____
3. Auscultated for bowel sounds; palpated patient's abdomen for distention, pain, and rigidity.	___	___	___	_____
4. Assessed patient's LOC and ability to follow instructions.	___	___	___	_____
5. Determined if patient had previous NG tube and which naris was used.	___	___	___	_____
6. Verified order for type of NG tube and whether tube is to be attached to suction or drainage bag.	___	___	___	_____
PLANNING				
1. Identified expected outcomes.	___	___	___	_____
2. Informed patient that procedure may make them gag and there will be a burning sensation in the nasopharynx, developed hand signal with patient.	___	___	___	_____
IMPLEMENTATION				
1. Identified patient using two identifiers.	___	___	___	_____
2. Placed patient in appropriate position, raised bed to comfortable working height.	___	___	___	_____
3. Placed bath towel over patient's chest, gave facial tissue to patient, allowed patient to blow nose if necessary, placed emesis basin within reach.	___	___	___	_____
4. Provided privacy.	___	___	___	_____
5. Washed bridge of nose with soap and water or alcohol.	___	___	___	_____
6. Stood on appropriate side of patient.	___	___	___	_____
7. Instructed patient to relax and breathe normally while occluding one naris then the other, selected naris with greater airflow.	___	___	___	_____
8. Measured distance to insert tube using either traditional or Hanson method.	___	___	___	_____

	S	U	NP	Comments
9. Marked length to be inserted with tape.	___	___	___	_____
10. Performed hand hygiene, applied clean gloves, curved appropriate length of tube around index finger and released.	___	___	___	_____
11. Lubricated end of tube with water-soluble lubricant.	___	___	___	_____
12. Alerted patient when procedure began.	___	___	___	_____
13. Initially instructed patient to extend neck back, inserted tube properly into naris.	___	___	___	_____
14. Passed tube along floor of nasal passage, applied pressure downward if resistance occurs.	___	___	___	_____
15. Rotated tube if continued resistance occurs, withdrew and tried other naris if necessary.	___	___	___	_____
16. Continued insertion of tube just past nasopharynx, allowed patient to relax, provided tissues and water, explained that next step requires patient to swallow.	___	___	___	_____
17. Placed tube above oropharynx; instructed patient to flex head forward, sip water, and swallow; advanced tube with each swallow.	___	___	___	_____
18. Withdrew or stopped advancement if patient coughed, gaged, or choked; instructed patient to breathe and sip water.	___	___	___	_____
19. Pulled tube back if patient continues to cough.	___	___	___	_____
20. Checked back of oropharynx if patient feels coiling behind throat, withdrew tube and reinserted if necessary.	___	___	___	_____
21. Advanced tube after patient relaxes until you reach tape, anchored tube to patient's cheek.	___	___	___	_____
22. Verified tube placement, checked agency policy for method.				
a. Asked patient to talk.	___	___	___	_____
b. Inspected posterior pharynx for presence of coiled tube.	___	___	___	_____
c. Placed towel under end of NG tube, attached syringe to end of tube, aspirated gastric contents, observed color.	___	___	___	_____
d. Used gastric pH paper to measure aspirate for pH.	___	___	___	_____
e. Obtained x-ray examination of chest and abdomen as ordered.	___	___	___	_____
f. Advanced tube if not in stomach, repeated steps to check tube position.	___	___	___	_____

	S	U	NP	Comments

23. Anchored tube.

   a. Clamped end of tube or connected tube to drainage bag or suction machine.

   b. Taped tube to nose, avoided putting pressure on nares.

     (1) Cut strip of tape, split down the middle halfway.

     (2) Applied tincture of benzoin to lower end of nose, allowed to dry, applied tape to nose, left split end free.

     (3) Wrapped split ends of tape around tube in opposite directions, applied tube fixation device instead if appropriate.

   c. Fastened end of NG tube to patient's gown properly, pinned rubber band to gown.

   d. Kept pigtail above level of stomach when using a Salem sump tube.

   e. Elevated head of bed if appropriate.

   f. Explained to patient that the sensation of the tube in the throat decreases over time.

   g. Removed and discarded gloves, performed hand hygiene.

24. Placed a mark where tube exits nose or measured length of tube from nares to connector and documented length of tube in patient's record.

25. Attached NG tube to suction as ordered.

26. NG tube irrigation:

   a. Performed hand hygiene, applied clean gloves.

   b. Checked for tube placement in stomach, clamped tube or reconnected connecting tube, removed syringe.

   c. Drew up normal saline into syringe.

   d. Clamped NG tube, disconnected from tubing, laid end of connection tubing on towel.

   e. Inserted tip of irrigating syringe into end of NG tube, removed clamp, held syringe properly, injected saline slowly, did not force solution.

   f. Checked for kinks in tubing if resistance occurred, turned patient onto left side, reported repeated resistance.

   g. Aspirated fluid after instilling saline, recorded any difference in output or intake.

	S	U	NP	Comments

h. Placed air into blue pigtail with Asepto syringe. ___ ___ ___ _____

i. Repeated irrigation if solution did not return. Reconnected NG tube to drain or suction. ___ ___ ___ _____

j. Removed and discarded gloves, performed hand hygiene. ___ ___ ___ _____

27. Removed NG tube.

a. Verified order to remove NG tube. ___ ___ ___ _____

b. Auscultated abdomen for presence of bowel sounds. ___ ___ ___ _____

c. Explained procedure to patient, reassured that removal is less distressing than insertion. ___ ___ ___ _____

d. Performed hand hygiene, applied clean gloves. ___ ___ ___ _____

e. Turned off suction, disconnected NG tube from drainage bag or suction, inserted air into lumen of NG tube with irrigating syringe, removed tape or fixation device, unpinned tube from gown. ___ ___ ___ _____

f. Stood on appropriate side of patient. ___ ___ ___ _____

g. Handed patient facial tissue, placed towel across chest, instructed patient to take and hold breath. ___ ___ ___ _____

h. Clamped or kinked tubing, pulled tube out into towel. ___ ___ ___ _____

i. Inspected intactness of tube. ___ ___ ___ _____

j. Measured amount of drainage, noted character of content, disposed of tube and drainage equipment appropriately. ___ ___ ___ _____

k. Cleaned nares, provided mouth care. ___ ___ ___ _____

l. Positioned patient comfortably, explained procedure for drinking fluids, instructed patient to notify you if nausea occurs. ___ ___ ___ _____

28. Cleaned equipment, returned to proper place, placed soiled linen in proper receptacle. ___ ___ ___ _____

29. Removed and discarded gloves, performed hand hygiene. ___ ___ ___ _____

EVALUATION

1. Observed amount and character of contents draining from NG tube, asked if patient feels nauseated. ___ ___ ___ _____

2. Auscultated for presence of bowel sounds, turned off suction while auscultated. ___ ___ ___ _____

	S	U	NP	Comments
3. Palpated patient's abdomen periodically; noted distention, pain, and rigidity.	___	___	___	_____
4. Inspected nares and nose.	___	___	___	_____
5. Observed position of tubing.	___	___	___	_____
6. Asked if patient feels sore throat or irritation in pharynx.	___	___	___	_____
7. Identified unexpected outcomes.	___	___	___	_____

RECORDING AND REPORTING

	S	U	NP	Comments
1. Recorded all pertinent information in the appropriate log.	___	___	___	_____
2. Recorded difference between saline instilled and gastric aspirate on I&O sheet, recorded amount and character of contents draining from NG tube every shift.	___	___	___	_____
3. Recorded removal of tube intact, patient's tolerance, and final amount and character of drainage.	___	___	___	_____

Student _____ Date _____

Instructor _____ Date _____

PERFORMANCE CHECKLIST SKILL 35-1 **POUCHING A COLOSTOMY OR AN ILEOSTOMY**

	S	U	NP	Comments

ASSESSMENT

1. Performed hand hygiene, applied gloves. ___ ___ ___ _____

2. Observed existing skin barrier and pouch for leakage, changed pouch at appropriate intervals, removed to fully observe stoma in case of opaque pouch. ___ ___ ___ _____

3. Observed amount of effluent in the pouch, emptied pouch properly if necessary, noted consistency of effluent, recorded I&O. ___ ___ ___ _____

4. Observed stoma for type, location, color, swelling, sutures, trauma, healing, or irritation; removed and disposed of gloves. ___ ___ ___ _____

5. Observed abdomen for best type of pouching system. ___ ___ ___ _____

6. Explored patient's attitude toward learning self-care, identified others who would be assisting patient after leaving the hospital. ___ ___ ___ _____

PLANNING

1. Identified expected outcomes. ___ ___ ___ _____

2. Explained procedure to patient, encouraged patient's interactions and questions. ___ ___ ___ _____

3. Assembled equipment, provided privacy. ___ ___ ___ _____

IMPLEMENTATION

1. Identified patient using two identifiers. ___ ___ ___ _____

2. Positioned patient properly, provided patient with mirror. ___ ___ ___ _____

3. Performed hand hygiene, applied clean gloves. ___ ___ ___ _____

4. Placed towel or waterproof barrier under patient and across patient's lower abdomen. ___ ___ ___ _____

5. Removed used pouch and skin barrier if necessary, used adhesive remover if necessary, emptied pouch and disposed of in appropriate receptacle, measured output if needed. ___ ___ ___ _____

6. Cleansed peristomal skin with warm water and washcloth, did not scrub, patted skin dry. ___ ___ ___ _____

	S	U	NP	Comments
7. Measured stoma.	___	___	___	_____
8. Traced pattern on pouch backing or skin barrier.	___	___	___	_____
9. Cut opening on backing or skin barrier, ensured opening was slightly larger than stoma.	___	___	___	_____
10. Removed protective backing from adhesive.	___	___	___	_____
11. Applied pouch over stoma, pressed into place around stoma and outside edges.	___	___	___	_____
12. Closed end of pouch, removed drape from patient.	___	___	___	_____
13. Removed gloves, performed hand hygiene.	___	___	___	_____

EVALUATION

	S	U	NP	Comments
1. Observed condition of skin barrier and adherence to abdominal surface.	___	___	___	_____
2. Observed appearance of stoma, peristomal skin, abdominal contours, and suture line during pouch change.	___	___	___	_____
3. Observed patient's and caregiver's willingness to view stoma and ask questions.	___	___	___	_____
4. Identified unexpected outcomes.	___	___	___	_____

RECORDING AND REPORTING

	S	U	NP	Comments
1. Recorded all pertinent information in the appropriate log.	___	___	___	_____
2. Recorded patient/family level of participation, teaching that was done, and response to teaching.	___	___	___	_____
3. Reported abnormal appearance of stoma, suture line, peristomal skin, or character of output to nurse in charge or health care provider.	___	___	___	_____

Student _____ Date _____

Instructor _____ Date _____

PERFORMANCE CHECKLIST SKILL 35-2 **POUCHING A UROSTOMY**

	S	U	NP	Comments
ASSESSMENT				
1. Performed hand hygiene, applied clean gloves.	___	___	___	_____
2. Observed existing barrier and pouch for leakage and length of time in place, change at appropriate intervals or if necessary.	___	___	___	_____
3. Observed urine in pouch or drainage bag, emptied pouch if necessary.	___	___	___	_____
4. Observed stoma for color, swelling, sutures, trauma, and healing of peristomal skin; assessed type of stoma; removed and disposed of gloves.	___	___	___	_____
5. Explored patient's attitude toward learning self-care, identified others who would be assisting patient after leaving the hospital.	___	___	___	_____
PLANNING				
1. Identified expected outcomes.	___	___	___	_____
2. Explained procedure to patient, encouraged patient's interaction and questions.	___	___	___	_____
3. Assembled equipment, provided privacy.	___	___	___	_____
IMPLEMENTATION				
1. Identified patient using two identifiers.	___	___	___	_____
2. Positioned patient appropriately, provided patient with a mirror.	___	___	___	_____
3. Performed hand hygiene, applied clean gloves.	___	___	___	_____
4. Placed towel or waterproof barrier under patient and across patient's lower abdomen.	___	___	___	_____
5. Removed used pouch and barrier, pulled pouch around stents and laid towel underneath when stents were present, emptied pouch and measured output, disposed of pouch in appropriate receptacle.	___	___	___	_____
6. Placed rolled gauze at stoma opening, maintained gauze at the stoma opening continuously during pouch measurement and change.	___	___	___	_____
7. Cleansed peristomal skin with warm water and washcloth, did not scrub, patted skin dry.	___	___	___	_____
8. Measured stoma, ensured opening was slightly larger than stoma.	___	___	___	_____

	S	U	NP	Comments
9. Traced pattern on pouch backing or barrier.	___	___	___	_____
10. Cut opening in pouch.	___	___	___	_____
11. Removed protective backing from adhesive surface.	___	___	___	_____
12. Applied pouch, pressed into place around stoma and outside edges, had patient hold hand over pouch.	___	___	___	_____
13. Used adapter to connect pouch to urinary bag.	___	___	___	_____
14. Removed drape from patient, removed gloves and performed hand hygiene.	___	___	___	_____

EVALUATION

	S	U	NP	Comments
1. Observed appearance of stoma, peristomal skin, and suture line.	___	___	___	_____
2. Evaluated character and volume of urinary drainage.	___	___	___	_____
3. Observed patient's and caregiver's willingness to view stoma and ask questions.	___	___	___	_____
4. Identified unexpected outcomes.	___	___	___	_____

RECORDING AND REPORTING

	S	U	NP	Comments
1. Recorded all pertinent information in the appropriate log.	___	___	___	_____
2. Recorded urinary output on I&O form.	___	___	___	_____
3. Recorded patient's and caregiver's reaction to stoma and level of participation.	___	___	___	_____
4. Reported abnormalities in stoma or peristomal skin and absence of urinary output to nurse in charge or health care provider.	___	___	___	_____

Student _____ Date _____

Instructor _____ Date _____

PERFORMANCE CHECKLIST SKILL 35-3 **CATHETERIZING A URINARY DIVERSION**

	S	U	NP	Comments
ASSESSMENT				
1. Observed for signs and symptoms of UTI.	___	___	___	_____
2. Obtained order for catheterization.	___	___	___	_____
3. Assessed patient's understanding of need for procedure and how procedure was done.	___	___	___	_____
PLANNING				
1. Identified expected outcomes.	___	___	___	_____
2. Assembled equipment, provided privacy.	___	___	___	_____
3. Explained procedure to patient, obtained specimen when patient was due to change pouch if using one-piece system.	___	___	___	_____
IMPLEMENTATION				
1. Identified patient using two identifiers.	___	___	___	_____
2. Positioned patient appropriately, draped towel across lower abdomen.	___	___	___	_____
3. Performed hand hygiene, put on clean gloves.	___	___	___	_____
4. Removed pouch, left barrier attached if patient uses two-piece system.	___	___	___	_____
5. Removed gloves, performed hand hygiene.	___	___	___	_____
6. Opened catheterization set or opened needed equipment and arranged on sterile barrier or placed gauze pad with lubricant on sterile field if did not use catheterization kit; applied sterile gloves.	___	___	___	_____
7. Had patient hold absorbent gauze wick on stoma if necessary.	___	___	___	_____
8. Cleansed surface of stoma with antiseptic, wiped off excess antiseptic with dry gauze.	___	___	___	_____
9. Removed lid from sterile specimen container.	___	___	___	_____
10. Lubricated tip of catheter, kept catheter sterile.	___	___	___	_____
11. Inserted catheter tip into stoma with dominant hand, did not force, placed distal end of catheter into specimen container, used gentle but firm pressure, had patient cough or turn slightly.	___	___	___	_____

	S	U	NP	Comments
12. Held container below level of stoma, waited long enough to get adequate amount of urine.	___	___	___	_____
13. Withdrew catheter properly, placed absorbent pad over stoma.	___	___	___	_____
14. Put lid on specimen container.	___	___	___	_____
15. Reapplied new pouch or reattached pouch if patient uses a two-piece system.	___	___	___	_____
16. Disposed of used pouch and equipment properly.	___	___	___	_____
17. Removed gloves, performed hand hygiene, labeled specimen in presence of patient, placed in biohazard bag, sent to laboratory at once.	___	___	___	_____

EVALUATION

	S	U	NP	Comments
1. Compared results of culture and sensitivity with expected findings.	___	___	___	_____
2. Instructed patient about signs of UTI.	___	___	___	_____
3. Identified unexpected outcomes.	___	___	___	_____

RECORDING AND REPORTING

	S	U	NP	Comments
1. Recorded time specimen collected; patient's tolerance; and appearance of urine, skin, and stoma.	___	___	___	_____
2. Reported results of laboratory test to nurse in charge or health care provider.	___	___	___	_____

Student _____ Date _____

Instructor _____ Date _____

PERFORMANCE CHECKLIST SKILL 36-1 **PREPARING A PATIENT FOR SURGERY**

	S	U	NP	Comments
ASSESSMENT				
1. Determined ability of patient to answer questions regarding health history and pending surgery.	___	___	___	_____
2. Collected nursing history; identified surgical risk factors, medications, and history of allergies.	___	___	___	_____
3. Performed physical examination, focused on body systems surgery will affect.	___	___	___	_____
4. Asked about patient's and family's knowledge and expectations of surgery and care.	___	___	___	_____
5. Reviewed patient's preoperative orders.	___	___	___	_____
6. Validated admission preparations were completed if necessary.	___	___	___	_____
7. Asked if patient had an advanced directive, placed in patient's record if so.	___	___	___	_____
PLANNING				
1. Identified expected outcomes.	___	___	___	_____
2. Explained procedure, allowed patient and family to ask questions and express concerns.	___	___	___	_____
IMPLEMENTATION				
1. Identified patient using two identifiers.	___	___	___	_____
2. Applied allergy/sensitivity band and others if applicable.	___	___	___	_____
3. Oriented patient to room or presurgical area.	___	___	___	_____
4. Acted as patient advocate as needed, witnessed consent form if allowed.	___	___	___	_____
5. Checked medical record, reviewed or completed preoperative checklist.	___	___	___	_____
6. Provided preoperative teaching.	___	___	___	_____
7. Maintained NPO status.	___	___	___	_____
8. Inserted IV and/or indwelling catheter if ordered.	___	___	___	_____
9. Provided for hygiene measures, ensured patient privacy, instructed patient to remove all clothes and to apply hospital gown and cap.	___	___	___	_____

	S	U	NP	Comments

10. Instructed patient to remove all headpieces, jewelry, and makeup; pinned religious medals to gown if policy permits; removed nail polish/acrylic nails as appropriate. ____ ____ ____ _____

11. Assisted patient in removing prostheses, documented items and location in appropriate log. ____ ____ ____ _____

12. Inventoried all items, gave to family member or secured in a locked area, had release form signed if necessary. ____ ____ ____ _____

13. Applied antiembolism stockings as ordered. ____ ____ ____ _____

14. Assessed vital signs immediately before going to OR. ____ ____ ____ _____

15. Assisted patient in voiding before receiving preoperative medication if necessary. ____ ____ ____ _____

16. Administered preoperative medications as ordered. ____ ____ ____ _____

17. Placed patient on bed rest with call light, informed patient not to get out of bed without assistance, allowed family to remain at bedside until patient was transferred to surgical area, maintained quiet and relaxing environment. ____ ____ ____ _____

EVALUATION

1. Had patient describe surgical procedure and benefits and risks. ____ ____ ____ _____

2. Compared assessment data with patient's baseline and expected normal levels. ____ ____ ____ _____

3. Had patient repeat preoperative instructions. ____ ____ ____ _____

4. Monitored patient for signs of anxiety, asked how patient and family were feeling. ____ ____ ____ _____

5. Identified unexpected outcomes. ____ ____ ____ _____

RECORDING AND REPORTING

1. Documented all preoperative assessment findings and preparations in the appropriate log. ____ ____ ____ _____

2. Documented patient's condition on transfer in appropriate log. ____ ____ ____ _____

3. Documented presence of any allergies/sensitivities on armband and in appropriate log. ____ ____ ____ _____

4. Recorded disposition of patient belongings. ____ ____ ____ _____

5. Reported lack of signed and witnessed consent form or failure of patient to remain NPO and action taken. ____ ____ ____ _____

6. Reported and recorded cultural practices and religious beliefs affecting care and any modification of care planned. ____ ____ ____ _____

470

Student _____ Date _____

Instructor _____ Date _____

PERFORMANCE CHECKLIST SKILL 36-2 **DEMONSTRATING POSTOPERATIVE EXERCISES**

	S	U	NP	Comments
ASSESSMENT				
1. Assessed patient's risk for postoperative respiratory complications.	___	___	___	_____
2. Auscultated lungs.	___	___	___	_____
3. Assessed properly patient's ability to deep breathe and cough.	___	___	___	_____
4. Assessed patient's risk for postoperative thrombus formation.	___	___	___	_____
5. Assessed patient's ability to move independently while in bed.	___	___	___	_____
6. Assessed patient's willingness and capability to learn exercises, noted relevant factors.	___	___	___	_____
7. Assessed family caregiver's willingness to learn and support patient postoperatively.	___	___	___	_____
8. Assessed patient's medical orders preoperatively and postoperatively.	___	___	___	_____
PLANNING				
1. Identified expected outcomes.	___	___	___	_____
2. Prepared equipment as needed.	___	___	___	_____
3. Prepared room for teaching.	___	___	___	_____
IMPLEMENTATION				
1. Taught diaphragmatic breathing properly:				
a. Assisted patient to comfortable position, used stool if necessary.	___	___	___	_____
b. Stood or sat facing patient.	___	___	___	_____
c. Instructed patient on how to place palms on rib cage, demonstrated if necessary.	S	U	NP	_____
d. Had patient take slow, deep breaths through nose while pushing abdomen against hands; explained that patient would feel movement of diaphragm.	___	___	___	_____
e. Had patient avoid using chest and shoulder muscles while inhaling.	___	___	___	_____
f. Had patient take slow, deep breath; hold; then exhale through mouth.	___	___	___	_____
g. Repeated breathing exercise appropriately.	___	___	___	_____

	S	U	NP	Comments

2. Taught PEP therapy and "huff" coughing:

   a. Set PEP device for setting ordered.

   b. Instructed patient to assume appropriate position, placed nose clip on patient's nose.

   c. Had patient place lips around mouthpiece, take full breaths, and exhale properly; repeated pattern appropriately.

   d. Removed device from mouth; had patient take slow, deep breath and hold.

   e. Instructed patient to exhale in forced "huffs."

3. Taught controlled coughing:

   a. Explained importance of maintaining position.

   b. Demonstrated coughing properly.

   c. Cautioned patient against clearing throat versus coughing.

   d. Taught patient to splint incision if necessary.

   e. Instructed patient to cough at appropriate intervals.

   f. Instructed patient to examine sputum for consistency, odor, amount, and color changes and to notify nurse if changes were noted.

4. Taught turning:

   a. Instructed patient to assume appropriate position on opposite side of the bed from turn.

   b. Instructed patient to place hand or pillow over incisional area.

   c. Instructed patient to straighten and flex legs appropriately.

   d. Had patient grab rail with opposite hand and pull self onto appropriate side.

   e. Instructed patient to turn at appropriate intervals or noted in chart that patient needs to be turned.

5. Taught leg exercises:

   a. Had patient assume proper position, demonstrated exercises properly.

	S	U	NP	Comments

b. Rotated each ankle in both directions, instructed patient to draw imaginary circles, repeated five times. ___ ___ ___ _____

c. Alternated dorsiflexion and plantar flexion properly, directed patient to feel calf muscles contract and relax, repeated five times. ___ ___ ___ _____

d. Performed quadriceps setting properly, repeated five times. ___ ___ ___ _____

e. Had patient raise each leg from bed surface properly, repeated five times. ___ ___ ___ _____

f. Had patient continue exercises at appropriate intervals. ___ ___ ___ _____

EVALUATION

1. Observed patient performing all exercises independently. ___ ___ ___ _____

2. Observed caregiver's ability to coach patient. ___ ___ ___ _____

3. Evaluated patient's chest excursion. ___ ___ ___ _____

4. Auscultated patient's lungs. ___ ___ ___ _____

5. Palpated calves for redness, warmth, swelling, and tenderness; assessed pedal pulses. ___ ___ ___ _____

6. Identified unexpected outcomes. ___ ___ ___ _____

RECORDING AND REPORTING

1. Recorded physical assessment findings in appropriate log. ___ ___ ___ _____

2. Reported and recorded any assessed complications and action taken. ___ ___ ___ _____

3. Recorded exercises demonstrated and patient's ability to perform independently in the appropriate log. ___ ___ ___ _____

4. Reported any problems to next nurse. ___ ___ ___ _____

Student _____ Date _____

Instructor _____ Date _____

PERFORMANCE CHECKLIST SKILL 36-3 **PERFORMING POSTOPERATIVE CARE OF A SURGICAL PATIENT**

	S	U	NP	Comments

ASSESSMENT

1. Phase I: Immediate recovery period:

   a. Received hand-off report from circulating nurse and anesthesia provider. ___ ___ ___ _____

   b. Reviewed surgeon's orders upon patient's arrival. ___ ___ ___ _____

   c. Considered type of procedure, restrictions to movement, and type of anesthesia. ___ ___ ___ _____

   d. Performed a thorough patient assessment; assessed patient's surgical site and drains, skin integrity, safety, and anxiety level. ___ ___ ___ _____

   e. Took vital signs at appropriate intervals. ___ ___ ___ _____

   f. Discharged patient from phase I based on appropriate assessment criteria. ___ ___ ___ _____

2. Phase II level of care: Convalescent period:

   a. Obtained phone report summarizing patient's current status. ___ ___ ___ _____

   b. Collected more detailed hand-off report upon patient's arrival at division. ___ ___ ___ _____

   c. Reviewed patient's chart for information pertaining to surgery, complications, and medical risks. ___ ___ ___ _____

   d. Reviewed postoperative medical orders. ___ ___ ___ _____

   e. Assessed patient and family's knowledge of expectations of surgical recovery. ___ ___ ___ _____

PLANNING

1. Identified expected outcomes. ___ ___ ___ _____

2. Prepared equipment as necessary at bedside, tested equipment for function. ___ ___ ___ _____

3. Explained to patient all procedures and rationale for each, included family if possible. ___ ___ ___ _____

	S	U	NP	Comments

IMPLEMENTATION

1. Phase I: Immediate recovery period:

   a. Performed hand hygiene.

   b. Attached oxygen tubing to regulator, hung IV fluids, checked flow rates, and attached pulse oximeter; connected drainage tubes to gravity drainage, suctioned as ordered; attached cardiac monitor; ensured catheter and bag were in drainage position and patent.

   c. Conducted ongoing assessment of vital signs at appropriate intervals, compared findings with patient's baseline, provided blankets as needed.

   d. Maintained patent airway:

      (1) Positioned patient properly.

      (2) Placed towel or pillow under patient's head, elevated head of bed and turned patient's head to side if needed, had emesis basin available.

      (3) Encouraged patient to cough and deep breathe on awakening and every 15 minutes.

      (4) Suctioned airway and oral cavity.

      (5) Had patient spit out oral airway once gag reflex returned, did not tape oral airway.

      (6) Avoided rapid position change for patient who had spinal anesthesia, encouraged fluid intake.

   e. Called patient by name, aroused patient gently if necessary, explained where patient was.

   f. Assessed circulatory perfusion. Palpated for skin temperature, tested for capillary refill.

   g. Monitored wound drainage:

      (1) Observed dressing and drains for bright red blood, looked for pooling of bloody drainage.

      (2) Inspected surgical area for swelling or discoloration, noted condition of dressing, marked dressing around drainage as well as the time, checked area at appropriate intervals, marked changes and noted vital signs.

	S	U	NP	Comments

(3) Reinforced pressure dressing, changed dressing if ordered, monitored condition of incision.

(4) Inspected condition and contents of drainage tubes and collecting devices, noted character and volume of drainage.

(5) Observed patency and intactness of urinary catheter system, noted volume and character of urine.

(6) Validated NG tube placement if present, irrigated per protocol.

(7) Continued monitoring of IV fluid rates, observed site for signs of infiltration.

h. Provided mouth care as patient awakened.

i. Continued to monitor and provide pain medication at appropriate times.

j. Encouraged patient to practice ankle circles and calf-pumping exercises.

k. Explained to patient about how he or she is progressing and if plans for transfer were being made.

l. Contacted surgeon for order to release to another unit once physiologic signs had stabilized, measured I&O before transfer.

2. Phase II level of care: Convalescent period:

a. Made final check of equipment setup, ensured bed was in highest position and wheels were locked.

b. Assisted PACU staff upon arrival, transferred patient to bed appropriately.

c. Attached existing oxygen tubing, hung IV fluids, checked flow rate, attached NG tube to suction, and placed catheter in drainage position once patient was transferred to bed.

d. Conducted complete assessment of all vital signs, compared findings with vital signs from recovery area and patient's baseline, continued monitoring as warranted.

e. Maintained patent patient airway:

(1) Positioned patient properly, kept head extended.

(2) Encouraged deep breathing and coughing using pillow as incisional splint.

	S	U	NP	Comments

f. Ensured drainage tubes were connected properly, validated correct placement of NG tube if present, irrigated as ordered and connected properly.

____ ____ ____ _____

g. Assessed patient's surgical dressing for intactness and presence and character of drainage, reinforced as ordered, inspected condition of wound without dressing.

____ ____ ____ _____

h. Assessed for bladder distention if patient did not have indwelling catheter, offered bedpan or urinal when necessary.

____ ____ ____ _____

i. Measured and recorded all sources of fluid I&O.

____ ____ ____ _____

j. Positioned patient for comfort, maintained airway and body alignment, avoided positioning on wound site.

____ ____ ____ _____

k. Encouraged patient to continue with leg exercises, did passive range of motion if necessary.

____ ____ ____ _____

l. Applied elastic stockings or pneumatic compression cuffs to lower extremities, attached compressor, explained cuffs to patient.

____ ____ ____ _____

m. Explained to patient that you have completed observations and family members would be entering, placed bed in lowest position and call light within reach, raised side rails as appropriate.

____ ____ ____ _____

n. Explained patient's status to family, described purpose of equipment, explained reason for observations and procedures.

____ ____ ____ _____

o. Gave family simple tasks to perform.

____ ____ ____ _____

p. Determined if pain medication was administered, asked patient to rate severity of pain, administered analgesic if vital signs remained stable, initiated PCA if ordered.

____ ____ ____ _____

q. Provided oral hygiene, repeated as needed.

____ ____ ____ _____

r. Performed measures as patient stabilizes over next hours or days:

(1) Had patient participate in postoperative exercises.

____ ____ ____ _____

(2) Encouraged use of incentive spirometer if ordered, judged efficacy of breathing pattern, charted level.

____ ____ ____ _____

(3) Began activity orders, assessed vital signs first time patient sat or stood.

____ ____ ____ _____

	S	U	NP	Comments
(4) Monitored bowel sounds per protocol, asked if patient had passed flatus.	——	——	——	————————
(5) Began dietary orders slowly, medicated with antiemetic if necessary, gave analgesic with antiemetic until patient was eating well.	——	——	——	————————
(6) Promoted normal voiding pattern, assessed bladder volume.	——	——	——	————————
(7) Monitored progress of wound healing, changed dressings as ordered.	——	——	——	————————
(8) Monitored and maintained wound drainage devices.	——	——	——	————————
(9) Monitored drainage for color, consistency, and amount at appropriate intervals, compared to previous assessment.	——	——	——	————————
s. Increased patient involvement in decision making and in any explanations.	——	——	——	————————
t. Taught patient and family signs of complications and techniques for wound care.	——	——	——	————————
u. Discussed with patient and family other plans for discharge.	——	——	——	————————
v. Prepared to make referral for home or convalescent care, obtained order from surgeon.	——	——	——	————————

EVALUATION

	S	U	NP	Comments
1. Compared vital sign assessment measurements with patient's baseline and normal levels.	——	——	——	————————
2. Measured patient's perception of pain after implementation of pain-relief measures.	——	——	——	————————
3. Monitored changes in surgical wound at least every shift.	——	——	——	————————
4. Monitored lung sounds following exercises.	——	——	——	————————
5. Auscultated bowel sounds at least each shift, asked patient if he or she had passed flatus.	——	——	——	————————
6. Monitored I&O balance for each shift.	——	——	——	————————
7. Discussed with patient general level of comfort and progress.	——	——	——	————————
8. Conducted appropriate physical assessments.	——	——	——	————————
9. Identified unexpected outcomes.	——	——	——	————————

	S	U	NP	Comments

RECORDING AND REPORTING

1. Documented all pertinent information in the appropriate log, continued documentation at appropriate intervals. ___ ___ ___ _____

2. Recorded vital signs, oxygen saturation, temperature, and I&O on appropriate flow sheets. ___ ___ ___ _____

3. Reported abnormal findings and signs of complications to nurse in charge and/or surgeon. ___ ___ ___ _____

Student _____ Date _____

Instructor _____ Date _____

PERFORMANCE CHECKLIST SKILL 37-1 **SURGICAL HAND ANTISEPSIS**

	S	U	NP	Comments

ASSESSMENT

1. Determined type and length of time for hand hygiene. ___ ___ ___ _____

2. Removed bracelets, rings, and watches. ___ ___ ___ _____

3. Inspected fingernails, removed nail polish and artificial or extended nails. ___ ___ ___ _____

4. Inspected condition of cuticles, hands, and fore-arms for presence of abrasions, cuts, or open lesions. ___ ___ ___ _____

PLANNING

1. Identified expected outcomes. ___ ___ ___ _____

IMPLEMENTATION

1. Donned surgical shoe covers, cap or hood, face mask, and protective eyewear. ___ ___ ___ _____

2. Performed a prescrub wash at beginning of work shift:

   a. Turned water on using foot or knee, adjusted temperature. ___ ___ ___ _____

   b. Wet hands thoroughly with water, applied soap. ___ ___ ___ _____

   c. Rubbed hands, covered all surfaces, washed for at least 15 seconds. ___ ___ ___ _____

   d. Rinsed well, dried hands thoroughly with disposable towel, discarded towel. ___ ___ ___ _____

3. Surgical hand scrub with sponge:

   a. Turned on water using foot or knee, cleaned properly under nails, rinsed hands and fore-arms under water. ___ ___ ___ _____

   b. Dispensed antimicrobial scrub agent, applied to hands and forearms using sponge. ___ ___ ___ _____

   c. Timed a 3- to 5-minute scrub; washed all sur-faces; kept hand elevated and elbow down; repeated for other hand, fingers, and arm. ___ ___ ___ _____

   d. Avoided splashing surgical attire, discarded sponges appropriately. ___ ___ ___ _____

   e. Rinsed hands and arms in running water, kept hands higher than elbows. ___ ___ ___ _____

	S	U	NP	Comments

f. Turned off water using foot or knee, backed into OR, held hands above elbows and away from surgical attire.   ____ ____ ____ _____

g. Approached sterile setup, grasped sterile towel, did not drip water on the sterile field.   ____ ____ ____ _____

h. Kept hands and arms above waist, dried one hand and elbow with one end of towel.   ____ ____ ____ _____

i. Used opposite end of towel to dry other hand.   ____ ____ ____ _____

j. Dropped towel into linen hamper or circulating nurse's hand.   ____ ____ ____ _____

4. Performed spongeless surgical hand scrub with alcohol-based hand-rub product:

a. Turned on water using foot or knee, cleaned properly under nails, rinsed hands and forearms under water, dried hands thoroughly with paper towel, turned off water.   ____ ____ ____ _____

b. Dispensed hand preparation, applied properly to hands and forearms.   ____ ____ ____ _____

c. Repeated application if indicated.   ____ ____ ____ _____

d. Rubbed thoroughly until dry, proceeded to OR to don gloves.   ____ ____ ____ _____

EVALUATION

1. Monitored patient postoperatively for signs of surgical site infection.   ____ ____ ____ _____

2. Identified unexpected outcomes.   ____ ____ ____ _____

Student _____ Date _____

Instructor _____ Date _____

PERFORMANCE CHECKLIST SKILL 37-2 **DONNING A STERILE GOWN AND CLOSED GLOVING**

	S	U	NP	Comments
ASSESSMENT				
1. Selected proper size and type of sterile gloves.	___	___	___	_____
2. Selected proper size and type of sterile surgical gown.	___	___	___	_____
PLANNING				
1. Identified expected outcomes.	___	___	___	_____
IMPLEMENTATION				
1. Donned sterile gown:				
a. Opened sterile gown and glove package on clean, dry, flat surface.	___	___	___	_____
b. Performed surgical hand antisepsis, dried hand thoroughly.	___	___	___	_____
c. Picked up gown grasping inside surface of gown at collar.	___	___	___	_____
d. Lifted folded gown upwards, stepped away from table.	___	___	___	_____
e. Located neckband, grasped inside front of gown just below neckband.	___	___	___	_____
f. Allowed gown to unfold with inside of gown toward body, did not touch outside of gown or allow gown to touch the floor.	___	___	___	_____
g. Slipped both arms into armholes with hands at shoulder level, did not allow hands to move through cuff opening, had circulating nurse pull gown over shoulders.	___	___	___	_____
h. Had circulating nurse tie neck and waist.	___	___	___	_____
2. Applied gloves using closed-glove method.				
a. Kept hands covered by gown cuffs and sleeves, opened sterile glove package.	___	___	___	_____
b. Grasped folded cuff of gloves for dominant hand with nondominant hand.	___	___	___	_____
c. Extended dominant forearm forward palm up, placed palm of glove against palm of hand.	___	___	___	_____
d. Grasped back of glove cuff with nondominant hand, turned glove cuff over end of dominant hand and gown cuff.	___	___	___	_____

	S	U	NP	Comments

e. Grasped top of glove and sleeve with nondominant hand, extended fingers into glove, ensured glove cuff covered gown cuff. ____ ____ ____ _____

f. Gloved nondominant hand in same manner, ensured fingers were fully extended into both gloves. ____ ____ ____ _____

3. Donned a wraparound gown:

a. Grasped sterile front flap or tab with gloved hands, untied. ____ ____ ____ _____

b. Passed sterile tab to a member of the team, kept gown tie in hand, turned as circulating nurse stood still. ____ ____ ____ _____

c. Turned to left covering back with extended gown flap, retrieved sterile tie from team member, secured both ties. ____ ____ ____ _____

EVALUATION

1. Monitored patient postoperatively for signs of surgical site infection. ____ ____ ____ _____

2. Identified unexpected outcomes. ____ ____ ____ _____

PERFORMANCE CHECKLIST PROCEDURAL GUIDELINE 38-1 **PERFORMING A WOUND ASSESSMENT**

	S	U	NP	Comments
PROCEDURAL STEPS				
1. Determined agency wound assessment tool, reviewed frequency of assessment, examined last wound assessment for comparison.	___	___	___	_____
2. Assessed comfort level or pain, identified symptoms of anxiety.	___	___	___	_____
3. Explained procedure of wound assessment to patient.	___	___	___	_____
4. Provided privacy, positioned patient, exposed only wound.	___	___	___	_____
5. Performed hand hygiene, formed cuff on waterproof biohazard bag, placed near bed.	___	___	___	_____
6. Applied clean gloves, removed soiled dressings.	___	___	___	_____
7. Examined dressings for quality of drainage, presence or absence of odor, quantity of drainage, discarded dressings in waterproof biohazard bag, discarded gloves.	___	___	___	_____
8. Performed hand hygiene, applied clean gloves.	___	___	___	_____
9. Inspected wound, determined type of wound healing.	___	___	___	_____
10. Used agency-approved assessment tool, assessed the following:				
a. Wound healing by primary intention:				
(1) Assessed anatomic location of wound on body.	___	___	___	_____
(2) Noted if wound margins were approximated or closed together.	___	___	___	_____
(3) Observed for presence of drainage.	___	___	___	_____
(4) Looked for evidence of infection.	___	___	___	_____
(5) Palpated along incision to feel a healing ridge.	___	___	___	_____

	S	U	NP	Comments

b. Wound healing by secondary intention:

    (1) Assessed anatomic location of wound on body.

    (2) Assessed wound dimensions properly, discarded measuring guide and applicator in trash bag.

    (3) Assessed for undermining, documented number of centimeters that area extends from wound edge.

    (4) Assessed extent of tissue loss.

    (5) Noticed tissue type including percentage of tissue intact and of granulation, slough, and necrotic tissue.

    (6) Noted presence of exudates, indicated amount.

    (7) Noted if wound edges were rounded toward the wound bed, described presence of epithelialization at wound edges.

    (8) Inspected periwound skin.

11. Reapplied dressings as per order; placed time, date, and initials on new dressing.

12. Reassessed patient's pain and level of comfort at wound site after dressing was applied.

13. Discarded biohazard bag, soiled supplies, and gloves properly; performed hand hygiene.

14. Recorded wound assessment findings, compared assessment with previous wound assessments.

Student _____   Date _____

Instructor _____   Date _____

PERFORMANCE CHECKLIST SKILL 38-1   **WOUND IRRIGATION**

	S	U	NP	Comments

ASSESSMENT

1. Reviewed order for irrigation and type of solution to be used.   ___ ___ ___ _____

2. Performed wound assessment, examined recent charted assessment of wound.   ___ ___ ___ _____

3. Assessed patient for history of allergies to antiseptics, medication, tapes, or dressing material.   ___ ___ ___ _____

PLANNING

1. Identified expected outcomes.   ___ ___ ___ _____

2. Administered analgesic 30 to 45 minutes before procedure if needed.   ___ ___ ___ _____

3. Educated patient and family about procedure.   ___ ___ ___ _____

IMPLEMENTATION

1. Identified patient using two identifiers.   ___ ___ ___ _____

2. Obtained supplies for irrigation and dressing, formed cuff on waterproof biohazard bag, placed near bed.   ___ ___ ___ _____

3. Provided privacy, performed hand hygiene, positioned patient properly.   ___ ___ ___ _____

4. Placed padding or towel on bed under area where irrigation would take place.   ___ ___ ___ _____

5. Exposed wound only.   ___ ___ ___ _____

6. Applied gown and goggles, applied sterile gloves and used sterile precautions.   ___ ___ ___ _____

7. Irrigated wound with wide opening:

   a. Filled syringe with irrigation solution.   ___ ___ ___ _____

   b. Attached 19-gauge angiocatheter or needle.   ___ ___ ___ _____

   c. Held syringe tip above upper end of wound and over area being cleansed.   ___ ___ ___ _____

   d. Flushed wound using continuous pressure until solution draining was clear.   ___ ___ ___ _____

8. Irrigated deep wound with small opening:

   a. Attached soft catheter to filled syringe.   ___ ___ ___ _____

   b. Inserted tip of catheter into opening.   ___ ___ ___ _____

	S	U	NP	Comments

c. Flushed wound using slow, continuous pressure. ___ ___ ___ _____

d. Pinched off catheter below syringe while in place. ___ ___ ___ _____

e. Removed and refilled syringe, reconnected to catheter, repeated until solution draining was clear. ___ ___ ___ _____

9. Cleansed wound with handheld shower:

   a. Performed hand hygiene, applied clean gloves, adjusted spray with patient seated, ensured water was warm. ___ ___ ___ _____

   b. Showered for 5 to 10 minutes. ___ ___ ___ _____

10. Obtained cultures after cleansing with nonbacteriostatic saline when indicated. ___ ___ ___ _____

11. Dried wound edges with gauze, dried patient. ___ ___ ___ _____

12. Applied appropriate dressing, labeled with time, date, and nurse's initials. ___ ___ ___ _____

13. Removed mask, goggles, and gown. ___ ___ ___ _____

14. Disposed of equipment and soiled supplies, removed gloves, performed hand hygiene. ___ ___ ___ _____

15. Assisted patient to comfortable position. ___ ___ ___ _____

EVALUATION

1. Had patient rate level of comfort. ___ ___ ___ _____

2. Monitored type of tissue in wound bed. ___ ___ ___ _____

3. Inspected dressing periodically. ___ ___ ___ _____

4. Evaluated periwound skin integrity. ___ ___ ___ _____

5. Observed for presence of retained irrigant. ___ ___ ___ _____

6. Identified unexpected outcomes. ___ ___ ___ _____

RECORDING AND REPORTING

1. Recorded all findings in appropriate log. ___ ___ ___ _____

2. Reported to health care provider any evidence of fresh bleeding, sharp increase in pain, retention of irrigant, or signs of shock immediately. ___ ___ ___ _____

Student _____ Date _____

Instructor _____ Date _____

PERFORMANCE CHECKLIST SKILL 38-2 **REMOVING SUTURES AND STAPLES**

	S	U	NP	Comments
ASSESSMENT				
1. Identified patient with need for suture or staple removal:				
a. Checked health care provider's order.	___	___	___	_____
b. Reviewed specific directions related to removal.	___	___	___	_____
c. Determined history of conditions that may pose risk for impaired wound healing.	___	___	___	_____
2. Assessed patient for history of allergies.	___	___	___	_____
3. Assessed patient's comfort level or pain.	___	___	___	_____
4. Assessed healing ridge and skin integrity of suture line for uniform closure, normal color, and absence of drainage and inflammation.	___	___	___	_____
PLANNING				
1. Identified expected outcomes.	___	___	___	_____
2. Explained to patient that suture removal was not usually painful but patient may feel tugging.	___	___	___	_____
IMPLEMENTATION				
1. Provided privacy.	___	___	___	_____
2. Identified patient using two identifiers.	___	___	___	_____
3. Positioned patient comfortably, exposed suture line, ensured direct lighting was on suture line.	___	___	___	_____
4. Performed hand hygiene.	___	___	___	_____
5. Placed cuffed waterproof disposal bag within easy reach.	___	___	___	_____
6. Prepared materials needed:				
a. Opened sterile kit.	___	___	___	_____
b. Opened antiseptic swabs, placed on inside surface of kit.	___	___	___	_____
c. Obtained gloves, sterile if necessary.	___	___	___	_____
7. Performed hand hygiene, applied clean gloves, removed dressing, discarded dressing and gloves in disposal bag.	___	___	___	_____
8. Inspected incision and suture line.	___	___	___	_____

	S	U	NP	Comments

9. Applied clean or sterile gloves as appropriate. ____ ____ ____ _____

10. Cleansed sutures or staples and healed incisions with antiseptic. ____ ____ ____ _____

11. Removed staples:

   a. Placed lower tip of extractor under first staple, closed handles to extract ends. ____ ____ ____ _____

   b. Controlled staple extractor carefully. ____ ____ ____ _____

   c. Moved staple away from surface when both ends were visible. ____ ____ ____ _____

   d. Dropped staple into refuse bag. ____ ____ ____ _____

   e. Repeated steps a to d until all staples were removed. ____ ____ ____ _____

12. Removed intermittent sutures:

   a. Placed gauze a few inches from suture line, held scissors and forceps appropriately. ____ ____ ____ _____

   b. Grasped knot with forceps, pulled while slipping tip of scissors under suture. ____ ____ ____ _____

   c. Snipped suture as close to skin as possible. ____ ____ ____ _____

   d. Grasped knotted end, pulled suture through from other side, placed removed sutures on gauze. ____ ____ ____ _____

   e. Repeated steps a to d until every other (alternating) suture was removed. ____ ____ ____ _____

   f. Observed healing level, determined whether remaining sutures were to be removed. ____ ____ ____ _____

   g. Stopped and notified health care provider if in doubt. ____ ____ ____ _____

13. Removed continuous and blanket stitch sutures:

   a. Placed gauze a few inches from suture line, held scissors and forceps appropriately. ____ ____ ____ _____

   b. Snipped first suture close to skin surface distal to knot. ____ ____ ____ _____

   c. Snipped second suture on same side. ____ ____ ____ _____

   d. Grasped knotted end, removed suture, placed suture on gauze compress. ____ ____ ____ _____

   e. Repeated steps a to d until entire line was removed. ____ ____ ____ _____

	S	U	NP	Comments

14. Inspected incision, ensured all sutures were removed, identified trouble areas, wiped suture line with antiseptic swab.

15. Applied Steri-Strips if any separation greater that two stitches or two staples wide.

    a. Cut strips to appropriate length.

    b. Removed backing, applied across incision.

    c. Instructed patient to take showers rather than soak in bathtub.

16. Applied light dressing, exposed to air if clothing would not come into contact, instructed patient about applying own dressing.

17. Discarded contaminated materials, removed and disposed of gloves.

18. Routed reusable items for sterilization, disposed of sharps properly, performed hand hygiene.

EVALUATION

1. Assessed site where sutures or staples were removed, inspected condition of soft tissues, looked for pieces of removed suture left behind.

2. Determined if patient had pain along incision.

3. Identified unexpected outcomes.

RECORDING AND REPORTING

1. Recorded all pertinent information in the appropriate log.

2. Reported if suture line separation, dehiscence, evisceration, bleeding, or purulent drainage occurred to health care provider immediately.

Student _____ Date _____

Instructor _____ Date _____

PERFORMANCE CHECKLIST SKILL 38-3 **MANAGING WOUND DRAINAGE EVACUATION**

	S	U	NP	Comments

ASSESSMENT

1. Identified presence, location, and purpose of closed wound drain and drainage system, assessed drainage on patient's dressing.

2. Identified number of wound drain tubes and what each was draining, labeled each drain tube.

3. Assessed if drain tube needed self-suction, wall suction, or no suction by checking orders.

4. Inspected system to determine presence of straight or Y-tube arrangement.

5. Inspected system to ensure proper functioning.

6. Ensured Penrose drain had a sterile safety pin in place, did not pull on drain while positioning gauze.

7. Identified type of drainage containers patient had.

PLANNING

1. Identified expected outcomes.

2. Explained procedure to patient.

IMPLEMENTATION

1. Provided privacy.

2. Performed hand hygiene, applied clean gloves.

3. Placed open specimen container or measuring graduate on bed between you and patient.

4. Emptied Hemovac or ConstaVac:

   a. Maintained asepsis while opening proper plug on port, tilted suction container in direction of plug, squeezed flat surfaces together, tilted toward measuring container.

   b. Drained contents into measuring container.

   c. Placed suction device properly on flat surface, pressed down until bottom and top were in contact.

   d. Held surfaces with one hand, cleaned opening and plug, replaced plug, secured suction device on patient's bed.

	S	U	NP	Comments

e. Checked device for reestablishment of vacuum, patency of drainage tubing, and absence of stress on tubing. ___ ___ ___ _____

5. Emptied Hemovac with wall suction:

   a. Turned off suction. ___ ___ ___ _____

   b. Disconnected suction tubing from Hemovac port. ___ ___ ___ _____

   c. Emptied Hemovac as described in step 4. ___ ___ ___ _____

   d. Cleansed port opening and end of suction tubing. ___ ___ ___ _____

   e. Set suction level appropriately or as prescribed. ___ ___ ___ _____

6. Emptied JP suction drain:

   a. Opened port on top of bulb-shaped reservoir. ___ ___ ___ _____

   b. Tilted bulb in direction of port, drained away from opening, emptied drainage into measuring container, cleansed end of port and plugged with alcohol. ___ ___ ___ _____

   c. Compressed bulb over drainage container, replaced plug immediately. ___ ___ ___ _____

7. Placed secure drainage system below site with safety pin on gown, ensured there was slack in tubing. ___ ___ ___ _____

8. Noted characteristics of drainage. ___ ___ ___ _____

9. Discarded soiled supplies, removed gloves, performed hand hygiene. ___ ___ ___ _____

10. Proceeded with dressing change and inspection of skin if indicated or ordered. ___ ___ ___ _____

11. Discarded contaminated materials, performed hand hygiene. ___ ___ ___ _____

EVALUATION

1. Observed for drainage in suction device. ___ ___ ___ _____

2. Inspected wound for drainage or collection of fluid under skin. ___ ___ ___ _____

3. Measured drainage, emptied drainage system, recorded on I&O form. ___ ___ ___ _____

4. Assessed patient's level of comfort. ___ ___ ___ _____

5. Identified unexpected outcomes. ___ ___ ___ _____

	S	U	NP	Comments

RECORDING AND REPORTING

1. Recorded all pertinent information in the appropriate log.

2. Recorded amount of drainage on I&O record.

3. Reported sudden change in amount of drainage, pungent odor of drainage or new signs of purulence, severe pain, or dislodgment of tube to health care provider immediately.

Student _____ Date _____

Instructor _____ Date _____

PERFORMANCE CHECKLIST SKILL 39-1 **APPLYING A DRESSING (DRY AND MOIST-TO-DRY)**

	S	U	NP	Comments
ASSESSMENT				
1. Asked patient to rate pain level and assess character of pain, administered analgesic if necessary.	___	___	___	_____
2. Assessed size, location, and condition of the wound; reviewed previous notes.	___	___	___	_____
3. Assessed patient's and caregiver's knowledge of purpose of dressing change.	___	___	___	_____
4. Assessed patient for allergies to antiseptics, tape, or latex.	___	___	___	_____
5. Assessed need, readiness, and willingness for patient or caregiver to participate in dressing wound.	___	___	___	_____
6. Reviewed medical orders for dressing change procedure.	___	___	___	_____
7. Identified patient with risk factors for wound healing problems.	___	___	___	_____
PLANNING				
1. Identified expected outcomes.	___	___	___	_____
2. Explained procedure to patient.	___	___	___	_____
IMPLEMENTATION				
1. Identified patient using two identifiers.	___	___	___	_____
2. Provided privacy.	___	___	___	_____
3. Positioned patient comfortably, draped to expose only wound site, instructed patient not to touch wound or supplies.	___	___	___	_____
4. Placed disposable waterproof bag within reach, folded top to make cuff, performed hand hygiene and put on clean gloves, applied necessary PPE.	___	___	___	_____
5. Removed tape, bandages, or ties properly, got permission to clip or shave hair if necessary, removed adhesive from skin.	___	___	___	_____

	S	U	NP	Comments

6. Removed dressing properly one layer at a time, observed appearance and drainage of dressing, avoided tension on drainage devices, kept soiled undersurface from patient's sight, freed dressing sticking to wound appropriately. ___ ___ ___ _____

7. Assessed condition of wound and periwound, used measuring guide or ruler to measure size of wound, palpated wound edges for bogginess or patient report of increased pain. ___ ___ ___ _____

8. Folded dressings with drainage inside, removed gloves inside out, folded gloves over dressing if appropriate, disposed of gloves and dressing appropriately, covered wound with sterile gauze, performed hand hygiene. ___ ___ ___ _____

9. Described appearance of wound and indications of healing to patient. ___ ___ ___ _____

10. Created sterile field on over-bed tray, poured prescribed solution in sterile basin. ___ ___ ___ _____

11. Cleansed wound:

   a. Applied clean gloves, used gauze or cotton ball with saline or antiseptic or sprayed wound with wound cleaner. ___ ___ ___ _____

   b. Cleaned from least to most contaminated area. ___ ___ ___ _____

   c. Cleaned appropriately around any drain. ___ ___ ___ _____

12. Used dry gauze to blot the wound dry. ___ ___ ___ _____

13. Applied antiseptic ointment properly if ordered, disposed of gloves, performed hand hygiene. ___ ___ ___ _____

14. Applied dressing:

   a. Dry dressing:

     (1) Applied clean gloves. ___ ___ ___ _____

     (2) Applied loose woven gauze as a contact layer. ___ ___ ___ _____

     (3) Applied split gauze around drain if present. ___ ___ ___ _____

     (4) Applied additional layers of gauze as needed. ___ ___ ___ _____

     (5) Applied thicker woven pad. ___ ___ ___ _____

	S	U	NP	Comments

b. Moist-to-dry dressing.

(1) Applied sterile gloves.

(2) Placed mesh or gauze in container of prescribed solution, wrung out excess solution.

(3) Applied moist mesh or gauze as a single layer onto wound surface, packed gauze into wound properly if necessary, ensured gauze did not touch peri-wound skin.

(4) Applied dry sterile gauze over moist gauze.

(5) Covered with ABD pad, Surgipad, or gauze.

15. Secured dressing properly with tape or Montgomery ties.

16. Disposed of all dressing supplies, removed PPE and disposed properly.

17. Labeled tape over dressing with initials, changed dressing date.

18. Assisted patient to comfortable position.

19. Performed hand hygiene.

EVALUATION

1. Observed appearance of wound for healing.

2. Asked patient to rate pain.

3. Inspected condition of dressing at least every shift.

4. Asked patient and/or caregiver to describe steps and techniques of dressing change.

5. Identified unexpected outcomes.

RECORDING AND REPORTING

1. Recorded all pertinent information in the appropriate log.

2. Reported unexpected appearance of wound drainage, accidental removal of drain, bright-red bleeding, or evidence of wound dehiscence or evisceration.

Student _____ Date _____

Instructor _____ Date _____

PERFORMANCE CHECKLIST SKILL 39-2 **APPLYING A PRESSURE BANDAGE**

	S	U	NP	Comments
ASSESSMENT				
1. Anticipated patients at risk for unexpected bleeding.	___	___	___	_____
2. Assessed location and condition of area where hemorrhage was expected.	___	___	___	_____
3. Assessed patient for allergies to antiseptics, tape, or latex; used other supplies if necessary.	___	___	___	_____
4. Assessed patient's anxiety level.	___	___	___	_____
5. Considered patient's baseline vital signs prior to onset of hemorrhage.	___	___	___	_____
PLANNING				
1. Identified expected outcomes.	___	___	___	_____
IMPLEMENTATION				
1. Identified external bleeding site, looked underneath patient with large abdominal dressings.	___	___	___	_____
2. Immediately applied manual pressure to site of bleeding.	___	___	___	_____
3. Sought assistance.	___	___	___	_____
4. Identified source of bleeding quickly.	___	___	___	_____
5. Elevated affected body part if possible.	___	___	___	_____
6. Continued to apply pressure as first nurse, while second nurse unwrapped roller bandage and cut tape appropriately.	___	___	___	_____
7. Covered bleeding area with multiple layers of gauze, applied pressure.	___	___	___	_____
8. Placed two adhesive strips appropriately over dressing with even pressure, secured tapes properly.	___	___	___	_____
9. Removed fingers, covered center area with third piece of tape.	___	___	___	_____
10. Continued reinforcing area with tape and applying pressure as needed.	___	___	___	_____

	S	U	NP	Comments
11. Applied roller gauze properly over pressure bandage, compressed over bleeding site, removed finger pressure and applied roller gauze over center, continued with figure-eight turns, secured end with two circular turns and adhesive.	___	___	___	_____

EVALUATION

	S	U	NP	Comments
1. Observed dressing for control of bleeding.	___	___	___	_____
2. Evaluated adequacy of circulation.	___	___	___	_____
3. Estimated volume of blood loss.	___	___	___	_____
4. Measured vital signs.	___	___	___	_____
5. Identified unexpected outcomes.	___	___	___	_____

RECORDING AND REPORTING

	S	U	NP	Comments
1. Reported details of incident to health care provider.	___	___	___	_____
2. Recorded interventions and patient's response in notes and vital signs flow sheet.	___	___	___	_____

Student _____ Date _____

Instructor _____ Date _____

PERFORMANCE CHECKLIST SKILL 39-3 **APPLYING A TRANSPARENT DRESSING**

	S	U	NP	Comments
ASSESSMENT				
1. Assessed location, appearance, and size of wound; reviewed previous nurses' notes.	___	___	___	_____
2. Reviewed health care provider's orders for frequency and type of dressing change.	___	___	___	_____
3. Assessed patient for allergies to antiseptics, tape, or latex.	___	___	___	_____
4. Asked patient to rate pain level and assessed character of pain, administered prescribed analgesic at the appropriate time.	___	___	___	_____
5. Assessed patient's knowledge of purpose of dressing.	___	___	___	_____
6. Assessed patient's risk for impaired wound healing.	___	___	___	_____
PLANNING				
1. Identified expected outcomes.	___	___	___	_____
2. Explained procedure to patient.	___	___	___	_____
3. Positioned patient comfortably, allowed access to dressing site.	___	___	___	_____
IMPLEMENTATION				
1. Identified patient using two identifiers per facility policy, compared identifiers with information on patient's ID bracelet.	___	___	___	_____
2. Provided privacy, kept body parts that did not require exposure draped.	___	___	___	_____
3. Exposed wound site, minimized exposure, instructed patient not to touch wound or supplies.	___	___	___	_____
4. Cuffed top of waterproof bag, placed within reach.	___	___	___	_____
5. Performed hand hygiene, applied clean gloves.	___	___	___	_____
6. Removed old dressing appropriately.	___	___	___	_____
7. Disposed of soiled dressing in waterproof bag, removed gloves inside out and disposed of in bag, performed hand hygiene.	___	___	___	_____

	S	U	NP	Comments
8. Prepared dressing supplies, used sterile supplies for new wounds.	___	___	___	_____
9. Poured prescribed solution over sterile gauze pads.	___	___	___	_____
10. Applied sterile gloves.	___	___	___	_____
11. Cleansed wound and periwound with gauze and saline or wound cleanser, cleansed from least to most contaminated.	___	___	___	_____
12. Patted skin around wound thoroughly dry with gauze.	___	___	___	_____
13. Inspected wound for tissue type, color, odor, and drainage; measured if indicated.	___	___	___	_____
14. Removed gloves, performed hand hygiene.	___	___	___	_____
15. Applied transparent dressing properly; applied clean gloves; labeled dressing with date, initials, and time of dressing change.	___	___	___	_____
16. Discarded soiled dressing materials properly, removed gloves inside out, discarded appropriately, performed hand hygiene.	___	___	___	_____
17. Assisted patient to comfortable position.	___	___	___	_____

EVALUATION

	S	U	NP	Comments
1. Inspected appearance of wound, amount of drainage, and size.	___	___	___	_____
2. Inspected periwound areas.	___	___	___	_____
3. Asked patient to rate pain.	___	___	___	_____
4. Identified unexpected outcomes.	___	___	___	_____

RECORDING AND REPORTING

	S	U	NP	Comments
1. Recorded appearance of wound, presence and characteristics of drainage or odor, noted patient response.	___	___	___	_____
2. Reported signs of infection to health care provider.	___	___	___	_____

Student _____ Date _____

Instructor _____ Date _____

PERFORMANCE CHECKLIST SKILL 39-4 **APPLYING HYDROCOLLOID, HYDROGEL, FOAM, OR ABSORPTION DRESSING**

	S	U	NP	Comments
ASSESSMENT				
1. Assessed for presence of allergies to antiseptics, tape, or latex.	___	___	___	_____
2. Inspected location, size, and condition of wound.	___	___	___	_____
3. Asked patient to rate pain and assess character of pain, administered prescribed analgesic at the appropriate time.	___	___	___	_____
4. Reviewed health care provider's orders for frequency and type of dressing change.	___	___	___	_____
5. Considered using customized shape or size of dressing.	___	___	___	_____
6. Assessed patient's knowledge of purpose of dressing, determined need to include caregiver in dressing wound.	___	___	___	_____
PLANNING				
1. Identified expected outcomes.	___	___	___	_____
2. Explained procedure to patient.	___	___	___	_____
3. Positioned patient comfortably to allow access to dressing site.	___	___	___	_____
IMPLEMENTATION				
1. Identified patient using two identifiers per agency policy, compared with information on patient's ID bracelet.	___	___	___	_____
2. Provided privacy.	___	___	___	_____
3. Exposed wound site, draped patient, instructed patient not to touch wound or supplies.	___	___	___	_____
4. Cuffed top of waterproof bag, placed within reach.	___	___	___	_____
5. Performed hand hygiene, put on clean gloves, applied appropriate PPE.	___	___	___	_____
6. Removed old dressing one layer at a time, noted amount and character of drainage, used caution to avoid tension on any drains.	___	___	___	_____

	S	U	NP	Comments

7. Disposed of soiled dressings in bag, removed clean gloves inside out, disposed of them in bag, covered wound with gauze, performed hand hygiene. ____ ____ ____ _____

8. Prepared sterile field on over-bed table. ____ ____ ____ _____

9. Poured saline over gauze or opened spray wound cleaner. ____ ____ ____ _____

10. Applied sterile gloves or used forceps to cleanse wound, removed gauze covering wound. ____ ____ ____ _____

11. Cleansed wound properly, cleansed around drain properly. ____ ____ ____ _____

12. Used gauze to blot dry the wound bed and skin around wound. ____ ____ ____ _____

13. Inspected appearance and condition of wound, measured wound size and depth. ____ ____ ____ _____

14. Removed glove, performed hand hygiene. ____ ____ ____ _____

15. Applied clean gloves. Applied dressing properly:

  a. Hydrocolloid dressings:

    (1) Selected proper size wafer. ____ ____ ____ _____

    (2) Applied hydrocolloid granules, impregnated gauze, or paste if necessary. ____ ____ ____ _____

    (3) Removed paper backing, placed over wound, avoided wrinkles, molded wafer to affected body part. ____ ____ ____ _____

    (4) Taped edges if necessary. ____ ____ ____ _____

    (5) Held dressing in place for appropriate time. ____ ____ ____ _____

    (6) Used nonallergenic tape to secure. ____ ____ ____ _____

  b. Hydrogel dressings:

    (1) Applied skin barrier wipe to skin that would come in contact with adhesive or gel. ____ ____ ____ _____

    (2) Applied gel into wound properly, covered with appropriate dressing. ____ ____ ____ _____

    (3) Cut hydrogel sheet containing glycerine so it extended over wound to intact skin; cut secondary dressing as needed. ____ ____ ____ _____

    (4) Secured dressing as necessary ____ ____ ____ _____

	S	U	NP	Comments

c. Foam dressings:

   (1) Knew removal and application characteristics of dressing.

   (2) Applied skin barrier to skin that would come in contact with adhesive.

   (3) Cut foam to proper size, verified orientation.

   (4) Covered foam dressing with secondary dressing if needed.

   (5) Cut secondary dressing as necessary.

d. Alginate dressing:

   (1) Cut sheet or rope to fit wound or packed into wound space.

   (2) Applied secondary dressing properly.

16. Discarded soiled dressing materials properly, removed gloves inside out, discarded in bags, performed hand hygiene.

17. Assisted patient to comfortable position.

EVALUATION

1. Inspected condition of wound and character of drainage.

2. Evaluated patient's level of comfort.

3. Asked patient or family to explain wound care method.

4. Identified unexpected outcomes.

RECORDING AND REPORTING

1. Recorded all pertinent information in appropriate log.

2. Graphed wound area or volume if wound was chronic.

3. Wrote date, time, and initials on dressing.

4. Reported signs of infection, necrosis, or deteriorating wound status to health care provider immediately.

Student _____ Date _____

Instructor _____ Date _____

PERFORMANCE CHECKLIST SKILL 39-5 **NEGATIVE-PRESSURE WOUND THERAPY**

	S	U	NP	Comments
ASSESSMENT				
1. Assessed location, appearance, and size of wound.	___	___	___	_____
2. Reviewed health care provider's orders for frequency of dressing change, amount of negative pressure, type of foam or gauze, and pressure cycle.	___	___	___	_____
3. Asked patient to rate level of pain, administered prescribed analgesic at appropriate time.	___	___	___	_____
4. Assessed patient's and caregiver's knowledge of purpose of dressing and whether they would participate in dressing wound.	___	___	___	_____
PLANNING				
1. Identified expected outcomes.	___	___	___	_____
2. Explained procedure to patient.	___	___	___	_____
3. Put system into "de-V. A. C." mode before removal of old dressings when using KCI V.A.C.	___	___	___	_____
IMPLEMENTATION				
1. Identified patient using two identifiers.	___	___	___	_____
2. Provided privacy.	___	___	___	_____
3. Positioned patient comfortably, draped to expose wound site only, instructed patient not to touch wound or supplies.	___	___	___	_____
4. Cuffed top of disposable waterproof bag, placed within reach.	___	___	___	_____
5. Performed hand hygiene, put on clean gloves, applied PPE if necessary.	___	___	___	_____
6. Followed directions for removal and replacement of NPWT unit, turned unit off:				
a. Raised tubing unit, engaged clamp on dressing tubing.	___	___	___	_____
b. Allowed drainage to flow from tubing into collector.	___	___	___	_____

	S	U	NP	Comments

c. Stretched transparent dressing to remove from skin. ____ ____ ____ _____

d. Removed old dressing properly, discarded in bag, kept soiled surfaces from patient's signs. ____ ____ ____ _____

7. Performed wound assessment; observed tissue area, tissue type, color, odor, and drainage within wound; measured length, width, and depth of wound. ____ ____ ____ _____

8. Removed and discarded gloves in waterproof bag, avoided having patient see old dressing because sight of wound may be upsetting, performed hand hygiene. ____ ____ ____ _____

9. Cleansed wound:

   a. Applied sterile gloves. ____ ____ ____ _____

   b. Cleansed wound properly, irrigated with solution if necessary, blotted periwound dry. ____ ____ ____ _____

10. Applied appropriate skin protectant to periwound skin. ____ ____ ____ _____

11. Filled any uneven skin surfaces with barrier product. ____ ____ ____ _____

12. Removed and discarded gloves, performed hand hygiene. ____ ____ ____ _____

13. Applied sterile or clean gloves as necessary. ____ ____ ____ _____

14. Applied NPWT properly:

   a. Prepared NPWT foam:

      (1) Checked wound measurement, selected appropriate foam dressing. ____ ____ ____ _____

      (2) Cut foam to appropriate size with sterile scissors, included tunnels and undermined areas. ____ ____ ____ _____

      (3) Instilled antimicrobial product or antibiotic in wound if necessary. ____ ____ ____ _____

   b. Placed foam in wound, ensured foam was in contact with entire wound base, counted number of foam dressings and documented in patient's chart. ____ ____ ____ _____

	S	U	NP	Comments

c. Applied NPWT transparent dressing over foam wound dressing:

(1) Trimmed dressing properly. ___ ___ ___ _____

(2) Applied transparent dressing, kept wrinkle-free. ___ ___ ___ _____

(3) Secured tubing of unit to transparent film, aligned tubing and drainage hole to ensure an occlusive seal, examined system to ensure seal was intact and therapy was working. ___ ___ ___ _____

15. Recorded initials, time, and date on new dressing. ___ ___ ___ _____

16. Assisted patient to comfortable position. ___ ___ ___ _____

17. Discarded gloves, disposed of dressing materials, performed hand hygiene. ___ ___ ___ _____

EVALUATION

1. Inspected condition of wound on ongoing basis, noted drainage and order. ___ ___ ___ _____

2. Asked patient to rate pain. ___ ___ ___ _____

3. Verified airtight dressing seal and correct negative pressure setting. ___ ___ ___ _____

4. Measured wound drainage output in canister on regular basis. ___ ___ ___ _____

5. Observed patient's or caregiver's ability to perform dressing change. ___ ___ ___ _____

6. Identified unexpected outcomes. ___ ___ ___ _____

RECORDING AND REPORTING

1. Charted EHR appearance of wound, characteristics of drainage, placement of NPWT, and patient response in appropriate log. ___ ___ ___ _____

2. Reported brisk, bright-red bleeding, poor wound healing, evisceration or dehiscence ___ ___ ___ _____

Student _____ Date _____

Instructor _____ Date _____

PERFORMANCE CHECKLIST PROCEDURAL GUIDELINE 39-1 **APPLYING GAUZE AND ELASTIC BANDAGES**

	S	U	NP	Comments
PROCEDURAL STEPS				
1. Reviewed patient's medical record for specific orders related to application of gauze and bandage.	___	___	___	
2. Identified patient using two identifiers.	___	___	___	
3. Observed adequacy of circulation properly, observed skin color and movement of body part to be wrapped.	___	___	___	
4. Assessed patient's level of comfort, administered analgesic at appropriate time if necessary.	___	___	___	
5. Applied clean gloves, inspected skin of area bandaged for alterations in integrity, paid close attention to areas over bony prominences.	___	___	___	
6. Inspected condition of wound for appearance, size, and presence and character of drainage; ensured if covered properly; reapplied dressing if necessary; removed clean gloves; performed hand hygiene.	___	___	___	
7. Assessed properly for size of bandage.	___	___	___	
8. Identified patient's and caregiver's knowledge level and ability to manipulate bandage if necessary.	___	___	___	
9. Provided privacy, positioned comfortably and properly in bed.	___	___	___	
10. Performed hand hygiene, applied clean gloves if drainage was present.	___	___	___	
11. Applied gauze or elastic dressing:				
a. Elevated dependent extremity before applying bandage.	___	___	___	
b. Ensured primary dressing was securely in place.	___	___	___	
c. Held bandage properly in dominant hand, held beginning layer at distal body part.	___	___	___	
d. Began with two circular turns, continued to transfer roll as you wrapped bandage.	___	___	___	

	S	U	NP	Comments

e. Applied bandage from distal point toward proximal boundary using appropriate turns, overlapped each layer properly.

f. Alternated ascending and descending turns over a joint.

g. Ensured bandage was snug and that primary dressing was positioned correctly.

h. Stretched bandage while unrolling, explained to patient reasoning for bandage.

i. Ended bandage with two circular turns, secured end to outside layer with tape or clips.

12. Applied elastic bandage over stump:

a. Elevated stump with pillow or assistance.

b. Secured bandage by wrapping twice around proximal end of stump or waist.

c. Made half turn perpendicular to edge.

d. Brought body of bandage over distal end of stump.

e. Continued to fold bandage over stump from distal to proximal.

f. Secured with metal clips, Velcro, or tape.

13. Removed gloves, performed hand hygiene.

14. Removed and reapplied elastic bandage at appropriate intervals.

15. Evaluated degree of tightness of bandage.

16. Evaluated distal circulation at appropriate intervals.

17. Observed mobility of extremity.

18. Evaluated bandage for wrinkles, looseness, and presence of drainage.

19. Had patient or caregiver demonstrate bandage application.

20. Recorded patient's baseline and postbandage application.

21. Recorded condition of wound or skin integrity if a dressing was present and type of bandage applied.

22. Reported any changes in neurologic or circulatory status to nurse in charge or health care provider immediately.

Student _____ Date _____

Instructor _____ Date _____

PERFORMANCE CHECKLIST PROCEDURAL GUIDELINE 39-2 **APPLYING AN ABDOMINAL BINDER**

	S	U	NP	Comments
PROCEDURAL STEPS				
1. Observed patient who needed support of thorax or abdomen; observed ability to breathe, cough, and turn independently.	___	___	___	_____
2. Reviewed medical record for order for binder.	___	___	___	_____
3. Identified patient using two identifiers.	___	___	___	_____
4. Inspected skin for alterations in integrity; observed for irritation, abrasion, and skin surfaces that rub against each other.	___	___	___	_____
5. Inspected any surgical dressing for intactness, presence of drainage, and coverage of incision; changed soiled dressings before applying binder.	___	___	___	_____
6. Determined patient's level of comfort, administered prescribed analgesic at appropriate time.	___	___	___	_____
7. Gathered necessary data regarding size of patient and appropriate binder to use.	___	___	___	_____
8. Determined patient's knowledge of purpose of binder.	___	___	___	_____
9. Provided privacy.	___	___	___	_____
10. Performed hand hygiene, applied clean gloves if necessary.	___	___	___	_____
11. Applied abdominal binder:				
a. Positioned patient properly.	___	___	___	_____
b. Assisted patient in rolling on side away from you while supporting abdominal incision and dressing, fanfolded far side of binder toward midline of binder.	___	___	___	_____
c. Placed binder flat on bed, fanfolded far side toward midline so patient could roll over.	___	___	___	_____
d. Placed fanfolded ends of binder under patient.	___	___	___	_____

	S	U	NP	Comments

e. Instructed patient in rolling over folded binder. ___ ___ ___ _____

f. Unfolded and stretched ends out smoothly on far side of bed, then near side. ___ ___ ___ _____

g. Instructed patient to roll back. ___ ___ ___ _____

h. Adjusted binder so patient was centered, used symphysis pubis and costal margins as lower and upper landmarks. ___ ___ ___ _____

i. Padded iliac prominences with gauze if necessary. ___ ___ ___ _____

j. Closed binder, pulled one end over patient's abdomen, pulled opposite end over and secured with fasteners, provided continuous wound support or comfort. ___ ___ ___ _____

12. Assessed patient's comfort level, adjusted binder as necessary. ___ ___ ___ _____

13. Removed gloves, performed hand hygiene. ___ ___ ___ _____

14. Asked patient to rate pain scale. ___ ___ ___ _____

15. Removed binder and surgical dressing to assess skin and wound characteristics at appropriate intervals. ___ ___ ___ _____

16. Evaluated patient's ability to ventilate properly at appropriate intervals, determined presence of impaired ventilation and potential pulmonary complications. ___ ___ ___ _____

17. Recorded all pertinent information in the appropriate log. ___ ___ ___ _____

18. Reported any complications to nurse in charge. ___ ___ ___ _____

19. Reported reduced ventilation to health care provider immediately. ___ ___ ___ _____

Student _____ Date _____

Instructor _____ Date _____

PERFORMANCE CHECKLIST SKILL 40-1 **APPLYING MOIST HEAT**

	S	U	NP	Comments

ASSESSMENT

1. Referred to health care provider's order for type of moist heat application, location and duration of application, desired temperature, and agency policies regarding temperature.

2. Assessed skin around area to be treated, performed neurovascular assessments for sensitivity to temperature and pain.

3. Referred to patient's medical record to identify contraindications to moist heat application.

4. Inspected wound for size, color, drainage, tenderness, and odor.

5. Assessed patient's blood pressure and pulse.

6. Assessed patient's mobility.

7. Assessed patient's level of comfort.

8. Assessed patient's and family member's understanding of application and related safety factors.

PLANNING

1. Identified expected outcomes.

2. Assembled and prepared equipment and supplies.

3. Explained steps of procedure and purpose to patient, described sensations patient would feel and precautions to prevent burning.

IMPLEMENTATION

1. Provided privacy.

2. Identified patient using two identifiers, compared with information on patient's ID bracelet.

3. Performed hand hygiene, applied clean gloves.

4. Placed waterproof pad under patient if appropriate.

	S	U	NP	Comments

5. Applied moist sterile compress:

   a. Positioned patient in comfortable, appropriate position; exposed patient properly, draped patient with bath blanket.

   b. Heated solution to desired temperature properly.

   c. Removed any dressing present, disposed of gloves and dressings in biohazard bag.

   d. Inspected condition of wound and surrounding skin.

   e. Performed hand hygiene.

   f. Prepared compress:

     (1) Opened sterile supplies, poured solution into sterile container.

     (2) Used sterile technique to immerse gauze into warmed solution.

     (3) Warmed solution if using portable heating source.

   g. Prepared aquathermia pad or heat pack.

   h. Applied sterile gloves or clean gloves.

   i. Picked up one layer of gauze, wrung out excess solution, applied to wound, avoided surrounding skin.

   j. Lifted edge of gauze to assess for redness.

   k. Packed gauze snugly if patient tolerated compress, covered all wound surfaces with compress.

   l. Covered moist compress with dry sterile dressing and bath towel, pinned or tied in place, removed and disposed of sterile gloves.

   m. Applied aquathermia, heat pack, or waterproof heating pad over towel; kept in place for desired duration.

   n. Changed warm compress using sterile technique as ordered if pad or heat pack was not used.

   o. Applied clean gloves; removed pad, towel, and compress; reassessed wound and condition of skin; replaced dry sterile dressing.

   p. Assisted patient to preferred comfortable position.

   q. Disposed of equipment and soiled compress, performed hand hygiene.

	S	U	NP	Comments

6. Sitz bath or warm soak to intact skin or wound: ___ ___ ___ _____

   a. Removed existing dressing, disposed of gloves and dressing properly, performed hand hygiene. ___ ___ ___ _____

   b. Inspected condition of wound and skin, paid attention to suture line. ___ ___ ___ _____

   c. Applied gloves and cleansed intact skin around open area when exudate was present, disposed of gloves, performed hand hygiene. ___ ___ ___ _____

   d. Filled bath with warmed solution, checked temperature. ___ ___ ___ _____

   e. Assisted patient to bathroom, immersed body part in bath, covered patient with bath blanket or towel as needed. ___ ___ ___ _____

   f. Assessed heart rate, ensured patient was not lightheaded and that call light was within reach. ___ ___ ___ _____

   g. Maintained constant temperature throughout soak. ___ ___ ___ _____

   h. Removed patient from soak, dried body thoroughly. ___ ___ ___ _____

   i. Drained solution from basin or tub, cleaned and placed in proper storage area, disposed of soiled linen and gloves, performed hand hygiene. ___ ___ ___ _____

EVALUATION

1. Inspected condition of body part or wound for evidence of healing. ___ ___ ___ _____

2. Asked patient to describe level of comfort, asked about any sensation of burning following treatment. ___ ___ ___ _____

3. Obtained vital signs, compared with baseline. ___ ___ ___ _____

4. Observed patient demonstrate application therapy and explain purpose. ___ ___ ___ _____

5. Identified unexpected outcomes. ___ ___ ___ _____

RECORDING AND REPORTING

1. Recorded and reported all pertinent information of procedure. ___ ___ ___ _____

2. Recorded preprocedure and postprocedure vital signs. ___ ___ ___ _____

3. Recorded any instructions given and patient's ability to explain and perform platform. ___ ___ ___ _____

Student _____ Date _____

Instructor _____ Date _____

PERFORMANCE CHECKLIST SKILL 10 2 **APPLYING DRY HEAT**

	S	U	NP	Comments
ASSESSMENT				
1. Referred to health care provider's order for location of application and duration of therapy.	___	___	___	_____
2. Assessed condition of skin and underlying tissue area where applying pad for skin integrity, color, temperature, sensitivity to touch, blistering, and excessive dryness.	___	___	___	_____
3. Asked patient to describe level of comfort, assessed ROM if necessary.	___	___	___	_____
4. Checked electrical plugs and cords for fraying or cracking.	___	___	___	_____
5. Determined patient's or family member's knowledge of procedure.	___	___	___	_____
PLANNING				
1. Identified expected outcomes.	___	___	___	_____
2. Prepared equipment and supplies.	___	___	___	_____
3. Explained procedure and precautions.	___	___	___	_____
IMPLEMENTATION				
1. Provided privacy.	___	___	___	_____
2. Identified patient using two identifiers, compared identifiers with patient's ID bracelet.	___	___	___	_____
3. Performed hand hygiene, positioned patient to expose area being treated.	___	___	___	_____
4. Applied aquathermia heating pad; covered area to be treated with bath towel, enclosed pad with pillowcase; secured with tape, tie, or gauze if needed; turned on aquathermia unit, checked temperature setting, applied commercially prepared heat pack properly.	___	___	___	_____
5. Monitored condition of skin over site at appropriate intervals, asked patient about sensation of burning.	___	___	___	_____
6. Removed pad at appropriate time and stored.	___	___	___	_____
7. Assisted patient in returning to preferred position, disposed of soiled linen, performed hand hygiene.	___	___	___	_____

	S	U	NP	Comments

EVALUATION

1. Inspected condition of skin for response to heat exposure, evaluated at appropriate interval.   ___ ___ ___ _____

2. Assessed ROM, asked patient to rate pain.   ___ ___ ___ _____

3. Observed patient or caregiver apply pad to be used in home.   ___ ___ ___ _____

4. Identified unexpected outcomes.   ___ ___ ___ _____

RECORDING AND REPORTING

1. Recorded type of application, temperature, duration of therapy, and patient's response in the appropriate log.   ___ ___ ___ _____

2. Described any instruction given and patient's success in demonstrating procedure.   ___ ___ ___ _____

3. Reported pain level, ROM of body part, skin integrity, color, temperature, sensitivity to touch, blistering, and dryness.   ___ ___ ___ _____

Student _____ Date _____

Instructor _____ Date _____

PERFORMANCE CHECKLIST SKILL 40-3 **APPLYING COLD**

	S	U	NP	Comments

ASSESSMENT

1. Referred to health care provider's order for type, location, and duration of application. ___ ___ ___ _____

2. Inspected condition or affected part, palpated area for edema. ___ ___ ___ _____

3. Considered time in which injury occurred. ___ ___ ___ _____

4. Asked patient to describe severity and character of pain. ___ ___ ___ _____

5. Performed neurovascular check, inspected surrounding skin for integrity, circulation, color, temperature, and sensitivity to touch. ___ ___ ___ _____

6. Assessed patient's understanding and awareness of procedure. ___ ___ ___ _____

PLANNING

1. Identified expected outcomes. ___ ___ ___ _____

2. Prepared equipment and supplies. ___ ___ ___ _____

3. Explained procedure and precautions. ___ ___ ___ _____

IMPLEMENTATION

1. Provided privacy, performed hand hygiene. ___ ___ ___ _____

2. Identified patient using two identifiers, compared with patient's ID bracelet. ___ ___ ___ _____

3. Positioned patient properly, exposed area to be treated, draped patient with blankets. ___ ___ ___ _____

4. Placed towel or pad under area you would treat. ___ ___ ___ _____

5. Applied clean gloves. ___ ___ ___ _____

6. Applied cold compress:

   a. Placed ice water in basin, tested temperature. ___ ___ ___ _____

   b. Submerged gauze into basin, wrung out excess moisture. ___ ___ ___ _____

   c. Applied compress to affected area, molded over site. ___ ___ ___ _____

   d. Removed, remoistened, and reapplied to maintain temperature as needed. ___ ___ ___ _____

	S	U	NP	Comments

7. Applied ice pack or bag:

   a. Filled bag with water, secured cap, inverted bag. ___ ___ ___ _____

   b. Emptied water, filled bag properly with ice chips and water. ___ ___ ___ _____

   c. Expressed excess air from bag, secured bag closure, wiped bag dry. ___ ___ ___ _____

   d. Squeezed or kneaded commercial ice pack. ___ ___ ___ _____

   e. Wrapped pack or bag with towel, applied over injury, secured with tape as needed. ___ ___ ___ _____

8. Applied commercial gel pack:

   a. Removed from freezer. ___ ___ ___ _____

   b. Wrapped in towel, applied over injury. ___ ___ ___ _____

   c. Secured with tape or gauze as needed. ___ ___ ___ _____

9. Applied electrically controlled cooling device:

   a. Ensured all connections were intact and temperature was set. ___ ___ ___ _____

   b. Wrapped cool-water flow pad in towel or pillowcase. ___ ___ ___ _____

   c. Wrapped cool pad around body part. ___ ___ ___ _____

   d. Turned device on and set correct temperature. ___ ___ ___ _____

   e. Secured with elastic wrap bandage, gauze roll, or ties. ___ ___ ___ _____

10. Removed gloves, disposed of properly. ___ ___ ___ _____

11. Check condition of skin at appropriate intervals:

   a. Used extra caution if area was edematous, assessed site more often. ___ ___ ___ _____

   b. Stopped if patient complained of burning sensation or skin began to feel numb. ___ ___ ___ _____

12. Applied clean gloves, removed compress or pad, dried any moisture. ___ ___ ___ _____

13. Assisted patient to comfortable position. ___ ___ ___ _____

14. Removed and disposed of supplies, emptied basin and dried, disposed of soiled linens and gloves, performed hand hygiene. ___ ___ ___ _____

	S	U	NP	Comments

EVALUATION

1. Inspected affected area for integrity, color, temperature, and sensitivity to touch; reevaluated at appropriate interval.

2. Palpated affected area for edema, bruising, and bleeding.

3. Asked patient to report pain level.

4. Observed patient apply cold application and explain risks of treatment.

5. Identified unexpected outcomes.

RECORDING AND REPORTING

1. Recorded procedure and patient's response in the appropriate log.

2. Describe instructions given and patient's success in demonstrating procedure.

3. Reported any sensations of burning, numbness, or unrelieved skin color changes to health care provider.

Student _____ Date _____

Instructor _____ Date _____

PERFORMANCE CHECKLIST SKILL 40-4 **CARING FOR PATIENTS REQUIRING HYPOTHERMIA OR HYPERTHERMIA BLANKETS**

	S	U	NP	Comments
ASSESSMENT				
1. Referred to health care provider's order, checked that patient's current body temperature indicated use of blanket.	___	___	___	_____
2. Assessed vital signs, neurologic status, mental status, and peripheral circulation.	___	___	___	_____
3. Verified that less intensive measures cannot return patient's body temperature to normal.	___	___	___	_____
4. Assessed patient's skin on chest and extremities, paid attention to bony prominences.	___	___	___	_____
PLANNING				
1. Identified expected outcomes.	___	___	___	_____
2. Explained procedure to patient.	___	___	___	_____
3. Positioned patient comfortably.	___	___	___	_____
4. Prepared blanket according to policy and instructions.	___	___	___	_____
IMPLEMENTATION				
1. Performed hand hygiene, applied clean gloves.	___	___	___	_____
2. Identified patient using two identifiers, compared with patient's ID bracelet.	___	___	___	_____
3. Applied lanolin and cold cream to patient's skin where it would touch blanket.	___	___	___	_____
4. Turned on blanket, observed that light was on, set pad temperature as desired.	___	___	___	_____
5. Verified that pad temperature limits were set safely.	___	___	___	_____
6. Covered blanket with thin sheet or bath blanket.	___	___	___	_____
7. Positioned blanket on top of patient properly, wrapped body parts as necessary.	___	___	___	_____
8. Lubricated rectal probe and inserted in patient's rectum.	___	___	___	_____

	S	U	NP	Comments

9. Positioned patient to protect from pressure ulcer development and impaired body alignment, kept linens free of perspiration and condensation.   ____   ____   ____   _____

10. Double-checked fluid thermometer on control panel before leaving.   ____   ____   ____   _____

11. Removed gloves, performed hand hygiene.   ____   ____   ____   _____

EVALUATION

1. Monitored patient's temperature and vital signs at appropriate intervals.   ____   ____   ____   _____

2. Evaluated automatic temperature control properly and at appropriate intervals.   ____   ____   ____   _____

3. Observed skin for burns, changes in color, and other signs of injury.   ____   ____   ____   _____

4. Observed patient for signs of shivering.   ____   ____   ____   _____

5. Determined patient's level of comfort.   ____   ____   ____   _____

6. Identified unexpected outcomes.   ____   ____   ____   _____

RECORDING AND REPORTING

1. Recorded baseline data.   ____   ____   ____   _____

2. Noted type of unit used; control settings; date, time, duration; and patient's tolerance of treatment.   ____   ____   ____   _____

3. Charted on temperature graphic repeated measurements of vital signs.   ____   ____   ____   _____

4. Reported any unexpected outcome to health care provider.   ____   ____   ____   _____

Student _____ Date _____

Instructor _____ Date _____

PERFORMANCE CHECKLIST SKILL 41-1 **HOME ENVIRONMENT ASSESSMENT AND SAFETY**

	S	U	NP	Comments
ASSESSMENT				
1. Reviewed risk factors that predispose patient to accidents in the home.	___	___	___	_____
2. Determined if patient had history of falls or other home injuries, used mnemonic SPLATT.	___	___	___	_____
3. Had patient who had a near fall or an actual fall maintain a fall diary.	___	___	___	_____
4. Conducted a TUG test properly.	___	___	___	_____
5. Determined if patient had fear of falling.	___	___	___	_____
6. Partnered with patient and family caregivers to conduct home safety assessment:				
a. Assessed front and back entrances.	___	___	___	_____
b. Assessed kitchen.	___	___	___	_____
c. Assessed bathroom.	___	___	___	_____
d. Assessed bedroom.	___	___	___	_____
e. Assessed living room/family room.	___	___	___	_____
f. Assessed other general house areas.	___	___	___	_____
g. Assessed general fire safety.	___	___	___	_____
h. Assessed general electric safety.	___	___	___	_____
i. Assessed carbon monoxide prevention.	___	___	___	_____
7. Assessed patient's financial resources, determined monthly income used for expenses.	___	___	___	_____
8. Assessed patient's and family caregiver's willingness to make changes, determined importance of functional independence for patient.	___	___	___	_____
PLANNING				
1. Identified expected outcomes.	___	___	___	_____
2. Prioritized environmental barriers that pose greatest risk.	___	___	___	_____
3. Recommended calling in reliable contractor if repairs were necessary.	___	___	___	_____

	S	U	NP	Comments

IMPLEMENTATION

1. General home safety:

    a. Provided direct light source in places where patient works. ___ ___ ___ _____

    b. Considered nonglossy finishes, had curtains or adjustable shades in other living areas. ___ ___ ___ _____

    c. Color coded controls of appliances. ___ ___ ___ _____

    d. Considered installing lazy Susans, pull-out drawers, or C-rings if necessary. ___ ___ ___ _____

2. Fall prevention steps:

    a. Painted edges of concrete stairs. ___ ___ ___ _____

    b. Installed treads on steps. ___ ___ ___ _____

    c. Rearranged furniture to open space. ___ ___ ___ _____

    d. Reduced clutter in living areas. ___ ___ ___ _____

    e. Secured all carpet, mats, and tiles; placed backing under rugs; removed rugs in dry areas. ___ ___ ___ _____

    f. Padded floor, used specialized tile that absorbs impact. ___ ___ ___ _____

    g. Used low-rise bed or mattress on the ground. ___ ___ ___ _____

    h. Installed extra electrical outlets, secured electrical cords against baseboards. ___ ___ ___ _____

    i. Installed nonskid surface in tub or shower, ensured floor was clean and dry. ___ ___ ___ _____

    j. Had grab bars installed in bathroom, allowed patient to select placement, ensured bar was different color than wall. ___ ___ ___ _____

    k. Had handrails installed along stairways, ensured stairways were well lit with switches at top and bottom of steps. ___ ___ ___ _____

    l. Installed appropriate lighting for outside walkways. ___ ___ ___ _____

    m. Kept a lighted phone accessible. ___ ___ ___ _____

    n. Installed motion sensor exterior lighting for walk/driveways. ___ ___ ___ _____

    o. Had patient use padding or clothing to cushion bony prominences. ___ ___ ___ _____

	S	U	NP	Comments

3. Prevented spread of infection:

   a. Instructed patient in cleaning practices.

   b. Instructed patient not to share utensils.

   c. Instructed patient to clean appliances and surfaces daily.

4. Fire safety:

   a. Had smoke detectors installed near each bedroom, in kitchen, and in basement of home; ensured detector was on each floor of home.

   b. Had patient select fire extinguisher that was easy to handle, asked patient to demonstrate proper use.

   c. Had area around furnace cleared of flammable items.

   d. Instructed patient to ensure space heater had an emergency shut off and that housing and electrical cords were intact.

   e. Had patient make appointments for furnace and chimney maintenance at appropriate times.

   f. Had patient check light bulb wattage in all fixtures.

   g. Had patient establish cooking routine that keeps him or her in the kitchen, ensure range was clean.

   h. Reviewed need to keep ashtrays clean and empty if necessary.

   i. Discouraged smoking in bed or chair or after taking medication that diminished alertness.

   j. Recommended patient install power strips for multiple devices.

5. Burn safety:

   a. Adjusted setting on hot water heater appropriately.

   b. Instructed patient to always turn cold water on first.

   c. Installed touch pads on lamps.

   d. Used color codes on faucets.

	S	U	NP	Comments

6. Carbon monoxide safety:

   a. Had condition of furnace venting checked annually.

   b. Cautioned patients against using gas stove of barbecue grill for heating inside.

   c. Had battery-operated carbon monoxide detector installed in home, checked batteries at appropriate times.

7. Firearm safety:

   a. Taught patient about dangers of guns in the home.

   b. Taught patient to install trigger locks, store guns in a locked cabinet, store ammunition separately, and store keys in a place inaccessible to children.

EVALUATION

1. Had patient and family member(s) identify safety risks revealed in home assessment.

2. Asked patient to discuss modification plans during follow-up, observed what changes had been implemented.

3. Asked if patient had experienced falls or other injuries in the home.

4. Reassessed for progression of dementia.

5. Identified unexpected outcomes.

RECORDING AND REPORTING

1. Retained copy of home safety assessment in patient's home care record.

2. Recorded any instruction provided, patient response, and changes made within environment in progress notes.

Student _____ Date _____

Instructor _____ Date _____

PERFORMANCE CHECKLIST SKILL 41-2 **ADAPTING THE HOME SETTING FOR PATIENTS WITH COGNITIVE DEFICITS**

	S	U	NP	Comments
ASSESSMENT				
1. Assessed patient over a short period of time, was sensitive to patient's sensory needs or disability.	___	___	___	_____
2. Ensured room was well lit with minimal noise or interruption, spoke clearly and in a normal tone.	___	___	___	_____
3. Asked patient to describe own level of health and ability to perform self-care skills.	___	___	___	_____
4. Asked how patient was doing with home management responsibilities.	___	___	___	_____
5. Assessed patient's medications and where patient stored them, had patient or caregiver keep list of medications, asked to see list.	___	___	___	_____
6. Determined if patient had family caregiver who assisted with self care or home management, assessed relationship and support given.	___	___	___	_____
7. Observed patient's dress, nonverbal expressions, appearance, and cleanliness.	___	___	___	_____
8. Observed immediate home environment.	___	___	___	_____
9. Completed Folstein's examination or SGDS if cognitive or mental status change was suspected.	___	___	___	_____
10. Observed for potentially hazardous behaviors if patient was suspected to be at risk for wandering.	___	___	___	_____
11. Assessed which current environmental strategies caregivers were using to deal with wandering.	___	___	___	_____
12. Assessed caregiver for signs of stress.	___	___	___	_____
PLANNING				
1. Identified expected outcomes.	___	___	___	_____
2. Referred family to occupational therapy, homemaker services, or respite care if patient had difficulty with self-care or fine-motor skills.	___	___	___	_____

	S	U	NP	Comments

3. Offered assistive devices to make bathing, dressing, writing, and feeding easier.
— — — _____

4. Considered patient's level of cognitive impairment when making changes to patient's living environment.
— — — _____

5. Determined best time of day for approaches that result in desired response.
— — — _____

IMPLEMENTATION

1. Helped create a list or post reminder notes if patient had difficulty remembering when to perform tasks, provided organized medication, recommended a wristwatch with an alarm.
— — — _____

2. Reduced steps it takes to complete tasks such as paying bills or bringing in groceries.
— — — _____

3. Helped patient and caregiver determine routine schedule for ADLs, posted a large calendar conspicuously.
— — — _____

4. Instructed caregiver to focus on patient's abilities rather than disabilities in modifying approaches.
— — — _____

5. Had caregiver assist in setting up activities so patient could complete tasks.
— — — _____

6. Discussed with patient, caregiver, and health care provider options for scheduling multiple medications.
— — — _____

7. Instructed caregiver in how to use simple and direct communication.
— — — _____

8. Placed clocks, calendars, and personal mementos throughout the home; enhanced the environment as necessary.
— — — _____

9. Had caregiver routinely orient patient to caregiver and activities.
— — — _____

10. Ensured patient had regular naps or rest.
— — — _____

11. Had caregiver support visits by family and friends, instructed caregiver in how to promote social interaction.
— — — _____

12. Provided safe place for a person to wander.
— — — _____

13. Used labels to cue and remind person.
— — — _____

14. Recommended family install door locks or guards.
— — — _____

15. Created calm, safe setting for patient's abilities.
— — — _____

16. Monitored patient for personal comfort.
— — — _____

	S	U	NP	Comments

17. Installed motion detector near an exit site with portable alarm that can accompany the caregiver. ___ ___ ___ _____

18. Considered need for full-time care assistance. ___ ___ ___ _____

EVALUATION

1. Asked patient to review activities completed during follow-up visits. ___ ___ ___ _____

2. Reviewed revised schedule for medication administration with patient and caregiver. ___ ___ ___ _____

3. Had caregiver keep track of doses patient took over a 1-week period. ___ ___ ___ _____

4. Asked caregiver to describe ways that would increase patient's success in completing tasks. ___ ___ ___ _____

5. Had caregiver show schedules of daily routines and review approaches used, observed environment for presence of reality-oriented cues. ___ ___ ___ _____

6. Had family caregivers describe options for minimizing wandering. ___ ___ ___ _____

7. Had family caregivers report number of occurrences of wandering. ___ ___ ___ _____

8. Identified unexpected outcomes. ___ ___ ___ _____

RECORDING AND REPORTING

1. Recorded assessment of patient's cognitive and mental status, recommended interventions, and patient's and caregiver's response in the appropriate log. ___ ___ ___ _____

2. Reported any change in patient's behavior that reflects a decline in cognitive or mental status to health care provider. ___ ___ ___ _____

Student _____ Date _____

Instructor _____ Date _____

PERFORMANCE CHECKLIST SKILL 41-3 **MEDICATION AND MEDICAL DEVICE SAFETY**

	S	U	NP	Comments
ASSESSMENT				
1. Assessed patient's sensory, musculoskeletal, and neurologic function.	___	___	___	_____
2. Assessed family caregiver assistance.	___	___	___	_____
3. Assessed patient's medication regimen and length of time patient had been receiving each drug,	___	___	___	_____
4. Asked patient to show you where medications were stored, looked at each container.	___	___	___	_____
5. Assessed temperature of storage area.	___	___	___	_____
6. Had patient describe daily schedule for drug administration and whether there were any problems.	___	___	___	_____
7. Asked to see where patient stored injection supplies and disposed of needles if necessary.	___	___	___	_____
8. Asked to see where glucose monitor, lancets, and strips were stored and how lancets were disposed of if necessary.	___	___	___	_____
PLANNING				
1. Identified expected outcomes.	___	___	___	_____
IMPLEMENTATION				
1. Educated patient and caregiver in principles to ensure medications were safe to use:				
a. Ensure medication was taken by patient for whom it was prescribed.	___	___	___	_____
b. Did not take medication older than a year old or past expiration.	___	___	___	_____
c. Did not place different medications in the same containers.	___	___	___	_____
d. Did not place medications in containers other than their original ones.	___	___	___	_____
e. Finished prescribed medication.	___	___	___	_____
f. Washed hands before and after administering medication.	___	___	___	_____

	S	U	NP	Comments
2. Recommended approaches for preparation of medications if necessary.	___	___	___	_____
a. Placed medications in screw-top container.	___	___	___	_____
b. Had pharmacy-type larger labels on medication containers.	___	___	___	_____
c. Had Braille labels placed on medication containers, if necessary.	___	___	___	_____
d. Introduced a color-coding system.	___	___		_____
e. Provided syringes with large numerals or a syringe magnifier.	___	___		_____
f. Offered spring-loaded needle insertion aid.	___	___	___	_____
g. Instructed caregivers in how to draw medication into syringe.	___	___	___	_____
3. Recommended approaches for medication and supply storage:				
a. Stored medications in a safe place.	___	___		_____
b. Kept liquid medications and parenteral drugs in a cool place.	___	___		_____
c. Kept medical supplies in airtight containers and in a cool place.	___	___	___	_____
d. Instructed patient and caregiver to use new needle with each medication administration.	___	___	___	_____
4. Reviewed proper techniques for disposal of medications, "sharps," and other supplies:				
a. Discarded unused or outdated drugs in a bag containing coffee grounds or kitty litter.	___	___	___	_____
b. Obtained sharps container.	___	___	___	_____
c. Cautioned against overfilling sharps container.	___	___	___	_____
d. Stored container in an area inaccessible to children.	___	___	___	_____
e. Disposed of soiled supplies in a separate, sealed, plastic bag; placed in second bag; discarded appropriately.	___	___	___	_____
f. Consulted local public health department or community regarding proper waste disposal.	___	___	___	_____

	S	U	NP	Comments

EVALUATION

1. Had patient/caregiver describe steps to ensuring safe medication. ___ ___ ___ _____

2. Observed patient/caregiver prepared and administered medication. ___ ___ ___ _____

3. Observed home setting for location of medication and supplies. ___ ___ ___ _____

4. Had patient describe how sharps and equipment were discarded. ___ ___ ___ _____

5. Did pill counts at appropriate intervals. ___ ___ ___ _____

6. Identified unexpected outcomes. ___ ___ ___ _____

RECORDING AND REPORTING

1. Recorded instructions and recommendation in the appropriate log, notified health care provider of unsafe situations. ___ ___ ___ _____

Student _____ Date _____

Instructor _____ Date _____

PERFORMANCE CHECKLIST SKILL 42-1 **TEACHING CLIENTS TO MEASURE BODY TEMPERATURE**

	S	U	NP	Comments
ASSESSMENT				
1. Assessed client's/caregiver's ability to manipulate and read thermometer, had client put on glasses if necessary.	___	___	___	_____
2. Assessed client's knowledge of normal temperature ranges, symptoms of fever and hypothermia, and client's risk for body temperature alterations.	___	___	___	_____
3. Assessed client's ability to determine appropriate type of thermometer to use.	___	___	___	_____
4. Assessed client's/caregiver's previous knowledge and experience in measuring temperature and maintaining thermometer, had client or caregiver perform demonstration if necessary.	___	___	___	_____
PLANNING				
1. Identified expected outcomes.	___	___	___	_____
2. Selected setting in home where client was most likely to measure temperature.	___	___	___	_____
3. Discussed and demonstrated normal temperature ranges, instructed caregiver to remain with patient if necessary.	___	___	___	_____
IMPLEMENTATION				
1. Demonstrated steps of thermometer preparation, insertion, and reading; provided rationale for steps.				
a. Performed hand hygiene, instructed caregiver to wear gloves and use thermometers appropriately.	___	___	___	_____
b. Had client/caregiver perform each step with guidance, did not rush him or her.	___	___	___	_____
c. Instructed client/caregiver in proper method for storing thermometer, selected a suitable storage location.	___	___	___	_____
2. Discussed common symptoms of fever.	___	___	___	_____

	S	U	NP	Comments

3. Discussed common signs and symptoms of hypothermia; explained risk factors; instructed clients to dress warmly in layers, avoid extreme cold, and ingest warm liquids.

4. Discussed importance of notifying health care provider when temperature elevations occur, reviewed common therapies for temperature reduction that are safe to perform at home.

5. Provided written guidelines for client's reference at appropriate level of health literacy.

6. Gave client/caregiver logbook to record temperature and time, instructed client to use record to report temperature to health care provider.

EVALUATION

1. Had client/caregiver demonstrate technique for temperature measurement.

2. Asked client/caregiver to identify normal temperature range and influences on readings, discussed safety implications.

3. Had client/caregiver describe common signs of fever and hypothermia and method for control.

4. Watched client/caregiver clean and store equipment.

5. Watched client/caregiver record values and times, reviewed logbook periodically to ensure correctness.

6. Identified unexpected outcomes.

RECORDING AND REPORTING

1. Recorded information taught and client's demonstration in home care record.

2. Recorded temperature in appropriate logs.

3. Reported high and low temperatures to health care provider.

PERFORMANCE CHECKLIST SKILL 42-2 **TEACHING BLOOD PRESSURE AND PULSE MEASUREMENT**

	S	U	NP	Comments
ASSESSMENT				
1. Assessed client's/caregiver's visual and auditory acuity and ability to use BP monitoring equipment, and feel pulse.	___	___	___	_____
2. Assessed client's/caregiver's knowledge of normal BP, pulse ranges, and symptoms and causes of high or low readings.	___	___	___	_____
3. Assessed client's/caregiver's knowledge of BP and pulse measure, medical issues that affect them, why awareness was important to client health.	___	___	___	_____
4. Assessed client's/caregiver's previous knowledge and experience in measuring blood pressure, had client or caregiver perform demonstration if appropriate.	___	___	___	_____
5. Assessed home environment for favorable place to measure BP and pulse.	___	___	___	_____
PLANNING				
1. Identified expected outcomes.	___	___	___	_____
2. Encouraged client or caregiver to perform measurements on routine schedule for long-term monitoring plan.	___	___	___	_____
3. Encouraged client to avoid exercise, caffeine, and smoking for 30 minutes before assessment.	___	___	___	_____
4. Had client or caregiver perform measurement in comfortable position and in warm, quiet environment.	___	___	___	_____
IMPLEMENTATION				
1. Blood pressure measurement:				
a. Discussed best sites for assessing BP, explained when not to apply cuff.	___	___	___	_____
b. Demonstrated steps for measuring BP:				
(1) Use of sphygmomanometer and stethoscope:	___	___	___	_____

	S	U	NP	Comments

(a) Taught palpation of artery, positioning and wrapping of cuff, placement of stethoscope, inflation and release of cuff, and listening for Korotkoff sounds. ___ ___ ___ _____

(b) Described sounds of measurement and relationship to observation of gauge during reading, cautioned client about level and time appropriate for cuff inflation. ___ ___ ___ _____

(c) Taught client or caregiver to routinely clean stethoscope properly. ___ ___ ___ _____

(2) Use of electronic BP monitor:

(a) Taught correct placement of cuff, use of equipment for proper cuff location, and procedure for changing batteries. ___ ___ ___ _____

2. Pulse measurement:

a. Discussed with client/caregiver best sites for assessing pulse. ___ ___ ___ _____

b. Demonstrated steps for palpating pulse properly. ___ ___ ___ _____

(1) Instructed in use of gentle pressure. ___ ___ ___ _____

(2) Instructed in use of clock with second hand. ___ ___ ___ _____

(3) Instructed to count for full 60 seconds, started with second hand at 12:00 position. ___ ___ ___ _____

3. Educated client about desired BP and pulse ranges, purposes for monitoring, and when to take measurements. ___ ___ ___ _____

4. Had client/caregiver attempt each skill on you or family member. ___ ___ ___ _____

5. Observed client demonstrate techniques on self, did not allow multiple repetitive BP attempts on any one limb. ___ ___ ___ _____

6. Taught client to monitor BP and pulse even if they remain in normal range. ___ ___ ___ _____

7. Provided client with printed instructions with guide or video demonstration of procedure if possible. ___ ___ ___ _____

	S	U	NP	Comments

8. Gave client log to record BP and pulse and time taken, instructed client to record whether medications that affect BP or pulse were taken, instructed client to use written record to report readings to health care provider.

9. Instructed client in proper care of equipment.

EVALUATION

1. Observed client or caregiver demonstrate technique for BP/pulse measurement on three different occasions, verified client adds information to log correctly.

2. Asked client if readings were within range and when to report abnormal readings to health care provider.

3. Asked client to describe reason for BP or pulse monitoring and any related medications or treatment.

4. Had client or caregiver demonstrate proper care of equipment.

5. Identified unexpected outcomes.

RECORDING AND REPORTING

1. Recorded teaching, client responses, and demonstration in the appropriate log.

2. Recorded BP and pulse in home care record and logbook.

3. Reported changes in readings of BP/pulse.

Student _____ Date _____

Instructor _____ Date _____

PERFORMANCE CHECKLIST SKILL 42-3 **TEACHING INTERMITTENT SELF-CATHETERIZATION**

	S	U	NP	Comments
ASSESSMENT				
1. Reviewed client's medical record; gathered information about voiding history, medical and surgical history, client's fluid intake, postvoid residual amount, and daily voiding routine.	___	___	___	_____
2. Assessed client's ability to perform CISC.	___	___	___	_____
3. Assessed client's/caregiver's knowledge about CISC, observed performance of CISC.	___	___	___	_____
PLANNING				
1. Identified expected outcomes.	___	___	___	_____
2. Selected setting that client/caregiver would most likely use when performing CISC	___	___	___	_____
3. Helped client/caregiver select proper catheter.	___	___	___	_____
IMPLEMENTATION				
1. Taught client/caregiver how to perform appropriate hand hygiene using soap and water.	___	___	___	_____
2. Helped client get comfortable in a place with adequate lighting.	___	___	___	_____
3. Taught client how to properly clean urethral meatus.	___	___	___	_____
4. Taught female client how to insert catheter:				
a. Helped client locate meatus.	___	___	___	_____
b. Lubricated tip of catheter with water-soluble jelly, rotated tip.	___	___	___	_____
c. Placed outflow end of catheter in urine collection container or toilet, inserted catheter tip into meatus until urine began to flow.	___	___	___	_____
5. Taught male client how to insert catheter:				
a. Lubricated tip of catheter with water-soluble jelly, rotated tip.	___	___	___	_____
b. Placed outflow end of catheter into urine collection container or toilet bowl, inserted catheter into meatus until urine began to flow.	___	___	___	_____

	S	U	NP	Comments
6. Instructed client to hold catheter in place while urine flowed.	___	___	___	_____
7. Taught client to remove catheter when urine flow stopped, performed hand hygiene.	___	___	___	_____
8. Gave client logbook to record amount of urine if needed.	___	___	___	_____
9. Instructed client to clean catheter with soap and water immediately; rinsed catheter, and allowed it to air dry, and stored it in dry towel or paper bag.	___	___	___	_____
10. Taught client to replace catheter at appropriate time.	___	___	___	_____

EVALUATION

	S	U	NP	Comments
1. Observed client/caregiver independently demonstrate technique for CISC.	___	___	___	_____
2. Asked client to identify plan for timing of CISC and steps to take when problems arise.	___	___	___	_____
3. Reviewed client's logbook, observed as client entered information.	___	___	___	_____
4. Identified unexpected outcomes.	___	___	___	_____

RECORDING AND REPORTING

	S	U	NP	Comments
1. Recorded the information taught, client's response, and demonstration in home care record.	___	___	___	_____
2. Recorded urine output in home care record and logbook.	___	___	___	_____
3. Reported signs and symptoms of UTIs and difficulty performing CISC.	___	U	NP	_____

Student _____ Date _____

Instructor _____ Date _____

PERFORMANCE CHECKLIST SKILL 42-4 **USING HOME OXYGEN EQUIPMENT**

	S	U	NP	Comments
ASSESSMENT				
1. Determined client's or caregiver's ability to use oxygen equipment correctly, assessed for appropriate use of equipment in home setting.	___	___	___	_____
2. Assessed home environment for adequate electrical service if oxygen concentrator was used.	___	___	___	_____
3. Assessed client's/caregiver's knowledge of purpose of oxygen and ability to observe for signs of hypoxia.	___	___	___	_____
4. Determined appropriate resource in community for equipment and assistance.	___	___	___	_____
5. Determined appropriate backup system in event of power failure, had space oxygen tank available.	___	___	___	_____
PLANNING				
1. Identified expected outcomes.	___	___	___	_____
2. Selected setting in home where client is most likely to use oxygen equipment.	___	___	___	_____
IMPLEMENTATION	___	___	___	_____
1. Instructed client/caregiver how to perform hand hygiene.	___	___	___	_____
2. Placed oxygen delivery system in appropriate environment.	___	___	___	_____
3. Demonstrated steps for preparation and maintenance of oxygen therapy:				
a. Compressed oxygen system:				
(1) Turned cylinder valve properly with wrench.	___	___	___	_____
(2) Checked pressure gauge on cylinder.	___	___	___	_____
(3) Stored wrench with oxygen tank.	___	___	___	_____
b. Oxygen concentrator system:				
(1) Plugged concentrator into appropriate outlet.	___	___	___	_____
(2) Turned on power switch.	___	___	___	_____

	S	U	NP	Comments

c. Liquid oxygen system:

   (1) Checked liquid system by reading dial on reservoir or tank.

   (2) Collaborated with DME provider to provide instruction in refilling ambulatory tank.

   (3) Taught to refill liquid oxygen tank:

     (a) Wiped both filling connectors clean.

     (b) Turned off flow selector of ambulatory unit.

     (c) Attached ambulatory unit to stationary reservoir properly.

     (d) Opened fill valve on ambulatory tank, applied pressure to top of stationary reservoir, stayed with unit while it filled.

     (e) Disconnected ambulatory unit from stationary reservoir when hissing changed and vapor cloud began to form.

     (f) Wiped both filling connectors clean.

4. Connected oxygen delivery device to oxygen delivery system.

5. Adjusted oxygen flow rate.

6. Had client/caregiver apply oxygen delivery device correctly, ensured client had two sets of delivery devices and tubing.

7. Instructed client not to change oxygen flow rate.

8. Had client/caregiver perform each step, provided written material for reinforcement or review.

9. Instructed client/caregiver to notify health care provider if signs of hypoxia or respiratory tract infection occurred.

10. Discussed emergency plans, had caregiver/client call 911 and notify health care provider and home care agency.

11. Instructed client in safe home oxygen practices.

	S	U	NP	Comments

EVALUATION

1. Monitored rate at which oxygen was delivered. ___ ___ ___ _____

2. Asked client/caregiver about ease or problems associated with home oxygen. ___ ___ ___ _____

3. Asked client/caregiver to state safety guidelines, emergency precautions, and emergency plan. ___ ___ ___ _____

4. Identified unexpected outcomes. ___ ___ ___ _____

RECORDING AND REPORTING

1. Recorded teaching plan and information provided in home care record. ___ ___ ___ _____

2. Communicated client's/caregiver's learning progress to other health care providers. ___ ___ ___ _____

3. Recorded oxygen delivery system, related supplies, and prescribed oxygen flow rate in home care record. ___ ___ ___ _____

4. Reported respiratory complications/concerns to health care provider. ___ ___ ___ _____

PERFORMANCE CHECKLIST SKILL 42-5   **TEACHING HOME TRACHEOSTOMY CARE AND SUCTIONING**

	S	U	NP	Comments
ASSESSMENT				
1. Assessed client's/caregiver's ability to perform tracheostomy care and suctioning properly.	___	___	___	_____
2. Assessed client's/caregiver's knowledge of need to perform tracheostomy care and suctioning.	___	___	___	_____
3. Observed client/caregiver performing complete tracheostomy tube care and suctioning.	___	___	___	_____
PLANNING				
1. Identified expected outcomes.	___	___	___	_____
2. Selected setting in home that was most likely to be used when completing tube care.	___	___	___	_____
3. Discussed and demonstrated proper position for procedure.	___	___	___	_____
IMPLEMENTATION				
1. For suctioning:				
a. Verified health care provider's orders for suctioning.	___	___	___	_____
b. Instructed client/caregiver on techniques for hand hygiene and application of clean gloves.	___	___	___	_____
c. Taught and demonstrated preparation and completion of tube suctioning, stressed technique for intermittent suction.	___	___	___	_____
d. Taught client/caregiver to suction nasal and oral pharynx and perform mouth care, encouraged client/caregiver to brush teeth and use mouth and lip moisturizer at appropriate intervals.	___	___	___	_____
e. Had client take deep breaths at end of procedure to reassess lungs.	___	___	___	_____
f. Disconnected suction catheter, discarded catheter appropriately or set aside to be disinfected, removed and disposed of gloves properly, performed hand hygiene.	___	___	___	_____

	S	U	NP	Comments

2. Tracheostomy care:

   a. Taught skills of tracheostomy care. ___ ___ ___ _____

   b. Instructed client/caregiver to apply clean gloves; demonstrated technique for cleaning reusable supplies properly, rinsed and dried supplies, stored supplies in plastic bag, labeled bag. ___ ___ ___ _____

   c. Had client/caregiver remove and discard gloves, performed hand hygiene. ___ ___ ___ _____

   d. Explained the procedure for disinfecting reusable supplies at appropriate intervals and using appropriate method. ___ ___ ___ _____

3. Had client/caregiver perform each step with guidance. ___ ___ ___ _____

4. Taught client/caregiver signs of stoma infection, respiratory tract infection, and transesophageal fistula. ___ ___ ___ _____

EVALUATION

1. Asked client to state signs of stoma or respiratory tract complications. ___ ___ ___ _____

2. Observed client/caregiver demonstrating technique for tracheostomy tube care and suctioning. ___ ___ ___ _____

3. Identified unexpected outcomes. ___ ___ ___ _____

RECORDING AND REPORTING

1. Recorded client instruction and accuracy of care delivered by client/caregiver. ___ ___ ___ _____

2. Developed system of recording home care for client/caregiver. ___ ___ ___ _____

Student _____ Date _____

Instructor _____ Date _____

PERFORMANCE CHECKLIST PROCEDURAL GUIDELINE 42-1 **CHANGING A TRACHEOSTOMY TUBE AT HOME**

	S	U	NP	Comments
PROCEDURAL STEPS				
1. Did not allow client to have anything by mouth or hold tube feedings for at least 1 hour before procedure.	___	___	___	_____
2. Explained procedure to client before tracheostomy was changed, had caregiver assist.	___	___	___	_____
3. Performed hand hygiene, applied clean gloves.	___	___	___	_____
4. Removed new tube from container, removed inner cannula, inserted obturator into outer cannula, attached clean ties to neck plate, checked integrity of cuff.	___	___	___	_____
5. Suctioned existing tracheostomy tube, had bag valve mask and face mask available.	___	___	___	_____
6. Had caregiver stabilize tracheostomy faceplate, loosened ties, deflated tracheostomy tube cuff.	___	___	___	_____
7. Had caregiver pull old tube out in same direction inner cannula would be removed, removed gloves, performed hand hygiene.	___	___	___	_____
8. Applied sterile gloves, pushed new tracheostomy properly through stoma, removed obturator, allowed air to flow, inserted inner cannula, locked in place.	___	___	___	_____
9. Secured new tracheostomy ties, inflated cuff, placed dressing around stoma if necessary.	___	___	___	_____

Student _____ Date _____

Instructor _____ Date _____

PERFORMANCE CHECKLIST SKILL 42-6   **TEACHING MEDICATION SELF-ADMINISTRATION**

	S	U	NP	Comments

ASSESSMENT

1. Assessed client's cognitive, sensory, and motor function.

2. Assessed resources client had in order to obtain medications.

3. Assessed client's learning readiness and ability to concentrate.

4. Assessed client's and caregiver's knowledge regarding medication therapy.

5. Assessed client's belief in need for medication therapy.

6. Assessed client's prescribed and OTC medications, included herbal supplements.

7. Assessed client's understanding of effects and interactions between prescribed medications and foods, OTC drugs, and herbal supplements.

8. Ensured caregiver knew client's drug allergies.

PLANNING

1. Identified expected outcomes.

2. Prepared environment for teaching session properly.

3. Prepared proper teaching materials.

4. Ensured client was wearing glasses or hearing aids if needed.

5. Consulted with health care provider to review medications and simplify regimen if possible.

6. Arranged teaching time to allow participation of family members.

	S	U	NP	Comments

IMPLEMENTATION

1. Instructed client/caregiver in importance of performing hand hygiene before medication administration. ___ ___ ___ _____

2. Presented information clearly and concisely. ___ ___ ___ _____

3. Provided frequent pauses so client/caregiver could ask questions and express understanding. ___ ___ ___ _____

4. Instructed client/caregiver on purpose of medications and desired effects, how medication works, schedules and rationale, side effects and relief from them, what to do if dose is missed, when to call health care provider, medication safety guidelines, and implications of not taking medication. ___ ___ ___ _____

5. Instructed client in appropriate route of medication delivery. ___ ___ ___ _____

6. Provided teaching sessions, planned several sessions if necessary, left instruction aids in home if possible. ___ ___ ___ _____

7. Provided teaching about OTC medications and herbal supplements. ___ ___ ___ _____

8. Provided client with charts, diagrams, learning aids, written information, and Internet resources. ___ ___ ___ _____

9. Offered assistance as client practiced preparing medication. ___ ___ ___ _____

10. Had pharmacy provide clear, large-print labels and teaching handouts if appropriate. ___ ___ ___ _____

11. Had pharmacy provide containers client can open independently. ___ ___ ___ _____

12. Facilitated arrangements for pharmacy to receive written prescriptions in a timely fashion, arranged for pharmacy to deliver medications to the home if necessary. ___ ___ ___ _____

EVALUATION

1. Asked client/caregiver to explain information about each drug. ___ ___ ___ _____

2. Identified client's problem-solving abilities. ___ ___ ___ _____

3. Had client/caregiver prepare doses for all prescribed medication. ___ ___ ___ _____

4. Asked client to verbalize any remaining questions regarding medication management. ___ ___ ___ _____

5. Identified unexpected outcomes. ___ ___ ___ _____

558

	S	U	NP	Comments

RECORDING AND REPORTING

1. Documented instruction provided and learning outcomes achieved by client in home record.

2. Developed client/caregiver recording mechanism of dosage schedules and self-monitoring of regimen.

3. Left phone number and directions about how to reach home care nurse if needed.

Student _____   Date _____

Instructor _____   Date _____

PERFORMANCE CHECKLIST SKILL 42-7   **MANAGING FEEDING TUBES IN THE HOME**

	S	U	NP	Comments
ASSESSMENT				
1. Assessed client's health status.	___	___	___	_____
2. Assessed client's/caregiver's physical, emotional, financial, and community resources.	___	___	___	_____
3. Assessed environmental conditions of home.	___	___	___	_____
4. Assessed client's/caregiver's understanding of purpose of enteral feedings and positive expected outcomes.	___	___	___	_____
5. Assessed client's/caregiver's understanding of storage and management of equipment and supplies as well as where and how to obtain supplies.	___	___	___	_____
6. Assessed client's/caregiver's ability to manipulate feeding equipment.	___	___	___	_____
PLANNING				
1. Identified expected outcomes.	___	___	___	_____
IMPLEMENTATION				
1. Had client/caregiver perform hand hygiene.	___	___	___	_____
2. Discussed purpose of enteral feeding and enhanced nutritional health.	___	___	___	_____
3. Assisted client/caregiver in determining feeding schedule that will maintain nutritional requirements and fit within client's or family's schedule.	___	___	___	_____
4. Had client/caregiver apply clean gloves, demonstrated how to identify placement of feeding tube.	___	___	___	_____
5. Observed client/caregiver in determining placement of nasally placed tube.	___	___	___	_____
6. Observed client/caregiver check for gastric residual volume, instructed to return aspirated contents to stomach if appropriate.	___	___	___	_____
7. Discussed use of medical asepsis in setting up and changing administration sets, mixing and refrigerating formula, limiting formula "hung," and maintaining and caring for bag.	___	___	___	_____

	S	U	NP	Comments
8. Instructed client/caregiver in how to position client properly for feeding or medications.	___	___	___	_____
9. Observed client/caregiver mixing, administering, and storing formulas; discussed flushing of tube.	___	___	___	_____
10. Observed client/caregiver administering medications and flushing tube.	___	___	___	_____
11. Discussed and observed use of infusion pump if necessary.	___	___	___	_____
12. Discussed measures to stabilize feeding tube in clients.	___	___	___	_____
13. Provided contact information for ordering equipment and supplies or whom to call in case of equipment failure.	___	___	___	_____
14. Discussed emergency plan and actions to take for signs and symptoms of aspiration.	___	___	___	_____
15. Discussed whom to contact and when for signs of diarrhea, constipation, or weight loss.	___	___	___	_____

EVALUATION

	S	U	NP	Comments
1. Asked client or caregiver to state purpose of home enteral nutrition therapy.	___	___	___	_____
2. Observed client/caregiver performing medical asepsis techniques, checking tube placement, aspirating residuals, administering medications, and using equipment.	___	___	___	_____
3. Asked client/caregiver to state measures used to prevent complications.	___	___	___	_____
4. Asked client/caregiver how to care for open formula cans.	___	___	___	_____
5. Asked client/caregiver about management of complications.	___	___	___	_____
6. Identified unexpected outcomes.	___	___	___	_____

RECORDING AND REPORTING

	S	U	NP	Comments
1. Recorded instructions given to client/caregiver and response in home care record.	___	___	___	_____
2. Recorded specifics of enteral feeding plan.	___	___	___	_____
3. Instructed client/caregiver in documentation needed.	___	___	___	_____

Student _____ Date _____

Instructor _____ Date _____

PERFORMANCE CHECKLIST SKILL 42-8 **MANAGING PARENTERAL NUTRITION IN THE HOME**

	S	U	NP	Comments
ASSESSMENT				
1. Assessed client's nutritional status and risk for malnutrition, identified signs of malnutrition, included measurement of vital signs.	___	___	___	_____
2. Assessed client's fluid and electrolyte levels, serum albumin, total protein, transferrin, prealbumin, triglycerides, and glucose levels.	___	___	___	_____
3. Assessed client's venous access device for edema, drainage, tenderness, and signs of inflammation; measured circumference and marked arm if necessary.	___	___	___	_____
4. Verified health care provider's orders for nutrients, vitamins, minerals, trace elements, electrolytes, and flow rate.	___	___	___	_____
5. Assessed client's/caregiver's anxiety level and readiness to learn.	___	___	___	_____
6. Assessed client's/caregiver's previous knowledge and experience in managing PN in the home, had client/caregiver perform return demonstration if able.	___	___	___	_____
PLANNING				
1. Identified expected outcomes.	___	___	___	_____
2. Selected setting in home where client was most likely to administer PN.	___	___	___	_____
IMPLEMENTATION				
1. Provided name and phone number of resources available if problems arise.	___	___	___	_____
2. Explained type of infusion, dosage, expected outcomes, and components of PN; explained that PN needs to be stored in refrigerator.	___	___	___	_____
3. Had client/caregiver perform each step with guidance, did not rush client.	___	___	___	_____
4. Instructed client/caregiver to inspect label of bag, ensured bag was not expired or leaking.	___	___	___	_____
5. Suggested taking PN solution out of refrigerator 30 to 60 minutes before scheduled infusion time.	___	___	___	_____

	S	U	NP	Comments
6. Explained need to inspect fluid in bag for color and precipitates.	___	___	___	_____
7. Performed hand hygiene, applied gloves; demonstrated how to attach IV tubing and filter, how to prime tubing, and how to load tubing into electronic infusion pump.	___	___	___	_____
8. Wiped CVC port with alcohol, showed how to flush CVC and connect tubing to port, used needleless system whenever possible.	___	___	___	_____
9. Explained how to determine appropriate rate of infusion and program infusion pump.	___	___	___	_____
10. Removed and disposed of gloves, performed hand hygiene.	___	___	___	_____
11. Explained how to disconnect tubing and flush CVC, ensured client/caregiver performed hand hygiene.	___	___	___	_____
12. Described appropriate use and storage of infusion pump and supplies, explained tubing replacement schedules.	___	___	___	_____
13. Assisted in developing plan for appropriate disposal of supplies.	___	___	___	_____
14. Demonstrated appropriate care of CVC site, discussed dressing changes and signs of infection.	___	___	___	_____
15. Taught client/caregiver about signs and symptoms indicating complications from PN therapy and when to call for help.	___	___	___	_____
16. Demonstrated use of self-blood glucose monitor, explained frequency of testing, normal glucose values, and what to do if values fell outside expected range.	___	___	___	_____
17. Provided client with logbook to record administration of PN, weights, I&O, and blood glucose levels.	___	___	___	_____
18. Helped client develop a plan to reorder supplies, an emergency plan, and a home safety plan.	___	___	___	_____

EVALUATION

	S	U	NP	Comments
1. Had client/caregiver independently demonstrate initiation, infusion, and discontinuation of PN infusion as well as CVC site care.	___	___	___	_____
2. Watched client clean and store PN, equipment, and supplies.	___	___	___	_____

	S	U	NP	Comments
3. Asked client/caregiver to identify expected outcomes.	___	___	___	_____
4. Had client/caregiver describe common signs of infection and other complications of PN.	___	___	___	_____
5. Watched client record information in logbook, reviewed book periodically.	___	___	___	_____
6. Identified unexpected outcomes.	___	___	___	_____

RECORDING AND REPORTING

	S	U	NP	Comments
1. Recorded information taught, client's response, and outcomes of PN therapy in home care record.	___	___	___	_____
2. Recorded appearance of CVC site, infusions, glucose monitoring results, client's weight in home documentation system (e.g., logbook).	___	___	___	_____

Student _____ Date _____

Instructor _____ Date _____

PERFORMANCE CHECKLIST SKILL 43-1 **URINE SPECIMEN COLLECTION: MIDSTREAM (CLEAN-VOIDED)**
URINE; STERILE URINARY CATHETER

	S	U	NP	Comments

ASSESSMENT

1. Assessed patient's or family's understanding of purpose of test and method of collection.

2. Assessed patient's ability to assist with urine specimen collection.

3. Assessed for signs of UTI.

4. Referred to agency procedures for collection methods.

PLANNING

1. Identified expected outcomes.

IMPLEMENTATION

1. Performed hand hygiene, checked labels and completed laboratory requisition for container.

2. Identified patient using two identifiers, compared with MAR on ID bracelet.

3. Provided privacy, allowed mobile patient to collect specimen in bathroom.

4. Collected clean-voided urine specimen:

   a. Applied clean gloves, gave patient supplies to clean perineum or assisted patient in cleansing perineum, removed and disposed of gloves.

   b. Opened package of commercial specimen kit aseptically.

   c. Applied sterile gloves.

   d. Poured antiseptic solution over cotton balls if necessary.

   e. Opened specimen container, maintained sterility of inside of container, placed cap properly.

   f. Assisted or allowed patient to cleanse perineum and collect specimen, informed patient antiseptic would feel cold.

	S	U	NP	Comments

(1) For male patient:

(a) Held penis with one hand, cleansed meatus properly, retracted foreskin if necessary, returned foreskin when done. ____ ____ ____ _____

(b) Rinsed area and dried if agency procedure indicates. ____ ____ ____ _____

(c) Had patient pass container through urine stream after patient initiated stream. ____ ____ ____ _____

(2) For female patient:

(a) Spread labia minora with fingers of nondominant hand or had patient assist. ____ ____ ____ _____

(b) Cleansed urethral area appropriately, used fresh swab for each fold. ____ ____ ____ _____

(c) Rinsed area and dried with cotton ball if agency procedure indicates. ____ ____ ____ _____

(d) Passed specimen container into urine stream after patient initiated stream. ____ ____ ____ _____

g. Removed specimen container before flow stopped and before releasing labia or penis, assisted with personal hygiene as appropriate. ____ ____ ____ _____

h. Replaced cap on container, touched only outside. ____ ____ ____ _____

i. Cleansed exterior of container, removed and disposed of gloves. ____ ____ ____ _____

5. Collected urine from indwelling urinary catheter:

a. Explained use of needleless syringe and that patient would not experience discomfort. ____ ____ ____ _____

b. Explained need to clamp catheter 10 to 15 minutes before obtaining specimen and that it could not be obtained from drainage bag. ____ ____ ____ _____

c. Performed hand hygiene, applied clean gloves, clamped drainage tubing below withdrawal site. ____ ____ ____ _____

d. Positioned patient properly, located port, cleansed port with disinfectant and allowed to dry. ____ ____ ____ _____

e. Attached needleless Luer-Lok syringe to port appropriately. ____ ____ ____ _____

568

	S	U	NP	Comments

f. Withdrew appropriate amount for culture for routine analysis.

g. Transferred urine from syringe to appropriate container.

h. Placed lid tightly on container.

i. Unclamped catheter, ensured urine was flowing freely.

6. Secured label to container, completed label properly.

7. Disposed of soiled supplies, removed discarded gloves, performed hand hygiene.

8. Sent specimen and requisition to laboratory within 20 minutes, refrigerated specimen if necessary.

EVALUATION

1. Inspected clean-voided specimen for contamination.

2. Assessed patient's urine C&S report for bacterial growth.

3. Observed urinary drainage system to ensure it was intact and patent.

4. Asked patient to describe midstream urine collection procedure.

5. Identified unexpected outcomes.

RECORDING AND REPORTING

1. Recorded collection of specimen in appropriate log.

2. Reported any abnormal findings to health care provider.

Student _____ Date _____

Instructor _____ Date _____

	S	U	NP	Comments

PROCEDURAL STEPS

1. Identified patient using two identifiers, compared with MAR and patient's ID bracelet.

2. Explained reason for specimen collection, how patient could assist, and that urine must be free of contaminants.

3. Placed collection container in bathroom, included can of ice if indicated; posted signs reminding of timed urine collection; ensured personnel in receiving area collected and saved urine if patient left unit.

4. Had patient drink two to four glasses of water about 30 minutes before times of collection.

5. Performed hand hygiene, applied clean gloves, discarded first specimen as test began, indicated time test began on requisition, ensured patient began test with empty bladder, began collecting all urine for designated time.

6. Measured volume of each voiding if I&O was to be recorded, placed all urine in labeled specimen bottles with appropriate additives.

7. Kept specimen bottle in refrigerator or ice in bathroom to prevent decomposition of urine unless instructed otherwise.

8. Encouraged patient to drink two glasses of water 1 hour before collection ended and empty bladder during last 15 minutes of collection period.

9. Performed hand hygiene, applied clean gloves, labeled specimen appropriately, attached requisition, sent to laboratory.

10. Removed signs, informed patient specimen collection period was complete.

Student _____ Date _____

Instructor _____ Date _____

PERFORMANCE CHECKLIST PROCEDURAL GUIDELINE 43-2 **URINE SCREENING FOR GLUCOSE, KETONES, PROTEIN, BLOOD, AND pH**

	S	U	NP	Comments
PROCEDURAL STEPS				
1. Identified patient using two identifiers, compared to MAR and information on ID bracelet.	___	___	___	_____
2. Determined if double-voided specimen was needed for glucose testing; asked patient to void, discard, and drink water if necessary.	___	___	___	_____
3. Performed hand hygiene, applied clean gloves, asked patient to collect fresh random urine specimen or removed specimen from catheter port.	___	___	___	_____
4. Immersed end of reagent strip into urine container, removed strip immediately and tapped against side of container to remove excess urine.	___	___	___	_____
5. Held strip in horizontal position.	___	___	___	_____
6. Time number of seconds on container, compared color of strip with color chart.	___	___	___	_____
7. Discussed test results with patient, removed and discarded gloves, performed hand hygiene.	___	___	___	_____
8. Recorded results immediately in appropriate log, reported reading to health care provider.	___	___	___	_____

Student _____ Date _____

Instructor _____ Date _____

	S	U	NP	Comments

ASSESSMENT

1. Assessed patient or family for understanding need for stool test.

2. Assessed patient's ability to cooperate with procedure and collect specimen.

3. Assessed patient's medical history for GI disorders.

4. Reviewed patient's medications for drugs that contribute to GI bleeding.

5. Referred to health care provider's orders for medication or dietary modifications before test.

PLANNING

1. Identified expected outcomes.

2. Explained procedure to patient or family member, discussed reason for collection and how patient could assist, explained that feces must be free of contaminants.

3. Arranged for any needed dietary or medication restrictions.

IMPLEMENTATION

1. Performed hand hygiene.

2. Identified patient using two identifiers, compared with MAR and patient's ID bracelet.

3. Applied clean gloves; obtained uncontaminated specimen in clean, dry container.

4. Used tip of wooden applicator to obtain small portion of feces.

5. Measured for occult blood:

   a. Performed Hemoccult slide test:

      (1) Opened flap of slide, applied thin smear of stool on paper in first box.

      (2) Obtained a second specimen from a different portion of stool, applied to second box of slide.

	S	U	NP	Comments

(3) Closed slide cover, turned slide over, opened cardboard flap, applied two drops of developing solution on each box of guaiac paper. ___ ___ ___ _____

(4) Read results at the appropriate time, noted color changes. ___ ___ ___ _____

(5) Disposed of test slide in proper receptacle. ___ ___ ___ _____

b. Performed test using Hematest tablets.

(1) Placed stool on guaiac paper and Hematest tablet on top of stool specimen, applied tap water, allowed to flow onto paper. ___ ___ ___ _____

(2) Observed color of paper at appropriate time. ___ ___ ___ _____

(3) Disposed of tablet and paper properly. ___ ___ ___ _____

6. Wrapped wooden applicator in paper towel, grabbed properly, removed gloves over wrapped applicator, disposed in proper receptacle, performed hand hygiene. ___ ___ ___ _____

EVALUATION

1. Asked patient to explain collection procedures. ___ ___ ___ _____

2. Noted color changes in guaiac paper. ___ ___ ___ _____

3. Noted character of stool specimen. ___ ___ ___ _____

4. Identified unexpected outcomes. ___ ___ ___ _____

RECORDING AND REPORTING

1. Recorded results of test and stool characteristics in appropriate log. ___ ___ ___ _____

2. Reported positive test results to health care provider. ___ ___ ___ _____

576

Student _____ Date _____

Instructor _____ Date _____

PERFORMANCE CHECKLIST SKILL 43-3 **MEASURING OCCULT BLOOD IN GASTRIC SECRETIONS (GASTROCCULT)**

	S	U	NP	Comments

ASSESSMENT

1. Assessed patient's or family members' understanding of need for test.

2. Assessed patient's medical history for bleeding or GI disorders.

3. Assessed patient's medical history for GI disorders.

PLANNING

1. Identified expected outcomes.

2. Explained procedure to patient or family, discussed why collection was necessary.

IMPLEMENTATION

1. Performed hand hygiene.

2. Identified patient using two identifiers, compared with MAR and patient's ID bracelet.

3. Verified NG tube placement.

4. Obtained specimen by disconnecting tube from suction or gravity drainage from tube, aspirated fluid properly from the tube.

5. Obtained sample of emesis from basin properly.

6. Performed Gastroccult test:

   a. Applied one drop of gastric sample to Gastroccult blood test slide properly.

   b. Applied two drops of developer solution over sample and one drop between positive and negative performance monitors.

   c. Verified that performance monitor turns blue in 30 seconds.

   d. Compared color of gastric sample with that of performance monitor at the appropriate time.

   e. Disposed of test slide, applicator, and syringe in proper receptacle; reconnected enteral tube to drainage system if needed; removed gloves; performed hand hygiene.

	S	U	NP	Comments

EVALUATION

1. Asked patient to explain reason for procedure. ___ ___ ___ _____

2. Noted changes in guaiac paper. ___ ___ ___ _____

3. Noted character of gastric secretions. ___ ___ ___ _____

4. Identified unexpected outcomes. ___ ___ ___ _____

RECORDING AND REPORTING

1. Recorded results of test and unusual characteristics of gastric contents in appropriate log. ___ ___ ___ _____

2. Reported positive test results to health care provider. ___ ___ ___ _____

Student _____ Date _____

Instructor _____ Date _____

PERFORMANCE CHECKLIST SKILL 43-4 **COLLECTING NOSE AND THROAT SPECIMENS FOR CULTURE**

	S	U	NP	Comments

ASSESSMENT

1. Assessed patient's understanding of purpose for procedure and ability to cooperate, obtained assistance if required. ___ ___ ___ _____

2. Inspected condition of nares and drainage from nasal mucosa and sinuses. ___ ___ ___ _____

3. Determined if patient experienced postnasal drip, sinus headache, tenderness, congestion, sore throat, or exposure to others with similar symptoms. ___ ___ ___ _____

4. Applied clean gloves, assessed condition of posterior pharynx. ___ ___ ___ _____

5. Assessed patient for signs of infection. ___ ___ ___ _____

6. Reviewed health care provider's orders to determine if nose, throat, or both cultures were needed. ___ ___ ___ _____

PLANNING

1. Identified expected outcomes. ___ U ___ _____

2. Planned to do culture at appropriate time. ___ ___ ___ _____

3. Explained procedure to patient or family, discussed reason for specimen collection and how patient can assist. ___ ___ ___ _____

4. Explained sensations patient may have felt during procedure. ___ ___ ___ _____

IMPLEMENTATION

1. Identified patient using two identifiers, compared with MAR and patient's ID bracelet. ___ ___ ___ _____

2. Asked patient to sit appropriately. ___ ___ ___ _____

3. Had swab ready to use. ___ ___ ___ _____

4. Collected throat culture:

   a. Performed hand hygiene, applied clean gloves. ___ ___ ___ _____

   b. Instructed patient to tilt head properly. ___ ___ ___ _____

   c. Asked patient to open mouth and say "ah," depressed tongue properly, illuminated with penlight as needed. ___ ___ ___ _____

	S	U	NP	Comments

    d. Inserted swab without touching lips, teeth, tongue, cheeks, or uvula.

    e. Swabbed tonsillar area properly, made contact with inflamed sites.

    f. Withdrew swab without touching oral structures.

5. Collected nasal culture:

    a. Performed hand hygiene, applied clean gloves.

    b. Encouraged patient to blow nose, check nostrils for patency, selected appropriate nostril.

    c. Had patient tilt head properly.

    d. Inserted nasal speculum properly.

    e. Passed swab into nostril until it reached portion of mucosa that was inflamed or containing exudates, rotated swab quickly.

    f. Removed swab without touching sides of speculum or nasal canal.

    g. Removed nasal speculum and placed in basin, offered patient facial tissue.

6. Inserted swab into culture tube, crushed ampule at bottom of tube with gauze to protect fingers.

7. Placed tip of swab into liquid medium, placed top securely on top of tube.

8. Attached completed identification label and requisition to culture tube in front of patient, noted if patient was taking antibiotic or if specific organism was suspected.

9. Enclosed specimen in plastic biohazard bag, sent to laboratory.

10. Returned patient to comfortable position, removed and disposed of gloves, performed hand hygiene.

EVALUATION

1. Checked laboratory record for results of culture test.

2. Asked patient to explain purpose of culture.

3. Identified unexpected outcomes.

	S	U	NP	Comments

RECORDING AND REPORTING

1. Described appearance of mucosal structures and recorded specimen collection in appropriate log.

2. Reported unusual test results to health care provider.

Student _____ Date _____

Instructor _____ Date _____

PERFORMANCE CHECKLIST SKILL 43-5 **OBTAINING VAGINAL OR URETHRAL DISCHARGE SPECIMENS**

	S	U	NP	Comments
ASSESSMENT				
1. Assessed patient understanding of need for culture and ability to cooperate with procedure.	___	___	___	_____
2. Performed hand hygiene; applied clean gloves; assessed condition of external genitalia and urethra, meatus, and vaginal orifice; observed for redness, swelling, tenderness, and discharge that was whitish; removed and discarded gloves; performed hand hygiene.	___	___	___	_____
3. Asked patient about dysuria, localized pruritus of genitalia, or lower abdominal pain.	___	___	___	_____
4. Gathered and recorded sexual history of patient if symptoms suggested STD.	___	___	___	_____
5. Referred to health care provider's order to determine if culture was to be vaginal or urethral.	___	___	___	_____
PLANNING				
1. Identified expected outcomes.	___	___	___	_____
2. Explained procedure to patient or family, discussed reason for collection and how patient could assist, instructed patient not to douche or urinate 1 hour before obtaining culture.	___	___	___	_____
IMPLEMENTATION				
1. Performed hand hygiene, applied clean gloves.	___	___	___	_____
2. Provided privacy.	___	___	___	_____
3. Identified patient using two identifiers, compared with MAR and patient's ID bracelet.	___	___	___	_____
4. Assisted patient to appropriate position, raised gown, draped body parts to be exposed properly.	___	___	___	_____
5. Directed light source onto perineum.	___	___	___	_____
6. Opened culture tube, held swab in dominant hand.	___	___	___	_____
7. Instructed patient to deep-breathe slowly.	___	___	___	_____

	S	U	NP	Comments

8. Obtained specimen properly:

   a. For female patient:

      (1) Separated labia to expose vaginal orifice.   ___   ___   ___   _____

      (2) Touched tip of swab into discharge pool or vaginal orifice, did not touch skin or mucosa.   ___   ___   ___   _____

      (3) Exposed urethral meatus, pulled labia minora upward and back.   ___   ___   ___   _____

      (4) Used clean swab, applied tip to meatus where discharge was visible, avoided touching labia.   ___   ___   ___   _____

   b. For male patient:

      (1) Grasped penis appropriately, gently retracted foreskin.   ___   ___   ___   _____

      (2) Held swab appropriately, applied to area of discharge.   ___   ___   ___   _____

      (3) Introduced swab into meatus if necessary.   ___   ___   ___   _____

      (4) Returned foreskin to natural position.   ___   ___   ___   _____

9. Returned each swab to culture tube, secured top.   ___   ___   ___   _____

10. Wrapped ampule with gauze if using commercial culture tube, crushed ampule, pushed tip into fluid medium.   ___   ___   ___   _____

11. Removed and discarded gloves, performed hand hygiene.   ___   ___   ___   _____

12. Labeled each culture tube with ID label, affixed requisition in front of patient.   ___   ___   ___   _____

13. Sent specimen immediately to laboratory or refrigerator.   ___   ___   ___   _____

14. Assisted patient to comfortable position, assisted with personal hygiene as needed, replaced gown, removed drape, discarded into appropriate receptacle.   ___   ___   ___   _____

EVALUATION

1. Reviewed laboratory results for evidence of pathogens.   ___   ___   ___   _____

2. Continued to monitor whether discharge was present and, if it was, observed color and amount.   ___   ___   ___   _____

3. Observed specimen for presence of feces.   ___   ___   ___   _____

4. Identified unexpected outcomes.   ___   ___   ___   _____

	S	U	NP	Comments

RECORDING AND REPORTING

1. Recorded types of cultures and date and time sent to laboratory.

2. Reported laboratory results to nurse in charge or health care provider.

Student _____ Date _____

Instructor _____ Date _____

PERFORMANCE CHECKLIST PROCEDURAL GUIDELINE 43-3 **COLLECTING A SPUTUM SPECIMEN BY EXPECTORATION**

	S	U	NP	Comments
PROCEDURAL STEPS				
1. Identified patient using two identifiers, compared with MAR and patient's ID bracelet.	___	___	___	_____
2. Provided opportunity to rinse mouth with water.	___	___	___	_____
3. Performed hand hygiene, applied clean gloves, provided sputum cup, instructed patient not to touch inside of container.	___	___	___	_____
4. Had patient take deep breaths with full exhalation then take full inhalation followed by a forceful cough, ensured sputum was expectorated directly into specimen container.	___	___	___	_____
5. Repeated until enough saliva had been collected.	___	___	___	_____
6. Secured lid on container, wiped outside of container with disinfectant.	___	___	___	_____
7. Offered patient tissues and mouth care, disposed of tissues properly.	___	___	___	_____
8. Removed and disposed of gloves, performed hand hygiene.	___	___	___	_____
9. Attached completed ID label and requisition to side of container.	___	___	___	_____
10. Enclosed specimen in biohazard bag.	___	___	___	_____
11. Sent specimen immediately to laboratory.	___	___	___	_____

Student _____ Date _____

Instructor _____ Date _____

PERFORMANCE CHECKLIST SKILL 43-6 **COLLECTING SPUTUM SPECIMEN BY SUCTION**

	S	U	NP	Comments
ASSESSMENT				
1. Checked health care provider's orders for type of analysis and specifications.	___	___	___	_____
2. Assessed patient's level of understanding or procedure and purpose.	___	___	___	_____
3. Assessed when patient last ate a meal or had tube feeding.	___	___	___	_____
4. Determined type of assistance needed by patient to obtain specimen.	___	___	___	_____
5. Assessed patient's respiratory status.	___	___	___	_____
PLANNING				
1. Identified expected outcomes.	___	___	___	_____
2. Explained procedure and purpose, instructed patient to breathe normally.	___	___	___	_____
IMPLEMENTATION				
1. Provided privacy.	___	___	___	_____
2. Identified patient using two identifiers, compared with MAR and patient's ID bracelet.	___	___	___	_____
3. Positioned patient properly.	___	___	___	_____
4. Performed hand hygiene, applied clean glove to nondominant hand, prepared suction device, determined if device was functioning properly.	___	___	___	_____
5. Connected tube to adapter on sputum trap, opened sterile water.	___	___	___	_____
6. Applied sterile glove to dominant hand or used clean glove.	___	___	___	_____
7. Connected sterile suction catheter to rubber tubing on sputum trap.	___	___	___	_____
8. Lubricated suction catheter tip with sterile water.	___	___	___	_____
9. Inserted suction catheter through appropriate tube without applying suction.	___	___	___	_____
10. Advanced catheter into trachea, warned patient to expect to cough.	___	___	___	_____

	S	U	NP	Comments
11. Applied suction appropriately as patient coughs.	—	—	—	_____
12. Released suction, removed catheter, turned off suction.	—	—	—	_____
13. Detached catheter from specimen trap, disposed of catheter in appropriate receptacle.	—	—	—	_____
14. Secured top on container, detached suction tubing and connected rubber tubing to plastic adapter.	—	—	—	_____
15. Wiped outside of container with disinfectant.	—	—	—	_____
16. Offered patient tissues, disposed of tissues in emesis basin or appropriate container.	—	—	—	_____
17. Removed and disposed of gloves, performed hand hygiene.	—	—	—	_____
18. Labeled with ID label on side of specimen container, placed specimen in appropriate container, attached requisition.	—	—	—	_____
19. Sent specimen immediately to laboratory or refrigerated.	—	—	—	_____
20. Offered patient mouth care if desired.	—	—	—	_____

EVALUATION

	S	U	NP	Comments
1. Observed patient's respiratory status throughout procedure, measured oxygen saturation if necessary.	—	—	—	_____
2. Noted anxiety or discomfort in patient.	—	—	—	_____
3. Observed character of sputum.	—	—	—	_____
4. Referred to laboratory reports for test results.	—	—	—	_____
5. Evaluated patient's ability to describe/demonstrate sputum collection process.	—	—	—	_____
6. Identified unexpected outcomes.	—	—	—	_____

RECORDING AND REPORTING

	S	U	NP	Comments
1. Recorded all pertinent information in appropriate log.	—	—	—	_____
2. Reported unusual sputum characteristics to nurse in charge or health care provider.	—	—	—	_____
3. Reported abnormal laboratory findings to health care provider, initiated isolation techniques if necessary.	—	—	—	_____
4. Noted on requisition if patient was receiving antibiotics.	—	—	—	_____

Student _____ Date _____

Instructor _____ Date _____

PERFORMANCE CHECKLIST SKILL 43-7 **OBTAINING WOUND DRAINAGE SPECIMENS**

	S	U	NP	Comments
ASSESSMENT				
1. Assessed patient's understanding of need to culture and ability to cooperate with procedure.	___	___	___	_____
2. Assessed patient for signs of fever, chills, or excessive thirst; noted if WBC was elevated.	___	___	___	_____
3. Asked patient about extent and type of pain at wound site, gave analgesic before dressing changes if necessary.	___	___	___	_____
4. Determined when dressing change was scheduled, performed wound assessment as part of procedure.	___	___	___	_____
5. Reviewed health care provider's orders for aerobic or anaerobic culture.	___	___	___	_____
6. Applied clean gloves, removed soiled dressings covering wound, applied sterile gloves to palpate wound, observed for signs of infection.	___	___	___	_____
PLANNING				
1. Identified expected outcomes.	___	___	___	_____
2. Determined and requested analgesic, administered as ordered and if needed.	___	___	___	_____
3. Explained reason for wound culture and how it would be collected.	___	___	___	_____
4. Explained that patient may feel tickling sensation.	___	___	___	_____
IMPLEMENTATION				
1. Provided privacy.	___	___	___	_____
2. Identified patient using two identifiers, compared with MAR and patient's ID bracelet.	___	___	___	_____
3. Performed hand hygiene, applied clean gloves, removed old dressing, assessed dressing for exudates and drainage, folded soiled dressing together and disposed of appropriately.	___	___	___	_____
4. Cleansed area around wound edges properly with antiseptic swab, removed old exudate.	___	___	___	_____
5. Discarded swab, removed and disposed of gloves, performed hand hygiene.	___	___	___	_____
6. Opened packages of culture tube and dressing supplies, applied sterile gloves.	___	___	___	_____

	S	U	NP	Comments

7. Obtained cultures:

   a. Aerobic culture:

      (1) Took swab from tube, inserted into wound in area of drainage, rotated swab gently, returned swab to tube, wrapped ampule in gauze, crushed ampule of medium, pushed swab into fluid.

   b. Anaerobic culture:

      (1) Took swab from culture tube, swabbed deeply into draining body cavity, rotated, returned swab to culture tube.

Or

      (2) Inserted syringe into wound, aspirated exudates, attached needle, expelled all air, and injected drainage into culture tube.

8. Placed specimen label on each culture tube in front of patient, indicated if patient was receiving antibiotics.

9. Sent specimen to laboratory immediately.

10. Cleaned wound per order, applied new sterile dressing, secured dressing appropriately.

11. Removed and disposed of gloves and soiled supplies appropriately, performed hand hygiene.

12. Assisted patient to comfortable position.

EVALUATION

1. Obtained laboratory report for results of culture.

2. Observed character of wound drainage.

3. Observed edges of wound for redness and bleeding.

4. Asked patient about purpose of wound culture.

5. Identified unexpected outcomes.

RECORDING AND REPORTING

1. Recorded all pertinent information in the appropriate log.

2. Reported evidence of infection to charge nurse and health care provider.

3. Recorded patient's tolerance of procedure and response to analgesics.

Student _____ Date _____

Instructor _____ Date _____

PERFORMANCE CHECKLIST SKILL 43 8 **COLLECTING BLOOD SPECIMENS AND CULTURE BY VENIPUNCTURE (SYRINGE AND VACUTAINER METHOD)**

	S	U	NP	Comments
ASSESSMENT				
1. Determined if patient understands purpose of procedure and ability to cooperate.	___	___	___	_____
2. Determined if special conditions need to be met before specimen collection.	___	___	___	_____
3. Assessed patient for possible risks associated with venipuncture, reviewed medication history.	___	___	___	_____
4. Assessed patient for contraindicated sites for venipuncture.	___	___	___	_____
5. Reviewed health care provider's orders for type of tests.	___	___	___	_____
PLANNING				
1. Identified expected outcomes.	___	___	___	_____
2. Explained procedure to patient, described purpose of tests, explained sensations patient would feel.	___	___	___	_____
IMPLEMENTATION				
1. Brought equipment to bedside and organized.	___	___	___	_____
2. Identified patient using two identifiers, compared with MAR and patient's ID bracelet.	___	___	___	_____
3. Provided privacy.	___	___	___	_____
4. Raised or lowered bed to comfortable height.	___	___	___	_____
5. Assisted patient to appropriate position.	___	___	___	_____
6. Applied tourniquet properly:				
a. Positioned tourniquet properly above site.	___	___	___	_____
b. Crossed tourniquet over patient's arm, placed over gown sleeve if appropriate.	___	___	___	_____
c. Held tourniquet between fingers, tucked loop between patient's arm and tourniquet.	___	___	___	_____
7. Did not keep tourniquet on patient longer than 1 minute.	___	___	___	_____
8. Asked patient to open and close fist *gently* several times, left fist clenched.	___	___	___	_____
9. Inspected extremity for best site.	___	___	___	_____

	S	U	NP	Comments
10. Applied clean gloves, palpated selected vein.	___	___	___	_____
11. Obtained blood specimen:				
a. Syringe method:				
(1) Had syringe with appropriate needle attached.	___	___	___	_____
(2) Cleansed venipuncture site properly with antiseptic, allowed to dry, used only appropriate antiseptic.	___	___	___	_____
(3) Removed needle cover, informed patient that "stick" lasts a few seconds.	___	___	___	_____
(4) Placed thumb or forefinger below site, pulled skin taut, stretched until vein was stabilized.	___	___	___	_____
(5) Held syringe and needle properly from arm bevel up.	___	___	___	_____
(6) Inserted needle into vein, stopped when "pop" was felt.	___	___	___	_____
(7) Held syringe, pulled back plunger.	___	___	___	_____
(8) Observed for blood return.	___	___	___	_____
(9) Obtained desired amount of blood, kept needle stabilized.	___	___	___	_____
(10) Released tourniquet.	___	___	___	_____
(11) Applied gauze without applying pressure, withdrew needle, applied pressure, checked for hematoma.	___	___	___	_____
(12) Activated safety cover, discarded needle in appropriate container.	___	___	___	_____
(13) Attached syringe to transfer device, attached tube, allowed vacuum to fill tube appropriately, removed and filled other tubes as appropriate, rotated tubes properly.	___	___	___	_____
b. Vacutainer system method:				
(1) Attached double-ended needle to Vacutainer tube.	___	___	___	_____
(2) Had proper tube resting inside Vacutainer device, did not puncture stopper.	___	___	___	_____
(3) Cleansed venipuncture site properly, allowed to dry.	___	___	___	_____

	S	U	NP	Comments

(4) Removed needle cover, informed patient that "stick" would only last a few seconds.

(5) Placed thumb and forefinger *below* site, pulled skin taut, stretched skin until vein stabilized.

(6) Held needle at appropriate angle from arm bevel up.

(7) Inserted needle into vein.

(8) Grasped Vacutainer securely, advanced specimen tube into needle of holder.

(9) Noted flow of blood into tube.

(10) Grasped Vacutainer firmly, removed tube, inserted additional tube as needed, rotated each tube back and forth properly.

(11) Released tourniquet after tubes were filled.

(12) Applied gauze pad over site without applying pressure, withdrew needle with Vacutainer.

(13) Applied pressure over site with gauze or antiseptic pad until bleeding stops, observed for hematoma, taped dressing securely.

(14) Disposed of syringe, needle, gauze and other supplies appropriately.

c. Blood culture:

(1) Cleansed site with antiseptic swab, allowed to dry.

(2) Cleaned tops of culture bottles properly, allowed to dry.

(3) Collected appropriate amount of venous blood from each venipuncture site.

(4) Activated safety guard, discarded needle, replaced with new sterile needle before injecting blood sample into culture bottle.

(5) Filled anaerobic bottle first if both aerobic and anaerobic cultures were needed.

(6) Mixed blood in each culture bottle.

	S	U	NP	Comments

d. CVC collection:

   (1) Selected appropriate port, turned off IV pumps, clamped lumens. ____ ____ ____ _____

   (2) Wiped all Luer-Lok caps or removed alcohol-impregnated cap, attached saline syringe to selected port, aspirated for blood return, flushed with saline, used appropriate-sized syringe. ____ ____ ____ _____

   (3) Wiped port with alcohol, attached syringe, aspirated 5 mL of blood and discarded, reclamped catheter, wiped port, attached Luer-Lok syringe, unclamped catheter, aspirated blood, reclamped catheter, removed syringe, cleansed catheter hub, attached Vacutainer with needle, inserted specimen tube, allowed tube to fill. ____ ____ ____ _____

   (4) For Vacutainer method, clamped catheter, attached needleless connecter to holder, placed blood tube into holder, disinfected cap, inserted needleless connection in cap, unclamped catheter, advanced blood tube into holder, allowed blood to fill tube, clamped catheter, discarded first tube in biohazard container, attached specimen tubes to Vacutainer with Luer-Lok adapted, unclamped catheter, obtained blood specimens. ____ ____ ____ _____

   (5) Clamped catheter, removed Vacutainer holder and needleless connection from cap, disinfected with alcohol. ____ ____ ____ _____

   (6) Attached prefilled NS syringe; flushed using push, pause method; ensured positive pressure for lumen; removed and locked lumen syringe properly. ____ ____ ____ _____

12. Checked tubes for sign of external contamination with blood, decontaminated if necessary. ____ ____ ____ _____

13. Removed gloves after specimen was obtained and spillage was cleaned. ____ ____ ____ _____

14. Assisted patient to comfortable position. ____ ____ ____ _____

15. Attached properly completed labels to each tube, affixed requisition in front of patient. ____ ____ ____ _____

	S	U	NP	Comments

16. Placed specimens in biohazard bag, sent to laboratory within 30 minutes.

17. Performed hand hygiene.

EVALUATION

1. Reinspected venipuncture site for homeostasis.

2. Determined if patient remained anxious or fearful.

3. Checked laboratory report for test results.

4. Asked patient to explain purposes of tests.

5. Identified unexpected outcomes.

RECORDING AND REPORTING

1. Recorded all pertinent information in appropriate log.

2. Reported any STAT or abnormal test results of health care provider.

Student _____ Date _____

Instructor _____ Date _____

PERFORMANCE CHECKLIST SKILL 43-9 **BLOOD GLUCOSE MONITORING**

	S	U	NP	Comments

ASSESSMENT

1. Assessed patient's understanding of procedure and purpose of blood glucose monitoring, determined if patient understood how to perform test and its importance in glucose control. ___ ___ ___ _____

2. Determined if specific conditions needed to be met before or after sample collection. ___ ___ ___ _____

3. Determined if risks exist for performing skin puncture. ___ ___ ___ _____

4. Assessed area of skin to be used as puncture site, inspected fingers and forearms for edema, inflammations, cuts, and sores; avoided areas of bruising and open lesions; avoided hand on side of mastectomy. ___ ___ ___ _____

5. Reviewed health care provider's orders for time or frequency of measurement. ___ ___ ___ _____

6. Assessed ability of patient to perform testing at home and to handle skin-puncturing device. ___ ___ ___ _____

PLANNING

1. Identified expected outcomes. ___ ___ ___ _____

2. Explained procedure and purpose to patient and family, offered opportunity to practice testing procedures, provided resources/teaching aids. ___ ___ ___ _____

IMPLEMENTATION

1. Identified patient using two identifiers, compared with MAR and patient's ID bracelet. ___ ___ ___ _____

2. Performed hand hygiene, instructed adult to perform hand hygiene, rinsed and dried. ___ ___ ___ _____

3. Positioned patient appropriately. ___ ___ ___ _____

4. Removed reagent strip from vial and cap, checked code on test strip vial, used proper test strips. ___ ___ ___ _____

5. Inserted strip into meter, did not bend strip. ___ ___ ___ _____

6. Removed unused reagent strip from meter; placed on clean, dry surface with test pad facing up. ___ ___ ___ _____

7. Matched code on screen with code from test strip vial, confirmed codes. ___ ___ ___ _____

	S	U	NP	Comments

8. Performed hand hygiene, applied clean gloves, prepared lancet device properly.   ___ ___ ___ _____

9. Obtained blood sample:

   a. Wiped finger or forearm with antiseptic, chose appropriate area for puncture site.   ___ ___ ___ _____

   b. Held area to be punctured in dependent position, did not massage finger site.   ___ ___ ___ _____

   c. Held tip of lancet against area of skin chosen for test site, pressed release button, removed device.   ___ ___ ___ _____

   d. Squeezed fingertip until round blood drop forms.   ___ ___ ___ _____

10. Obtained test results.

   a. Ensured meter was still on, brought test strip to drop of blood, ensured adequate sample was obtained.   ___ ___ ___ _____

   b. Read glucose test result on the screen.   ___ ___ ___ _____

11. Turned meter off; disposed of test strip, lancet, and gloves in proper receptacle.   ___ ___ ___ _____

12. Performed hand hygiene.   ___ ___ ___ _____

13. Discussed test results with patient, encouraged questions and participation.   ___ ___ ___ _____

EVALUATION

1. Reinspected puncture site for bleeding and tissue injury.   ___ ___ ___ _____

2. Compared glucose meter reading with normal levels and previous results.   ___ ___ ___ _____

3. Asked patient to discuss procedure.   ___ ___ ___ _____

4. Asked patient to explain test results and perform next reading.   ___ ___ ___ _____

5. Identified unexpected outcomes.   ___ ___ ___ _____

RECORDING AND REPORTING

1. Recorded procedure and glucose level in appropriate log, took action for abnormal range.   ___ ___ ___ _____

2. Described patient response in notes.   ___ ___ ___ _____

3. Described explanations or teaching provided in notes.   ___ ___ ___ _____

4. Recorded and reported abnormal blood glucose levels.   ___ ___ ___ _____

600

Student _____ Date _____

Instructor _____ Date _____

PERFORMANCE CHECKLIST SKILL 43-10 **OBTAINING AN ARTERIAL SPECIMEN FOR BLOOD GAS MEASUREMENT**

	S	U	NP	Comments
ASSESSMENT				
1. Assessed factors that influence ABG measurements including hyper- or hypoventilation and body temperature.	___	___	___	_____
2. Identified medications that may influence ABG measurement.	___	___	___	_____
3. Assessed respiratory status.	___	___	___	_____
4. Reviewed criteria for choosing site for ABG sample:				
a. Assessed collateral blood flow with Allen test.	___	___	___	_____
b. Assessed accessibility of vessel.	___	___	___	_____
c. Assessed tissue surrounding artery.	___	___	___	_____
d. Assessed that arteries were not directly adjacent to veins.	___	___	___	_____
5. Assessed arterial sites (radial, brachial, and femoral arteries) for use in obtaining specimen.	___	___	___	_____
6. Reviewed baseline ABG values for patient.	___	___	___	_____
7. Determined patient's knowledge about ABG procedure.	___	___	___	_____
PLANNING				
1. Identified expected outcomes.	___	___	___	_____
2. Prepared heparinized syringe properly.	___	___	___	_____
3. Explained steps and purpose of procedure to patient.	___	___	___	_____
IMPLEMENTATION				
1. Identified patient using two identifiers, compared with MAR and patient's ID bracelet.	___	___	___	_____
2. Performed hand hygiene.	___	___	___	_____
3. Palpated selected site with fingertips.	___	___	___	_____
4. Elevated patient's wrist with small pillow, asked patient to extend fingers downward, stabilized artery with hyperextension of wrist.	___	___	___	_____
5. Applied clean gloves, cleaned area of maximal impulse with alcohol or antiseptic, allowed to dry.	___	___	___	_____

	S	U	NP	Comments
6. Held gauze pad with same fingers used to palpate artery.	___	___	___	_____
7. Used corner of gauze pad to point to site.	___	___	___	_____
8. Held needle bevel up, inserted at appropriate angle, prepared patient for painful stick.	___	___	___	_____
9. Stopped advancing needle at appropriate time.	___	___	___	_____
10. Allowed arterial pulsations to pump appropriate amount of blood into syringe.	___	___	___	_____
11. Held gauze pad over puncture site, withdrew syringe and needle, activated safety guard over needle.	___	___	___	_____
12. Applied pressure over and proximal to puncture site with pad.	___	___	___	_____
13. Maintained continuous pressure for appropriate time.	___	___	___	_____
14. Inspected site visually for signs of bleeding or hematoma formation.	___	___	___	_____
15. Palpated artery below or distal to puncture site.	___	___	___	_____
16. Took syringe, removed safety needle, discarded in biohazard container, attached filter cap to syringe or covered tip with gauze to dispel air.	___	___	___	_____
17. Removed gloves, performed hand hygiene.	___	___	___	_____
18. Placed ID label on syringe in front of patient, placed syringe in cup of crushed ice, attached requisition to sample.	___	___	___	_____
19. Sent sample to laboratory immediately.	___	___	___	_____

EVALUATION

1. Inspected puncture site and area distal for complications.	___	___	___	_____
2. Reviewed results of sample as soon as possible.	___	___	___	_____
3. Identified unexpected outcomes.	___	___	___	_____

RECORDING AND REPORTING

1. Recorded all pertinent information in the appropriate log.	___	___	___	_____
2. Reported ABG results to health care provider.	___	___	___	_____
3. Reported patient's FiO_2 and any ventilator settings.	___	___	___	_____
4. Recorded results of test in nurses' notes.	___	___	___	_____

Student _____ Date _____

Instructor _____ Date _____

PERFORMANCE CHECKLIST SKILL 44-1 **INTRAVENOUS MODERATE SEDATION DURING A DIAGNOSTIC PROCEDURE**

	S	U	NP	Comments
ASSESSMENT				
1. Verified type of procedure scheduled and procedure site with patient.				
2. Verified that a preprocedure medication reconciliation and H&P examination were completed.				
3. Verified that informed consent was obtained at an appropriate time.				
4. Assessed patient's past history if adverse reaction to IV sedation.				
5. Verified patient's ASA Physical Status Classification.				
6. Assessed patient for risk factors increasing likelihood of adverse event.				
7. Assessed patient's history for substance abuse or liver/kidney disease.				
8. Verified patient has not ingested food or fluids for at least 4 hours.				
9. Determined if patient was allergic to latex, antiseptic, tape, or anesthetic solutions.				
10. Assessed patient's level of understanding of procedure.				
11. Assessed baseline vital signs.				
12. Determined patient's height and weight.				
13. Assessed patient's baseline status via agency's scoring system.				
PLANNING				
1. Identified expected outcomes.				
2. Explained to patient that sedation would cause relaxation and amnesia but he or she would be awake during the procedure, taught patient nonverbal signals if necessary.				
3. Explained that close monitoring does not mean that there were problems.				
4. Explained to patient major steps of procedure.				
5. Positioned patient as needed for procedure.				

	S	U	NP	Comments

IMPLEMENTATION

1. Identified patient using two identifiers, compared with MAR and patient's ID bracelet.   ___ ___ ___ _____

2. Established peripheral IV access.   ___ ___ ___ _____

3. Monitored heart rate and SpO_2 continuously during diagnostic procedure; monitored airway patency, respiratory rate and depth, blood pressure, and LOC and responsiveness; kept oxygen and suction equipment nearby.   ___ ___ ___ _____

4. Observed for verbal and nonverbal evidence of pain, grimacing, or eye opening.   ___ ___ ___ _____

5. Assessed level of sedation using appropriate scale.   ___ ___ ___ _____

6. Repositioned patient as needed without interrupting.   ___ ___ ___ _____

EVALUATION

1. Monitored patient throughout the procedure using the Ramsay Sedation Scale.   ___ ___ ___ _____

2. Used Aldrete score after procedure, monitored LOC, respiratory rate, oxygen saturation, blood pressure, heart rate and rhythm, and pain score.   ___ ___ ___ _____

3. Asked patient to repeat back what he or she understands regarding procedure or any postprocedure patient instructions.   ___ ___ ___ _____

4. Had patient's driver explain postprocedure education and sign appropriate documents.   ___ ___ ___ _____

5. Identified unexpected outcomes.   ___ ___ ___ _____

RECORDING AND REPORTING

1. Documented vital signs, SpO_2, end-tidal CO_2, and sedation level at the appropriate times.   ___ ___ ___ _____

2. Recorded all pertinent information in the appropriate log.   ___ ___ ___ _____

3. Reported any respiratory distress, cardiac compromise, or unexpected altered mental status to health care provider immediately.   ___ ___ ___ _____

4. Documented discharge teaching, medication reconciliation, discontinuation of IV access, final/discharge assessment, and who/how discharged.   ___ ___ ___ _____

Student _____ Date _____

Instructor _____ Date _____

PERFORMANCE CHECKLIST SKILL 44-2 **CONTRAST MEDIA STUDIES: ARTERIOGRAM (ANGIOGRAM), CARDIAC CATHETERIZATION, AND INTRAVENOUS PYELOGRAM**

	S	U	NP	Comments
ASSESSMENT				
1. Verified type of procedure scheduled and procedure site with patient.	___	___	___	_____
2. Verified that informed consent was obtained at appropriate time.	___	___	___	_____
3. Determined if patient was taking anticoagulants, aspirin, or nonsteroidal medication.	___	___	___	_____
4. Assessed patient for history of allergies and previous reaction to contrast agent, notified cardiologist or radiologist if necessary.	___	___	___	_____
5. Reviewed medical record for contraindications.	___	___	___	_____
6. Assessed patient's bleeding and coagulation status.	___	___	___	_____
7. Obtained vital signs and peripheral pulses.	___	___	___	_____
8. Assessed patient hydration status.	___	___	___	_____
9. Assessed patient's level of understanding of procedures.	___	___	___	_____
10. Determined type of arteriogram scheduled, verified details if necessary.	___	___	___	_____
11. Determined and documented last time of ingested food, drink, or medications.	___	___	___	_____
12. Reviewed health care provider's order for preprocedure medications, hydration, antihistamines, and IV sedation.	___	___	___	_____
PLANNING				
1. Identified expected outcomes.	___	___	___	_____
2. Explained to patient purpose of procedure and what would happen.	___	___	___	_____
3. Removed all patient's jewelry and metal objects.	___	___	___	_____
4. Completed appropriate preprocedure preparation for IVP or cardiac catheterization.	___	___	___	_____
5. Verified availability of emergent cardiac surgery if necessary and patient's ASA classification	___	___	___	_____

	S	U	NP	Comments

IMPLEMENTATION

1. Identified patient using two identifiers, compared identifiers patient's ID bracelet, verified type of procedure scheduled and procedure site with patient.

2. Had patient empty bladder before procedure.

3. Prepared cardiac monitor and/or end-tidal CO_2 monitor.

4. Performed hand hygiene, applied appropriate PPE.

5. Provided IV access using large-bore cannula, removed gloves.

6. Monitored vital signs, SpO_2, end-tidal CO_2; palpated peripheral pulses for arterial procedures.

7. Told patient that he or she may experience chest pain and severe hot flash during injection of dye.

8. Applied necessary PPE, draped patient leaving puncture site exposed.

9. Anesthetized skin overlying arterial puncture site.

10. Observed patient for signs of anaphylaxis if iodinated dye was used.

11. Assisted with measuring cardiac volumes and pressure for cardiac catheterization.

12. Monitored levels of sedation and LOC if appropriate.

13. Kept extremity immobilized for 2 to 6 hours, used orthopedic bedpan if necessary, emphasized need to lie flat for 6 to 12 hours, encouraged patient to drink 1 to 2 L of fluid.

EVALUATION

1. Evaluated patient's body position and comfort during procedure.

2. Monitored vital signs and oxygen saturation, assessed for signs of cardiac complications at appropriate intervals.

3. Monitored for complications:

   a. Performed neurovascular checks properly, used a Doppler ultrasonic stethoscope if necessary.

   b. Assessed vascular access site for bleeding and hematoma.

606

	S	U	NP	Comments

c. Auscultated heart and lungs, compared with preprocedure findings.

d. Observed patient for possible delayed reaction to iodine.

4. Evaluated level of sedation, LOC, and SpO_2; used Aldrete Scale.

5. Assessed postprocedure laboratory values.

6. Had patient rate discomfort on pain scale.

7. Identified unexpected outcomes.

RECORDING AND REPORTING

1. Recorded patient's status; recorded any drainage from puncture site, appearance of dressing, and condition of the puncture site.

2. Reported problems to health care provider if necessary.

PERFORMANCE CHECKLIST SKILL 44-3 **ASSISTING WITH ASPIRATIONS: BONE MARROW ASPIRATION/ BIOPSY, LUMBAR PUNCTURE, PARACENTESIS, AND THORACENTESIS**

	S	U	NP	Comments

ASSESSMENT

1. Verified type of procedure scheduled, purpose, and procedure site with patient and medical record.

2. Verified that informed consent was obtained at an appropriate time.

3. Reviewed medical record for contraindications.

4. Determined patient's ability to assume position and stay still, discussed need for premedication with health care provider.

5. Obtained vital signs, SpO_2/end-tidal CO_2 value, and weight; obtained abdominal girth measurement if necessary; assessed lower extremity movement, sensation, and muscle strength.

6. Instructed patient to empty bladder.

7. Assessed patient's coagulation status.

8. Determined whether patient was allergic to antiseptic, latex, or anesthetic solutions.

9. Assessed patient's level of understanding of procedure.

10. Assessed baseline pain level.

PLANNING

1. Identified expected outcomes.

2. Explained steps of skin preparation, anesthetic injection, needle insertion, and position required.

3. Premedicated for pain if ordered.

4. Verified recent chest x-ray examination.

IMPLEMENTATION

1. Identified patient using two identifiers per agency policy, compare with patient's ID bracelet.

2. Performed hand hygiene.

3. Set up sterile tray or opened supplies.

	S	U	NP	Comments

4. Took "Time-Out" to verify patient's name, type of procedure, and procedure site with patient and team.

5. Assisted patient in maintaining correct position, reassured patient while explaining procedure.

6. Explained to patient that pain might occur when lidocaine was injected and that pressure might occur when tissue or fluid was aspirated.

7. Assessed patient's condition during procedure including respiratory status, vital signs, and complaints of pain.

8. Noted character of aspirate.

9. Properly labeled specimen in presence of patient, transported to laboratory in proper container, labeled specimens in order of collection.

10. Assisted with pressure over insertion site and application of gauze after needle was removed.

11. Removed PPE, discarded appropriately, performed hand hygiene.

EVALUATION

1. Monitored LOC, vital signs, and SPO_2/end-tidal CO_2 at appropriate intervals.

2. Inspected dressing over puncture site for signs of infection, inspected area under patient for bleeding.

3. Evaluated pain score.

4. Measured abdominal girth and respirations following a paracentesis, compared with preprocedure assessments.

5. Identified unexpected outcomes.

RECORDING AND REPORTING

1. Recorded all pertinent information in the appropriate log.

2. Reported changes in vital signs, unexpected pain, or excessive drainage to health care provider immediately.

Student _____ Date _____

Instructor _____ Date _____

PERFORMANCE CHECKLIST SKILL 44-4 **ASSISTING WITH BRONCHOSCOPY**

	S	U	NP	Comments

ASSESSMENT

1. Verified type of procedure scheduled and procedure site with patient.

2. Verified that informed consent was obtained at the appropriate time.

3. Assessed patient's history for inability to tolerate interruption of high-flow oxygen if necessary.

4. Obtained baseline vital signs, SpO_2 and end-tidal CO_2 values.

5. Assessed type of cough, sputum produced, and heart and lung sounds.

6. Determined purpose of procedure.

7. Determined whether patient was allergic to local anesthetic.

8. Assessed need for preprocedure medication.

9. Assessed time patient last ingested food, fluids, or medications.

10. Assessed patient's level of understanding of procedure.

PLANNING

1. Identified expected outcomes.

2. Administered atropine, opioid, or antianxiety agent 30 minutes before procedure.

3. Explained procedure to patient.

4. Removed and safely stored patient's dentures/eyeglasses.

IMPLEMENTATION

1. Identified patient using two identifiers according to agency policy, compared with information on patient's ID bracelet.

2. Assessed current IV access or established new access.

	S	U	NP	Comments
3. Assisted patient to assume appropriate position.	___	___	___	_____
4. Took "Time-Out" to verify patient's name, type of procedure, and procedure site with patient and team.	___	___	___	_____
5. Performed hand hygiene, applied PPE, positioned tip of suction catheter for easy access to patient's mouth.	___	___	___	_____
6. Instructed patient not to swallow the local anesthetic, provided emesis basin.	___	___	___	_____
7. Assisted patient throughout procedure with explanations, verbal reassurance, and support.	___	___	___	_____
8. Assessed patient's pulse, BP, respirations, SpO_2, end-tidal CO_2, and breathing capacity; observed degree of restlessness, capillary refill, and color of nail beds.	___	___	___	_____
9. Noted characteristics of suctioned material.	___	___	___	_____
10. Wiped patient's mouth and nose to remove lubricant with gloved hand after bronchoscope was removed.	___	___	___	_____
11. Instructed patient not to eat or drink until gag reflex had returned, tested for presence of gag reflex properly.	___	___	___	_____
12. Removed protective equipment, discarded, and performed hand hygiene.	___	___	___	_____

EVALUATION

	S	U	NP	Comments
1. Monitored vital signs, SpO_2, and end-tidal CO_2.	___	___	___	_____
2. Observed character and amount of sputum.	___	___	___	_____
3. Observed respiratory status closely, palpated for facial or neck crepitus.	___	___	___	_____
4. Assessed for return of gag reflex.	___	___	___	_____
5. Asked patient to describe postprocedure normal and abnormal symptoms.	___	___	___	_____
6. Identified unexpected outcomes.	___	___	___	_____

RECORDING AND REPORTING

	S	U	NP	Comments
1. Recorded all pertinent information in the appropriate log, documented time of gag reflex return.	___	___	___	_____
2. Reported bleeding, respiratory distress, or changes in vital signs to health care provider immediately, reported results of procedure to appropriate health care personnel.	___	___	___	_____

Student _____ Date _____

Instructor _____ Date _____

PERFORMANCE CHECKLIST SKILL 44-5 **ASSISTING WITH GASTROINTESTINAL ENDOSCOPY**

	S	U	NP	Comments

ASSESSMENT

1. Verified type of procedure scheduled and procedure site with patient.

2. Verified that informed consent was obtained prior to administering sedation.

3. Determined if GI bleeding was present; observed character of emesis, stool, and NG tube drainage for frank blood.

4. Obtained vital signs and SpO_2/end-tidal CO_2 values.

5. Determined purpose of procedure.

6. Verified that patient was NPO for at least 8 hours for endoscopy of upper GI tract.

7. Verified patient followed a clear liquid diet and completed any ordered bowel-cleansing regimen for lower GI studies.

8. Assessed patient's level of understanding and previous experience with procedure.

PLANNING

1. Identified expected outcomes.

2. Explained steps of procedure, included sensations to expect, administered preprocedure medication.

IMPLEMENTATION

1. Identified patient using two identifiers per agency policy, compared with information on patient's ID bracelet.

2. Performed hand hygiene, applied PPE.

3. Removed patient's eyeglasses, dentures, or other dental appliances.

4. Took "Time-Out" to verify patient's name, procedure, and site with patient and team.

5. Ensured IV line was patent, administered IV sedation as ordered.

6. Assisted patient to assume proper position, applied appropriate drape.

	S	U	NP	Comments

7. For upper GI procedures:

   a. Assisted health care provider in spraying the nasopharynx and oropharynx with local anesthetic. ⎯ ⎯ ⎯ _____

   b. Administered atropine if ordered. ⎯ ⎯ ⎯ _____

   c. Positioned suction cannula for easy access in the patient's mouth. ⎯ ⎯ ⎯ _____

8. For lower GI procedures: _____

   a. Prepared lubricant for fiber optic endoscope. ⎯ ⎯ ⎯ _____

9. Assisted patient throughout procedure by anticipating needs, telling patient what was happening, and suctioning if necessary. ⎯ ⎯ ⎯ _____

10. Placed tissue specimen in proper containers, sealed as needed, dated and initialed all containers. ⎯ ⎯ ⎯ _____

11. Assisted patient to return to comfortable position. ⎯ ⎯ ⎯ _____

12. Assisted in disposing of equipment and performing hand hygiene. ⎯ ⎯ ⎯ _____

13. Informed patient not to eat or drink until gag reflex returned. ⎯ ⎯ ⎯ _____

EVALUATION

1. Monitored vital signs and SpO_2 at appropriate intervals. ⎯ ⎯ ⎯ _____

2. Assessed for level of sedation and LOC. ⎯ ⎯ ⎯ _____

3. Asked patient to describe level of comfort, observed for pain. ⎯ ⎯ ⎯ _____

4. Evaluated emesis or aspirate for frank of occult blood. ⎯ ⎯ ⎯ _____

5. Assessed for return of gag reflex, provided oral hygiene. ⎯ ⎯ ⎯ _____

6. Asked patient to state postprocedure dietary and activity limitations. ⎯ ⎯ ⎯ _____

7. Identified unexpected outcomes. ⎯ ⎯ ⎯ _____

RECORDING AND REPORTING

1. Recorded all pertinent information in the appropriate log. ⎯ ⎯ ⎯ _____

2. Reported onset of bleeding, abdominal pain, dyspnea, and vital sign changes to health care provider. ⎯ ⎯ ⎯ _____

Student _____ Date _____

Instructor _____ Date _____

PERFORMANCE CHECKLIST SKILL 44-6 **OBTAINING AN ELECTROCARDIOGRAM**

	S	U	NP	Comments
ASSESSMENT				
1. Verified type of EKG ordered.	___	___	___	_____
2. Determined rationale for obtaining ECG.	___	___	___	_____
3. Assessed patient's level of understanding of procedure.	___	___	___	_____
4. Assessed patient's ability to follow directions and remain still in position.	___	___	___	_____
PLANNING				
1. Identified expected outcomes.	___	___	___	_____
2. Provided privacy.	___	___	___	_____
IMPLEMENTATION				
1. Identified patient using two identifiers per agency policy, compared with information on patient's ID bracelet.	___	___	___	_____
2. Performed hand hygiene.	___	___	___	_____
3. Removed or repositioned clothing to expose only patient's chest and arms.	___	___	___	_____
4. Placed patient in appropriate position.	___	___	___	_____
5. Instructed patient to lie still without talking.	___	___	___	_____
6. Cleansed and prepared skin, clipped chest hair if necessary.	___	___	___	_____
7. Applied self-sticking electrode, used pressure only on the perimeter, attached leads appropriately to chest and extremities.	___	___	___	_____
8. Turned on machine, entered required demographic information into computer, obtained tracing:				
a. Entered patient's name and record number for simultaneous 12-channel recording, repositioned leads as needed, documented any chest pain experienced.	___	___	___	_____
b. Applied electroconductive gel to over V_1 to V_6 locations, recorded lead tracing appropriately for three- or five-lead recording.	___	___	___	_____

	S	U	NP	Comments

c. Applied limb electrodes for continuous interpretation/monitoring, applied electroconductive gel over location for single chest lead, maintained either two or four limb electrodes.

9. Disconnected leads, wiped off excess paste from chest, marked where leads were placed if necessary.

10. Delivered ECG tracing appropriately, provided any previous tracings.

EVALUATION

1. Documented if patient experienced chest discomfort.

2. Identified unexpected outcomes.

RECORDING AND REPORTING

1. Recorded pertinent information in appropriate log.

2. Reported arrhythmias or chest pain to health care provider immediately.

616